LIFE ON THE LINE

Life on the Line

*Ethics, Aging, Ending Patients' Lives,
and Allocating Vital Resources*

John F. Kilner

WILLIAM B. EERDMANS PUBLISHING COMPANY
GRAND RAPIDS, MICHIGAN

Unless otherwise indicated, Scripture quotations in this volume are taken from the HOLY BIBLE: NEW INTERNATIONAL VERSION. Copyright © 1973, 1978, 1984 by the International Bible Society. Used by permission of Zondervan Bible Publishers.

Some of the material in this book appeared in different form in a variety of journal articles written by the author. The author and publisher gratefully acknowledge permission to use these materials in this book:

"A Pauline Approach to Ethical Decision-Making," *Interpretation* 43 (October 1989): 366-79.

"A Needy World — A Needed Word: Scarce Medical Resources and the Christian Story," *Asbury Theological Journal* 41 (Fall 1986): 23-58.

"Age Criteria in Medicine," *Archives of Internal Medicine* 149 (October 1989): 2343-46 (copyright 1989, American Medical Association).

"Age as a Basis for Allocating Lifesaving Medical Resources," *Journal of Health Politics, Policy and Law* 13 (Fall 1988): 405-23.

"Ethics to Live By," *Catalyst* 18 (March 1992): 4-5.

"The Ethical Legitimacy of Excluding the Elderly When Medical Resources Are Limited," *Annual of the Society of Christian Ethics* (1988): 179-203.

Who Lives? Who Dies? New Haven: Yale University Press, 1990.

To Suzanne Kilner,
such a beautiful testimony to
God's life, love, and joy

Introduction:
The Challenge at Hand

Anyone who pays health insurance premiums knows. Anyone who has no health insurance also knows. The cost of health care is skyrocketing beyond our means. We do what we can to make the best of available resources, but we are gradually realizing that we are not doing enough. Perhaps if we had different national and international priorities, we might be able to redirect substantial resources away from less worthy pursuits to health care. And if people were more careful than they are, we could eliminate substantial wasteful expenditures on health care. But even if we do devote greater energies to obtaining the needed health care resources, there will come a time when we have to face our limitations responsibly.

We are all affected by resource limitations at both a personal and a social level.[1] Many patients and their families have personally experienced the overwhelming financial burden of severely debilitating or terminal illness. The pressure to let patients die rather than sustain lives of questionable quality or length is immense. In this context, so-called active

1

euthanasia or mercy killing may appear relatively humane. Confusion arises as those in a position to make the important decisions are motivated not only by a desire to respect patients' wishes that meaningless suffering be avoided but also by a desire to save money. How can one safely navigate such a moral quagmire?[2]

Socially we are compelled to look for ways to decide who will be eligible for certain types of health care and who will not. We observe, for instance, that elderly people require a great deal of health care. If they can be ruled less eligible, the savings potential is enormous. So the results of a study of patient selection criteria involving 453 medical directors throughout the United States is not surprising: when health care resources become limited, the primary effect on patient selection is that elderly people are judged to be less eligible for care.[3] Other social groups such as poor persons and those who are unproductive are also predictably disadvantaged.[4] Is such a situation morally acceptable?

In this book I describe a way to grapple with the personal and social predicaments that arise in the face of death. While Christians, Jews, and people of other religious communities may make common cause on the issues addressed here, my approach is explicitly Christian. More specifically, it is rooted in the Bible, which has been the most authoritative guide to Christian living throughout the history of the church. Yet it is an approach that can operate quite well in a religiously and ethically pluralistic society, as I show in Chapter 2. The book should be of interest to all those concerned about biblical, Christian, and other theological ways of thinking about ethical issues. I have especially tried to speak to ethicists, theologians, clergy, and students in ethics, medical ethics, and biblical theology courses, but I think that health care professionals looking for an explicitly Christian way to address the ethical issues they repeatedly confront will also find this book helpful. So will politicians and others who want to understand better the ways that people's views on health care policy issues may be shaped by religious convictions. The topics addressed in the second and third sections of the book should be of particularly widespread interest, since most of us will someday have to deal with the death of a loved one or be called upon to counsel or care for someone who needs expensive health care resources.

This reference to "us" raises an important matter of terminology that needs clarification at this point. The intended audience of ethical teaching in the Bible is typically a particular group of people who have (or at least have professed) a faith in God. So it is difficult to refer to what various biblical writers say to "us" without assuming at least a professed biblical faith on the part of all readers of this book. I do not make such an assumption. Accordingly, I will often use generic and third-person terms (people, they, her or his) to refer to the audiences that the biblical materials address. While technically correct, though, this approach alone would miss the spirit of the way that these materials point all people to the God of the Bible. To reflect this spirit, I will periodically use the first-person plural (we, us) throughout as a reminder that the biblical writings at least in some indirect way address us all.

While this book draws on various biblical materials, it is situations such as the following that more immediately have prompted its writing:

Statistically, Bill was classified as a poor, 67-year-old Latino man. More importantly, he was known to friends and family alike as an energetic and loving person. By either account, he had heart problems. Different forms of treatments had been attempted, but they had only temporarily stalled the developing disease.

Recently Bill's condition had begun to deteriorate rapidly. His lungs as well as his heart were seriously compromised. Upon hospitalization, Bill was found to have a form of pneumonia that proved resistant to treatment. Three times he had to be placed on a respirator to maintain breathing while the pneumonia was treated. Each time he was progressively weaker after the respirator was removed, and each treatment was less effective than the previous one in combating the pneumonia. Gradually the disease did such damage that Bill began to experience frequent chest pain and he looked progressively worse.

In light of Bill's deteriorating condition and the family's evident concern, Bill's physician called a meeting to discuss continued treatment. The family's pastor joined Bill's wife and three children for this meeting at their request. The physician explained to the family her inability to arrest the progress of the heart and lung deterioration. When asked if a heart or heart-lung transplant had been considered at any point in the course of treatment, the physician indicated that Bill was not a good transplantation candidate "for a variety of medical, economic, and social reasons." The physician went on, together with the pastor, to help the family to envision the suffering that both they and Bill would experience during Bill's final weeks.

At this point two questions arose. Should Bill be resuscitated if his heart stopped? Should he be placed on a respirator again if his lungs deteriorated further? Knowing that these actions would extend Bill's life a week or two at most, the family opted for what the physician termed "passive involvement" (i.e., no treatment except to provide comfort) should the need for such emergency actions arise. One of Bill's daughters was so moved by the suffering that lay ahead for all that she inquired about the possibility of so-called "active euthanasia" — painlessly inducing her father's death right away for his and the family's sake. While the physician acknowledged that this could easily be done using intravenous potassium chloride or a similar drug, she refused to consider this possibility.

At the same meeting the physician, family, and pastor also considered whether or not to discuss the preferred course of passive involvement with Bill himself. Bill had consistently maintained his determination to overcome his illness. Bill's wife in particular felt that Bill would maintain this attitude to the end — for the family's as well as his own sake — but that he would in fact appreciate the physician deciding not to prolong the dying process. Everyone present agreed. So it was decided not to discuss the matter with Bill. The physician proceeded to order that no emergency measures be taken to maintain Bill's life and that his pain be aggressively controlled.

Shortly thereafter Bill's condition began to deteriorate rapidly. Three days following the meeting of caregivers, his heart stopped beating. No attempt was made to revive him. During Bill's final days, his wife and children were increasingly disturbed by the sight of him wasting away and his inability to communicate meaningfully with them. Nevertheless, while comfort care was continued to the end, no steps were taken to speed up Bill's death.

The patient, family, pastor, physician, and others involved in this situation were besieged with a host of questions: How should the patient's wishes be ascertained, and what weight should they be given? Should death be battled relentlessly or be actively sought? Should suffering be avoided at all costs? Is suicide or "euthanasia" an option? When can treatment ethically be withheld? Should the patient's quality of life be taken into account? What factors are legitimate to consider in assessing whether or not Bill should have received an organ transplant — his age? his ability to pay? his gender? the cultural group to which he belongs? the likelihood that treatment will provide a lasting benefit? the amount of family support he can count on? his value to others? Should expensive, high-tech treatment be readily available in a world where so many go without basic health care?

Such questions emerging from life experiences are what occasion the substance of this book. Part I is as much a response to this experience as are Parts II and III. It provides some ethical tools for the kind of careful consideration that is necessitated by questions of life and death. Much of the reflection informing Parts II and III actually preceded the formulation of Part I and made me aware of the need for such a formulation.

The three chapters that constitute Part I of this book are devoted to describing in some detail an ethics that is identifiably Christian. Of broad interest will be the opening section of Chapter 1 and all of Chapter 3, in which I outline my approach and elaborate its significance for the rest of the book. Those interested in a more detailed demonstration of how the approach is at work in the ethical reflection of Paul and Jesus will find it in the remainder of Chapter 1 and the first half of Chapter 2. In the second half of Chapter 2, I compare the approach with three outlooks popular today — perspectives that focus on consequences, principles, and virtue — and I examine the place of a Christian approach in a non-Christian world.

In the second part of the book I take up some of the more personal ethical issues arising in the face of death. In Chapter 4 I document the growth of support for life-ending decisions, identify the key ethical questions involved, and explore the importance of acting in accordance with the patient's wishes. In Chapter 5 I discuss the ethics of a situation in which a patient or caregiver chooses a course of treatment that directly causes the patient's death. In Chapter 6 the focus is on decisions to forgo treatment and to let an illness take its fatal course. This section of the book concludes with a chapter in which I discuss especially difficult situations, such as the permanently unconscious patient whose quality of life some would judge to be essentially nonexistent and the steadily declining elderly patient whose elaborate treatment is financially destroying her or his family.

In the third section of the book I more directly examine the social context within which decisions to provide lifesaving resources are made.[5] I begin in Chapter 8 by documenting the limited availability of certain resources, noting the growing prevalence of age criteria for excluding elderly people from some treatments and describing some biblical perspectives on elderly persons and health care. I also offer a critical evaluation of the medical reasons being given for the use of age criteria in health care. In Chapter 9 I probe the nonmedical reasons given for the use of these same criteria. Chapter 10 features medical and nonmedical critiques of other ethically dubious criteria. I conclude this section of the book by proposing six ethical criteria for patient selection in contradistinction to the more objectionable criteria that are coming to the fore in this era of unavoidable resource limitations.

Throughout the book I have attempted to steer a course between two dangerous temptations. On one side has always loomed the temptation to assume a posture of certainty about what "the Bible as a whole" says God's will is. On the other side has lurked the temptation to deny that there is a unified voice about anything in the Scriptures. I have attempted to probe the biblical materials to discover the extent to which there is a unified voice present — ever wary of the inability of any individual to hear that voice with complete accuracy because of biases, self-centeredness, and other blinders. Men and women bring crucial differences in experience and consciousness to the task of listening to the "biblical word," as do the representatives of different ethnic and economic groups.[6] We need to pledge ourselves to an ongoing communal effort both to understand better what the biblical materials were meant to communicate about God's will when they were written and to discern how the Bible speaks to the situation today. In this spirit, I make periodic references not to "my approach" or "the biblical approach" but to "the described approach." This book is not merely an expression of my own views or a comprehensive account of all that the Bible has to say about health care ethics; rather, it represents one attempt to describe what a way of thinking shaped by the biblical writings might look like in the context of some crucial issues in health care today.

The ideas presented in the pages that follow have already been significantly refined through the years by many insightful responses to presentations I have given at various universities (Harvard, Yale, Brown, Kentucky, Loma Linda) and in numerous professional settings (the American Hospital Association, Chicago; the National Kidney Foundation, Washington, D.C., and Ann Arbor; the Society of Health and Human Values, Chicago; the American Society of Nephrology, Washington, D.C.; the American College of Health Care Executives, Orlando; the Society of Christian Ethics, Atlanta; the Evangelical Lutheran Church of America, Chicago; the Christian Holiness Association, Columbus, Ohio; the Cleveland Clinic, Cleveland; Children's Hospital, Boston; Rush-Presbyterian-St. Luke's Hospital, Chicago; Istituto Scientifico H San Raffaele, Milan, Italy). I am more grateful than I can say for these responses and for the rich experiences I received working with patients and caregivers as hospital ethicist at St. Joseph Hospital in Lexington, Kentucky, and as director of the ethics grand rounds program at the University of Kentucky Medical Center. I also want to express a special appreciation to "Bill" and his caregivers for their openness in speaking about their struggles, described earlier.

My involvement in the Integrative Lecture Series at Asbury Theological Seminary and the Staley Lecture Series at Ft. Wayne Bible College has also provided occasions for extremely helpful dialogue on issues I deal with in this book. Similarly, co-chairing the medical ethics section of the Society of Christian Ethics has put me in touch with many profound and devout leaders who have enriched my thinking greatly. Gracious colleagues, students, and church congregations too numerous to list have contributed as well to the shaping of this book. I have great appreciation for each one. I would, though, like to express a special word of thanks to Arthur Dyck, Stephen Mott, Sissela Bok, George MacRae, Andrew Lincoln, Gerald Winslow, Nancy Cummings, Richard Boone, Elizabeth Collins, Harriet Cook, and Rose Luciano for their unique contributions to the development and writing of this book. To Christine Pohl in particular goes my deepest gratitude for her insightful paragraph-by-paragraph review of the entire text. The American Academy of Religion, Asbury Theological Seminary, and the Park Ridge Center for the Study of Health, Faith, and Ethics also deserve a special word for their gracious financial support during the writing of this book, as do Eerdmans' Jon Pott and Tim Straayer for their superb editorial assistance.

As I emphasize at the conclusion of the book, the questions addressed here are complex and interrelated. They are among the most important that we will ever confront as individuals and as societies. If faith is to make any difference in how people live, surely it must have something to say when life itself is at stake.

PART I

LIVING ETHICALLY

PART II

ENDING PATIENTS' LIVES

CHAPTER 4

The Patient's Wishes

Seventy percent of those alive in the United States today will at some point be faced with a decision about whether or not to provide lifesaving medical care for themselves or family members.[1] Over two-thirds of all physicians have already been involved in such decisions with their patients.[2] In many of these predicaments the option of intervening to end a painful or seemingly useless existence also presents itself. How are such difficult situations to be faced?

Even talking about these questions is hard, because it reminds people of their own mortality. Some are frightened by uncertainty about what lies beyond death. For such individuals an assurance of eternal life can hold particular significance. However, for many people the most distressing fear lies not in death itself but in the dying process — and with good reason. Most people have heard about, if not personally witnessed, patients in their final days or weeks attached to various machines. In their dying they are isolated from loved ones, and it appears that their suffering is only being prolonged.

Although we might prefer not to think about such matters, we cannot avoid them. In fact, there is mounting evidence that people do not necessarily want all that medicine has to offer when their end is near. A U.S. poll, for example, has shown that 70 percent of the population would want to have their life-support systems removed should they lapse into an irreversible coma.[3] As early as 1983 a U.S. presidential commission reflected an emerging national consensus regarding the acceptability of forgoing life-sustaining treatment under certain circumstances.[4] In the years since, studies have appeared documenting the frequency with which patients choose to withdraw from such treatment.[5]

Researchers have also documented lesser but growing support for active intervention to bring about death under certain circumstances. In California, for instance, 68 percent of the people already supported such active intervention in 1983 (as compared with 94 percent in support of allowing treatment refusal at that time).[6] More recent polls show similar figures.[7] Nationwide support in the United States for terminating life in some situations appears to run closer to 50-60 percent, according to public opinion polls.[8] However, there is some evidence indicating that this figure may be overstated. Shortly before the November 1991 Washington state referendum on legalizing physician-assisted suicide, for example, polls indicated that 61 percent of populace supported legalization. However, legalization was defeated when only 46 percent voted for the measure.

Medical opinion seems to be more cautious, as indicated by the controversies in medical circles stirred up by published reports of medically induced deaths and announcements of medical devices to enable patients to commit suicide.[9] Nevertheless, at least one prestigious medical panel has concluded that physician assistance of patients in committing suicide "is certainly not rare" and is to be commended in some circumstances.[10] Surveys of physicians in such locations as Colorado and San Francisco have found about two-thirds of those questioned favoring the option of intentionally ending a patient's life in some situations.[11]

Support for terminating life in the face of poor medical prognosis, though, is hardly limited to the present day or to the United States. There has been support for such action throughout history and around the globe.[12] An example of another country in which support for so-called active euthanasia is great today is the Netherlands. About three quarters of the Dutch public has supported this practice for years under limited conditions. More recently the figure has increased to 82 percent.[13] Physician support is also substantial; estimates and studies suggest that thousands of patients are killed by physicians annually. The Dutch Medical Association has even proposed guidelines for the performing of euthanasia.[14] While causing the death of a patient remains illegal in the Netherlands, a government-appointed Commission on Euthanasia and the court system have both expressed support for the practice when strict conditions such as the clearly expressed wishes of the patient are satisfied.[15] Late in 1991 the Dutch Committee to Investigate the Medical Practice concerning Euthanasia released official annual figures documenting the practice of euthanasia in the Netherlands. Actions were taken (or omitted) with the intent to end patients' lives, with patients' permission, in 10,615 cases.[16]

Not all euthanasia in the Netherlands takes place with the expressed consent of the patient, however. The official report just cited documents 14,691 cases in which actions were taken (or omitted) with the intent to end patients' lives — without patients' permission. In a significant number of these cases, the patients had complete mental capability.[17] At least two other studies have documented a significant number of similar cases; in one study, 41 percent of nearly three hundred responding physicians admitted performing euthanasia without the request of the patient.[18] The Royal Dutch Society of Medicine has acknowledged that decisions regarding euthanasia in the case of mentally incompetent patients may need to be made by persons other than the patients themselves.[19] Opinion polls also suggest that as many as three quarters of the Dutch public may support involuntary euthanasia in some situations.[20] Are the Dutch unique in their support of ending life under certain (especially voluntary) circumstances? Opinion polls in various countries suggest not.[21]

The possibility of making decisions that shorten life, then, appears to be a matter of interest to most people. However, of all groups in society, elderly people have the most at stake. They are the group most frequently facing end-of-life treatment decisions. They also require a disproportionately large amount of medical resources, so the larger society also has a financial stake in how long their treatment continues.

A Matter of Definition

How can elderly people — or anyone — be protected from unwanted and unhelpful treatment without a significant risk of wrongly being denied needed treatment? The way forward is hindered by the confusion surrounding the term *euthanasia*. Does euthanasia include all of the actions referred to in the paragraphs above or only to some of them? The term has in fact been used — modified by such adjectives as *active, passive, voluntary*, and *involuntary* — to refer to them all. Its most common meaning is the equivalent of active euthanasia: taking some action that is itself the medical cause of someone's death.

This variable usage may be enough to undermine its usefulness as a term. However, there are also other reasons to avoid it. Those opposed to active euthanasia resist lumping it together with other such potentially acceptable measures as discontinuing useless treatment, arguing that the differences are more significant than the similarities between the two categories.[22] The common use of *euthanasia* to describe the killing of Jews, those disabled or politically undesirable, and others deemed "unworthy to live" in Nazi Germany also has probably tarnished the word beyond practical use.[23]

The central ethical question, then, is not whether euthanasia (whatever that term means) is ethically justifiable. Rather, the many measures affecting the exact timing and other details of a person's death have to be sorted out and assessed ethically. There are two basic questions that will prove useful in doing this: (1) Is the patient willing? and (2) Is death intended?

It is important to distinguish these questions from the categories commonly applied to the term *euthanasia*. Such categories are descriptive rather than ethical (in the normative sense) and so tend to obscure important ethical distinctions. The first question, regarding willingness, is somewhat related to the common distinction between "voluntary" and "involuntary" euthanasia. Euthanasia is voluntary when people choose it for themselves and involuntary when others choose it for them. The relevant ethical issue, however, is whether the decision is made in accordance with the patient's wishes. This issue remains at the heart of ethical considerations regardless of whether the patient is capable of making a medical treatment decision, as we will see.

The second question, regarding intention, is somewhat related to the common distinction between "active" and "passive" euthanasia. This distinction may also be misleading in the context of ethical analysis, in that it tends to obscure the relevant ethical issue. What matters ethically, according to the described perspective, is whether the treatment decision intends the patient's death. Active euthanasia by definition intends the patient's death, for it entails an action, such as an injection of potassium chloride, which itself is the medical cause of death. Because of its consistent intention, active euthanasia provides a convenient context for exploring the notions of intention, death, and suffering (which are discussed in Chapter 5).

Passive euthanasia is somewhat more ambiguous ethically. It involves the withholding or discontinuing of medical treatment such that the medical condition is allowed to take its course and become the medical cause of death. We will consider different forms of passive involvement (again, the term *euthanasia* is confusing) in Chapter 6. We will then turn to a consideration of the terminal/nonterminal distinction and several related issues in Chapter 7, since we can generally get a much better sense of whether death is intended by a given course of action if we can determine whether the patient would have lived significantly longer had treatment been provided.

Models of Relationship

As important as the above clarifications are, however, we have to do much more than just define words and concepts if we want to formulate patterns of how to live morally in the face of death. One area of special concern is the relationship between patients and caregivers (physicians, nurses, other health professionals, social workers, chaplains, family, friends, and others). Treatment decisions are profoundly influenced by the model of this relationship assumed by the patient and the caregiver — particularly the physician. Four models warrant special attention.[24]

1. *The War Model.* This model envisions the caregiver as a warrior engaged in a battle to defend the patient-victim. The caregiver's fundamental goal is victory over death.

2. *The Family Model.* This model envisions the caregiver as a surrogate parent whose chief concern is the good of the patient.

3. *The Contract Model.* In its simplest form, this model envisions the caregiver as a professional who enters into some sort of explicit contract with a patient, promising to provide

health-care services in exchange for some sort of compensation. The fundamental notion here is the autonomy of both parties to the contract.

4. *The Covenant Model.* This model focuses on a range of mutual commitments between the caregiver and the patient, drawing on the biblical notion of covenant. We can think of these commitments in terms of the ethical guides we considered in Chapter 3 and, within the context of those guides, the general welfare of all those involved. Respect for the freedom of the parties involved is part of the picture, but it is just one aspect of an approach that also champions an essential commitment to life, truth, justice, and the well-being of both the patient and the caregiver.

While the first three models are all based on important insights, each also carries an inherent danger so long as it is the only model out of which one operates. For example, the war model does answer the desire patients have for somebody who will fight on their behalf. However, if this commitment on the part of the caregiver becomes an all-consuming drive, it actually might serve to thwart the patient's desires by augmenting the agony of the dying process. Similarly, the family model answers the desire patients have for somebody to look out for their best interests in a confusing and overwhelming situation. But if in the course of providing treatment the caregiver fails to take patients' values and judgments seriously, patients may perceive treatment as onerous regardless of how well-intentioned it is, and may well question whether the decisions being made are in fact in their best interests. Finally, the contract model answers the patient's desire that the caregiver invite her or him to participate in decision making about treatment and provide the kind of information that such decision making requires. But it remains an open question in the vastly complicated context of modern medicine whether the mere provision of information is sufficient to ensure that patients can make truly voluntary decisions based on genuine understanding of their condition and all the implications of the various treatments available.

The covenant model of the caregiver-patient relationship seeks to draw on the positive insights of each of the other three models. Each of the three seeks to address an important ethical concern, and yet their narrow focus on these concerns blind them to other compelling ethical considerations and render them potentially destructive. By drawing on an overarching ethical commitment, the covenant model offers checks and balances to ensure that the concerns that drive the other three models work together with one another rather than at cross purposes.

Problems in the caregiver-patient relationship arise not only as a result of deficiencies inherent in a given model but also as a result of the conflicts in expectations that crop up when the patient and the caregiver are committed to different models. Consider, for example, what happens when patients are committed to the family model while caregivers are committed to the contract model. Patients expect caregivers to make the difficult decisions for them, while caregivers assume they are fulfilling their obligation by providing patients with the necessary information and then leaving them to decide how they want to proceed. In such a situation, patients will likely feel that they are not being cared for adequately. Or, consider the converse situation, in which patients are committed to the contract model while caregivers are committed to the family model. Caregivers proceed in good conscience to lay out courses of treatment for patients without any significant discussion. The patients, who are very much interested in getting as much information as possible from their caregivers so that they can make their own decisions about treatment, will naturally feel frustrated and angry about being left out of the decision-making process.

It is vitally important for medical caregivers to discern what model or models of relationship both they and their patients consider to be in force. Conflicts like the two just noted need to be brought into the open and discussed early on — if possible before treatment is undertaken. Patients and caregivers are much more likely to reach agreement regarding some of the toughest decisions to begin or to end treatment when they share expectations.

The Mentally Capable Patient

In light of this clarification of some of the essential terms and the basic relationship between the patient and the caregiver, we can now proceed to look at the first of the two basic ethical questions identified earlier: Is the patient willing? This question is important for a variety of reasons, some of which are suggested by the predicament of Bill in the case described in the Introduction. At issue, for instance, is one of the basic ethical guides we investigated in Chapter 3: freedom. In few areas of life is freedom more important than in the area of health care — particularly lifesaving health care. This is a context in which the patient's basic well-being and even life is in jeopardy. The patient, more than anyone else, will bear the burden of the results of any decisions made. One might think that a physician could assess the quality of a patient's life and the burdensomeness of treatment with reasonable accuracy. However, much evidence suggests that such is not the case, because of the difference between the patient's and the physician's point of view.[25] So it should not be surprising that there is such widespread support in medical circles for limiting treatment to those who want it.[26]

Every reasonable effort should be made, then, to ascertain the patient's wishes when a vital treatment decision must be made. And yet freedom in the biblical context (see Chapter 3) requires more than this. It is not the case that every course of treatment the patient might choose will be as morally sound as every other simply because the patient chooses it. A variety of considerations must come into play. Nevertheless, freedom does entail that even an otherwise sound decision will not be completely moral if it is not in accordance with the wishes of the patient, as best those can be ascertained.

Ascertaining the patient's wishes regarding treatment is easiest when the patient is capable of expressing them. Under such circumstances caregivers are supposed to seek what is referred to as the patient's "informed consent." The standard of informed consent was developed because of the need to protect patients from medical decisions that are not truly in their best interests and to give them a genuine voice in decisions about treatment that will, after all, affect them much more than their caregivers. However, from the perspective of the described approach, there are two problems with "informed consent": the word *informed* and the word *consent.*

The word *consent* is problematic in this context because it suggests that the patient is involved in the decision-making process only to the extent of agreeing with the course of treatment being proposed by the caregiver. Giving the patient an opportunity to agree is better than leaving treatment decisions solely to the discretion of the caregiver. However, the intent of the concept of informed consent would be better served if we used some more neutral term — *decision*, perhaps, or *decision-making* — in place of *consent.*

The idea of "*informed* consent" is also problematic. The mere fact that a caregiver provides a patient with information hardly ensures that the patient will then be able to reach a morally sound decision on the basis of that information. For a decision to be moral, four conditions must be satisfied: (1) the patient must have the capacity to make the decision; (2) the patient must be able to decide voluntarily, free from coercion; (3) the patient must receive sufficient information to make a good decision; and (4) the patient must come to a genuine understanding of the nature and implications of the proposed treatment.

1. *Capacity.* The first condition for moral decision making is that the patient must have the ability to make such decisions. *Competence* is the legal term traditionally used to distinguish those who have this ability from those who do not. While many also use this legal term in discussions about moral decision making, I prefer the term *capacity*, since it emphasizes that the moral considerations at stake may well involve more than just what is legally required. Also, the term *capacity* does a better job of suggesting that there are degrees of decision-making ability than does the term *competence.* A patient might well be able to handle certain kinds of decisions but not other kinds. There are various techniques for ascertaining the capacity of patients, but three general standards apply in any case. Patients have capacity to the degree that they can understand the relevant information, reflect on it in accordance with their values, and communicate their wishes. Since capacity is the norm, it should be assumed unless its absence can be demonstrated.[27]

2. *Voluntariness.* The second condition for moral decision making is that patients must be able to reach a decision free from coercion. Patients are typically subject to many subtle forms of coercion beyond the prospect of the harm they face if they fail to consent to proposed treatment. They tend to be weak and vulnerable as a result of their illness. They are dependent on their caregivers for their very lives and well-being. Normally patients will not risk the displeasure of their caregivers by disagreeing with them unless the caregivers explicitly give them the freedom to express their own preferences. Sometimes caregivers have strong views about the need for a proposed treatment. While there is room for persuasion, the line between persuasion and coercion is easily crossed. Caregivers have an obligation to remember and periodically affirm the patient's responsibility for the decision and the freedom to make it.

3. *Information.* Only when the conditions of capacity and voluntariness are satisfied does it make sense to talk about the third condition for moral decision making, information, which is central to the concept of informed consent. Sufficient information is indeed essential, for without it the freedom of patients is undermined. If they are not presented with information about all of the treatment alternatives available to them, patients may consent to treatment, but they cannot be said to have really chosen freely. Caregivers who withhold complete information (regardless of their intent in doing so) thereby violate not only the basic ethical guide of freedom but also that of truth. In effect, they deceive patients, who naturally assume that they are making decisions — regarding personal and family matters as well as treatment — on the basis of an assessment of all available options. Nevertheless, there is evidence that the consent of patients to treatment is frequently based on inadequate information.[28]

What constitutes adequate information? Some standards have evolved from years of experience. For example, patients typically want to know about all viable options for treatment and the potential benefits and harms of each of them. Patients are not all alike, however, and it is generally agreed that they should also explicitly be given the opportunity to ask questions and to request additional information.

4. *Understanding.* The fourth condition necessary for moral decision making is that there be genuine understanding on the part of the patient. The manner in which information is conveyed is very important. After all, even the best information will not do patients much good if it is presented in such a way that they cannot grasp its essential implications. Such misunderstanding is a real possibility given the complexities of modern diagnoses and treatment options. This is an area in which the moral virtues of the caregiver can be decisive. Caregivers need such fruit of the Spirit as patience, faithfulness, and gentleness (Gal. 5:22-23). They need to speak

in meaningful language, avoiding medical jargon and explaining the risks of medical procedures by analogy to risks in everyday life. Caregivers must also allow patients the time they need to come to grips emotionally with what may be very distressing options.

Once patients have reached decisions, caregivers should seek to determine their level of understanding by asking them what led them to choose the course they did. Such queries are appropriate not only from the physician directing treatment but from anyone else concerned about a patient's well-being. If a patient cannot answer these questions, then some probing is called for in order to determine whether the decision was in fact based on genuine understanding.

Two implications of moral decision making are worth noting at this point. First, the decision belongs to the patient and not to the family. It is tempting for caregivers to tell bad news to the family rather than to the patient. This temptation is particularly strong when a caregiver is operating out of the war model and finds it difficult to admit defeat to the patient. Families, though, should insist that the caregiver convey to the patient any information that is shared with them. The caregiver's covenant is with the patient, not with the family.

Second, the caregiver should presume that patients want to be the decision makers unless they explicitly say that such is not the case. Most patients do in fact want the information they need to make important end-of-life decisions and to resolve problems in relationships with people and with God. Accordingly, patients should ordinarily be kept fully informed. The desire to spare patients suffering in the face of death by withholding information from them is understandable but misguided. It not only violates the ethical guides of freedom and truth but also betrays a misunderstanding of the role of suffering in our lives.[29]

Nevertheless, just as there must be some latitude for patients to make bad decisions, so they must be allowed to make the usually bad choice of allowing someone else to make major treatment decisions for them. Studies have shown that some patients distinctly prefer that treatment decisions be made by their physicians or family members.[30] In such a case it is crucial that the four conditions for moral decision making be satisfied in relation to this choice not to choose and that the patient designate the surrogate decision maker. It is appropriate for caregivers to try to convince patients to make their own decisions, but they must take care to ensure that such attempts to persuade do not cross the line and become coercion, lest the condition of voluntariness be violated.

The Mentally Incapable Patient

When the patient does not have the necessary decision-making capacity as we have defined it, then someone other than the patient must make treatment decisions. Even in such circumstances the wishes of the patient should remain the controlling ethical consideration. However, determining what these wishes are is likely to be problematic. Morally speaking, the patient's most recent relevant statements should be considered binding as long as they satisfy the conditions of capacity, voluntariness, information, and understanding. Broad recognition that such statements have been made and that these conditions have been met will more likely be achieved if the statements have been written down in the form of a living will that is signed and witnessed.

In theory, a living will is simply a statement of a patient's wishes regarding treatment should a situation arise in which he or she cannot communicate those wishes. The vast majority of state legislatures in the United States have legalized living wills. And even in the absence of relevant legislation, courts have held that living wills provide convincing evidence of patients' wishes that should be given great weight in decisions about treatment. There is significant support for living wills in Christian circles as well. In fact, the American Protestant Health Association and the Catholic Health Association of the United States have designed model living wills for Christians, complete with statements of faith.[31]

Despite such support, surveys in the United States indicate that only about 10 percent of respondents have actually signed living wills.[32] There are probably several reasons why this figure is so low. Many people know little about living wills. Others fear that they necessarily promote dying rather than living by making it easier for caregivers to end treatment. This problem is compounded by the notoriously vague language of many living wills. They are simply unable to address the specifics of all possible future circumstances. So the generalities that result provide wide latitude for discontinuing treatment that the patient might actually want. Ironically, vague language may also greatly delay acting on the patient's wishes because of legal problems such as demands for court rulings and fears of malpractice suits. The ability of relatively healthy patients to predict their own wishes in future situations of severe illness is also commonly questioned.[33]

In order to avoid many of these difficulties, some people have endorsed the use of surrogate decision makers rather than living wills. Although fewer states have adopted the durable power of attorney for health care than have legalized the living will, the number is rapidly growing. Legislation permitting a durable power of attorney allows patients to designate the person who will make treatment decisions for them if they lose their capacity for doing so. As with the living will, the patient's wishes remain the governing consideration, but the serious problem of vague language is overcome because there is a designated person who can make clear decisions in any situation.

The durable power of attorney, by itself, does have some limitations. There are no guarantees that the surrogate decision maker will have much information regarding the patient's wishes in the situation at hand. Accordingly, a so-called "advance directive" that combines a living will and a durable power of attorney may be the most effective means of ensuring that treatment decisions are made in accordance with the wishes of a mentally incapacitated patient. Various models of such combined documents have been developed.

One of the most detailed models combines a living will and durable power of attorney together with a statement about what organs the person is willing to donate after death. The living will portion of the document describes four of the most common scenarios in which difficult decisions have to be made. Those filling out the document are asked to indicate, in each scenario, for each of twelve common medical interventions, whether they would want the intervention, would not want it, are undecided, or would prefer a trial period with the intervention.[34]

There are, however, two difficulties with this advance directive. The first concerns the organ donation provision. While organ donation is important, linking it with the termination of treatment in this way is probably counterproductive for both. One of the major reasons that people resist signing organ donor cards is that they fear that a need for their organs might induce caregivers to cease treatment too soon. Linking organ donation and treatment termination in the same document tends to augment that fear and discourage people from choosing either provision.[35]

A second difficulty with this four-scenario advance directive is that the living will portion requires the patient to prescribe treatment in a wide range of situations — something that many people feel untrained to do well. Even were they to complete this form — perhaps with the aid of a physician — only a limited number of situations would be addressed explicitly. Other situations could well arise that the living will fails to address. Accordingly, the American Medical Association has developed an advance directive in which the living will section takes a simpler and yet more comprehensive approach.[36] Instead of involving patients in prescribing treatments, it asks them to identify their goals for their own health care. They can indicate, for instance, whether they want to receive *any* medical treatment that will keep them alive or whether they prefer to receive only those life-sustaining treatments that will restore or maintain certain capabilities. In the latter case, the patient identifies which capabilities are important enough to warrant life-sustaining treatment (e.g., the capability to leave the hospital and live without being attached to a machine, or merely the capability both to understand what others are saying to them and to be able to respond in some way, as by squeezing a hand, blinking, or the like).

While the living will and surrogate decision-maker provisions of an advance directive are both potentially helpful, their usefulness is limited unless their relationship to each other is carefully spelled out in the directive itself. We might take a first step toward clarity by specifying that the surrogate's interpretation of the patient's wishes is definitive except for any particular limitations that the patient notes. Such documents typically assume — and sometimes make explicit — that the surrogate is to make decisions in accordance with the patient's wishes, not on the basis of the surrogate's assessment of what is in the patient's best interests. However, evidence suggests that people vary greatly regarding the degree to which they would want their wishes overridden if doing so were in their best interests.[37] Accordingly, it is important that the patient indicate whether explicit provisions of the living will may be disregarded if the surrogate judges that it is in the patient's best interests to do so. If such disregarding is to be allowed, the patient should specify whether all or only certain provisions of the living will may be disregarded.

Other means for giving the designated decision maker access to the detailed wishes of the patient are also to be welcomed. One such vehicle is the so-called "values history." It extends the living will by recording not only specific treatment preferences but also the values that guide the patient in formulating such preferences. Analogous to the medical histories that are routinely taken on patients, values histories provide surrogate decision makers with the frame of reference they need to identify patients' likely wishes in situations they could not have anticipated.[38]

Admittedly, the kinds of documents I have been describing do make it easier to discontinue or refuse treatment and, ultimately, to die. However, such decisions are not necessarily disrespectful of life (see Chapter 6). Moreover, as we have seen, God has granted us the freedom to make bad decisions about our lives. The documents we are examining here do not expand that freedom; they merely affirm it.

These documents cannot remove all ambiguity as to the patient's wishes. Yet they do serve to reduce the ambiguity considerably, and in that way they provide a morally preferable alternative to disregarding those wishes. They serve not only to safeguard the patient's freedom but also to spare those charged with making a decision about treatment (usually family members) from having to make agonizing choices. They do not have to decide whether treatment should be discontinued if the patient has already spoken on this issue. Evidence suggests that many surrogate decision makers will not decline even the most useless and burdensome medical interventions if the patients for whom they are speaking have not explicitly indicated their wishes about such matters.[39]

It is easiest by far to treat patients in accordance with their wishes if they are capable of expressing them or have indicated them in advance. So people should take the initiative even before becoming terminally ill to complete at least something like the combined document described above. The U.S. Patient Self-Determination Act, which became law near the end of 1991, is designed to encourage exactly that. Patients are asked if they have completed or would like to complete an advance directive at the time of admission to health care facilities that receive some federal funds — which includes most hospitals and nursing homes.[40] Churches could provide an important service to their members by helping them to think through the issues and act appropriately.

Nevertheless, there will probably remain many situations in which mentally incapable patients will not have expressed their wishes in advance regarding treatment. Even in such cases, the primary ethical concern should be to act in accordance with patients' wishes. So the best persons to make treatment decisions will be those most likely to know what patients' wishes would be.

While courts of law have differed about whether family members, the courts themselves, or some other agent or combination of agents are the best surrogate decision makers, health care has traditionally looked to family members because of their familiarity with and commitment to "their own." While affirming the importance of family, the biblical materials add the observation that "family" includes the entire people of God.[41] If a believer's biological family does not respect the will of God, then other believers may become the primary family when important decisions must be made.[42] (Of course, a non-Christian family is not likely to defer to a believer when treatment decisions must be made unless the patient has designated that believer in advance as the appropriate decision maker through a durable power of attorney.) For a Christian biological family, how much more readily can the church be a source of great support and counsel.

If at all possible, then, the wishes of the patient should be respected. However, even family members are not always in a position to know what patients would want in unanticipated situations, particularly if the patients involved are infants or very young children.[43] When there is such uncertainty, it should be honestly acknowledged by all concerned.

Decision makers are then left with the responsibility of making the treatment decisions that are most clearly God-centered, reality-bounded, and love-impelled. As we have seen, the God-centered dimension has many implications, such as the importance of seeking God's wisdom through prayer, God's written word, and other believers. The reality-bounded dimension adds the proviso that all decisions made must be within the bounds of God-created realities, including the moral guides that flow from them. Finally, the love-impelled dimension directs people, within these bounds, to make that decision which is the most beneficial (or least burdensome) for those affected by it — primarily the patient. In the chapters that follow we will focus on the specific content of such decisions as well as on the process by which they are made and the type of person who makes them.

CHAPTER 5

Taking Someone's Life

Hardly a week goes by, it seems, without a news item discussing patients' decisions to kill themselves or some physician's willingness to do it for them. A medical resident allegedly ends the life of a young woman suffering from cancer and writes an article about the event, "It's Over, Debbie," in the *Journal of the American Medical Association*. Dr. Jack Kevorkian facilitates the death of Janet Adkins using a "suicide machine," is charged with murder (though not convicted), later helps others to end their lives using an "improved" version of the machine, and publishes the popular book *Prescription: Medicide*. Derek Humphrey also publishes a book, *Final Exit* — a how-to manual on suicide that quickly vaults to the top of the New York *Times* bestseller list. Meanwhile, Dr. Timothy Quill writes an article in the *New England Journal of Medicine* detailing how he has enabled his patient Diane to commit suicide. The entire state of Washington wrestles with legalizing physician-assisted suicide, narrowly defeating the measure, and similar debates rage in California and other states.[1] Bill's caregivers (see the Introduction) and countless others in similar predicaments reach conflicting conclusions.

What does the described approach have to say about

this debate? We have seen that one crucial question to ask about any vital treatment decision is whether such treatment is in accordance with the patient's wishes. Now we must turn to a second crucial question: Is death the intended outcome of the treatment decision?

I have been arguing that a Christian outlook is characterized by a commitment to life — a commitment that involves not merely a way of acting but also a way of being. It shapes who people are and how they think as well as what they do. So a Christian ethical analysis will be concerned not simply with whether people's actions actually cause death but also with whether they intend to cause death by their actions and why that is their intention.

Distinctions are necessary, then, between actions (what people do), intentions (what they decide to do), and motivations (why they decide to do it). Ideally all three work together in harmony with the divine purpose. Motivations are formed as part of overall character, and in turn they often (though not always) shape intentions, which in turn often shape actions. Nevertheless, in a fallen world the three can become separated, and we have to distinguish among them in order to pinpoint the location of the problem.

Motivation is notoriously difficult to assess in other people. It is difficult enough to assess in oneself. According to the described perspective, however, we are all responsible before God not merely to do the right things but also to do them for the right reasons. We have been created by God to be holy in all aspects of our being, which comprises more than just our physical bodies. If we were merely physical, then only actions would matter. But we are more, and motivations are as significant ethically as actions. As Jesus explains in Matthew 5, internal dispositions have great ethical significance before God. Proper motivation, however, is not enough. Even well-meaning actions can be quite hurtful and can violate the God-centered, reality-bounded, or love-impelled dimensions of moral action.

So while we should undertake moral action out of a desire to affirm life and other relevant God-given considerations, the action itself and what it is intended to accomplish also matter greatly. In this chapter I want to focus on the decision to take a patient's life, generally with medical assistance (so-called "active euthanasia"). The defining characteristic here is the medical cause of death, whether people are ending their own lives or the lives of others. Something is intentionally done, such as injecting potassium chloride, which becomes the cause of death. In other words, whatever the motivation for the action may be, the intention — expressed in a specific action — is the patient's death.

It is my contention that intending the death either of oneself or another necessarily runs counter to the understanding of God's will embodied in the approach to ethics being described here. To understand why this is so, it will be necessary to gain some perspective on two critical topics, death and suffering.

Death

According to the Bible, every person has an important choice to make — the choice between life and death (see, e.g., Deut. 30:15-20; Prov. 8:35-36; Jer. 21:8; Matt. 7:13-14; Rom. 8:6; 1 John 3:14-15). The choice is far more cosmic than a particular decision about whether to have a specific medical treatment; it is a choice between two basic orientations that encompass all aspects of existence.

The choice goes back to the very beginning of the human race, as described in Genesis 2. God provides the means for sustaining life (v. 16) and warns that death will come if people seek provision outside of those means (v. 17). There appears to be no attempt to limit the issue to physical or nonphysical life and death, probably because this distinction is foreign to the holistic perspective of Genesis. God's warning is disregarded, and so the curse of death is pronounced in Genesis 3 (v. 19). More specifically, Adam and Eve are separated from the tree of life — the source that would have sustained their lives forever had they not disobeyed (vv. 22-24).

This turns out to be only the first in a series of limitations that God placed on people's lives because of their disobedience. Initially God restricted their lives from "forever" to a limited (albeit long) period in Genesis 3. According to Genesis 5, this period was many hundreds of years. However, Genesis 6:3 suggests that human disobedience continued to alienate people from God, resulting in a further physical manifestation of that alienation: the shortening of their lives to about 120 years. By the time the psalmist wrote Psalm 90, this physical deterioration, so intimately related to the degeneration of the relationship between people and God, appears to have reduced life expectancy to 70-80 years (v. 10). Interestingly enough, most religions of the world recognize human disobedience as the original cause of human deterioration and death (physical and nonphysical).[2]

Taking their cue from the origin of death, other writers in the Bible portray death as something in direct opposition to the nature and purposes of God (and of people in that they are created in the image of God). For example, in the Old Testament death is portrayed as the "king of terrors" (Job 18:14), aptly associated with the "valley of the shadow" (Ps. 23:4). In the final day, when the disgrace of God's people is removed, death will be swallowed up and all tears will be wiped away (Isa. 25:7-8).

New Testament pictures are similar. Jesus sends out the twelve to announce the nearness of "the kingdom of heaven" and to demonstrate it by healing the sick, driving out demons, and raising the dead (Matt. 10:5-8). Sickness, demons, and death are antithetical to the nature of God's reign. Paul picks up the multidimensional perspective on death characteristic of Genesis, interweaving physical and nonphysical dimensions of death in his reflections on death. Death first came to humanity because of human disobedience, and it is an "enemy" that will ultimately be destroyed by Christ (Rom. 5:12; 1 Cor. 15:20-26, 54-55). As other writers add, death is a tool of the devil (Heb. 2:14) that can persist only as long as the devil does (Heb. 2:14; Rev. 20:10-14). In the end, God will again live with people as originally intended in Genesis 2–3, and so "there will be no more death" (Rev. 21:3-4).

In a pervasive and profound sense, then, death is an enemy of God and people that is intimately bound up with human disobedience. Recognizing this, the wise woman of Tekoa in 2 Sam. 14, prompted by Joab, encourages King David to side with God. In a world scarred by death, God works for life and reconciliation, she observes, rather than for death and separation (v. 14). David — like any person after God's own heart — should be devoted to fostering life rather than acting in a way that aligns him with death.

Various critics have raised objections to this sort of understanding of death. The least substantial of these has to do with what would have happened if people had never disobeyed God and had never died. The earth, it is objected, would have become hopelessly overrun with people. Such an assertion, though, is based on mere speculation, except for its certainty that God's plan for humanity could not have forestalled this problem. However, there are numerous possibilities. God may have intended to fill an ever-expanding universe with people. Alternatively, God may have intended to change physical life to nonphysical life periodically, either on an individual basis as was done with Enoch (Gen. 5:24; Heb. 11:5) and Elijah (2 Kings 2:10-12), or on a group basis as will be done with believers who are still physically alive at Christ's return (1 Cor. 15:50-53). Such speculation is best avoided, except to affirm that God must have had some viable alternative to death, since human death does not appear to have been God's original intention.

A second objection holds that only "spiritual" (i.e., non-physical) death was introduced by human disobedience and that physical death was an intended part of human creation from the beginning.[3] To be sure, some of the biblical passages dealing with death do have a context in which the nonphysical dimension is most apparent. That is not always the case, however, and even when it is, the association with physical death is not disavowed. The very ambiguity of many passages dealing with death suggests that the biblical authors were more impressed with the profound commonality of different dimensions of life and death than with their differences.

The debate over whether physical or nonphysical death is the result of human disobedience needs to give way to a more comprehensive view — truer to the complete biblical witness as well as Christian tradition[4] — that both have resulted from disobedience. The drive to separate fundamentally the physical and nonphysical aspects of life and death indicates more a nonbiblical dualism than the well-integrated perspective of the Bible.[5]

Why, then, does God restore life eternally in a nonphysical but not in a physical sense? Such a dichotomy again indicates a misreading of the present relationship of death to life. According to the described perspective, both physical and nonphysical life have been contaminated by human disobedience, and so death, followed by resurrection to new life, is necessary in relation to both. We must not only die physically but must also die to the "old self" in a broader spiritual sense in order to be "born again" to new life (Rom. 6:3-4; John 3:3-7). Similarly, eternal life is not only a continuation of the "soul," or nonphysical life, but also of the body, albeit not a strictly physical body (1 Cor. 15:35-44 — and recall the earlier speculation that translation to some such body may have been part of God's plan from the start).

Critics contend that if God had physical death in view when warning that Adam would die when he ate from the forbidden tree, then God was wrong and the serpent was right (Gen. 2:17; 3:4). Adam ate, but he did not die physically. Such reasoning, however, misses the point of divine warnings throughout the Bible. God repeatedly says that certain actions will produce certain consequences. From the context it often sounds as though the consequences will be immediate. They do occur, but sometimes not until much later. So with Adam's physical death. His disobedience ensured that it would occur, though it occurred in God's timing. God's people have often struggled with the delayed fulfillment of God's statements and come to the conclusion that God's "today" may be a much longer period of time, as people count time (see, e.g., Ps. 90:4; 2 Pet. 3:8).

The Genesis text has also been misread with regard to the conclusion of God's curse upon Adam, "dust you are and to dust you will return" (3:19). Those who support the second objection — the claim that physical death was an intended part of human creation from the beginning — understand this pronouncement as a mere restatement of God's original plan. However, the text does not support such a reading. Genesis 3:14-18 is divided into three parts: the curses on the serpent, Eve, and Adam. All of the statements in the verses directed to the serpent (vv. 14-15) and Eve (v. 16) are parts of the curse resulting from their disobedience. So it is likely that the same is true in the similar verses directed to Adam (vv. 17-19). In fact, verses 17-19 are introduced with God's words "because you listened to your wife and ate from the tree about which I commanded you . . . ," and hence the implication is that all that God says will happen to Adam here (including death) will happen as a result of Adam's disobedience.

Some critics have also raised a third type of objection — that physical death may fundamentally be something good rather than an enemy, as when death provides a release from suffering. But those who press this argument fail to recognize that God can bring good things out of bad without making the bad things themselves good. One might as well object that suffering is a good gift of God that one should sometimes strive for — in that it, too, can produce good effects. Critics are not prone to accept this view of suffering, preferring to see the good effects of suffering as the result of God's redemptive work in the midst of something bad that is not God's fault.[6]

A view of death as something bad out of which God can bring good effects would be more consistent and truer to the biblical texts. The very existence of death and suffering is a testimony to the disobedience of the human race as a whole, not to God's goodness; nevertheless, God can work these evils to good ends. As I have already argued, God's work in the midst of something that is an evil does not change the moral character of that evil. To recognize this is to take a God-centered rather than a human-centered approach. Even Paul recognized that death could be beneficial, especially for the believer, but he left the timing of his own death to God, who knew better than he its many implications (Phil. 1:21-26).

A variation of the assertion that death is good holds that death is generally to be welcomed because it is a "normal" or "natural" part of life. However, sickness is also "normal," and destructive hurricanes are "natural," and yet few are inclined to welcome them. Most people recognize that "what is" is not necessarily the same as "what ought to be." To welcome such evils — and death as well — is to undermine the significance of the life that they destroy. "Normalizing" death may also stifle in an unhealthy manner the experiencing and expressing of uncertainty and fear commonly associated with meeting an enemy face to face.[7]

To refuse to accept physical death as "normal" or "good" does not entail embracing another extreme: death as disaster. To embrace this view would not only be to overlook Christ's victory over death and the opportunity for eternal life but would involve an idolatrous worship of physical life itself. In this present world, death is essentially unavoidable, as the psalmists and other biblical writers observe. So it is important that we reckon with it in the context of God's larger purposes. Death is both enemy and destiny, both penalty and promise, both cross and resurrection.[8] It is necessarily a real evil, the result of rebellion against God, but it is something over which God's love did, does, and will triumph. As we will see, too benign a view of death may lead to too hasty an abandonment of a God-guided commitment to life, while too desperate a view of death may result in too prolonged a dying process.

Suffering

Before turning directly to such implications, however, it is important to clarify some matters surrounding the issue of suffering. The topic of suffering is vast and will always remain something of a mystery. While we can formulate a limited understanding of suffering in general, we need to be prepared, with Job, to settle for incomplete explanations of what is occurring in any given instance of suffering. The answer to a sufferer's quest for deeper understanding may take the shape of a fuller account of God and the appropriateness of trusting God even in the midst of suffering rather than a fuller accounting of the reasons for that suffering (see Job 40–42).[9]

There are two generalizations about suffering, however, that are commonly accepted today and can shape people's approach to health care in profound ways. One is that suffering is an unqualified evil; the other is that suffering should be removed at all costs. Both of these generalizations are in sharp conflict with the described Christian outlook and need to be examined critically.

Consider first the notion that suffering is unqualifiedly evil. It is true that suffering is not portrayed in the Bible as something good in itself and therefore to be sought. Nevertheless the inference that it has no value is misguided, for God can use it powerfully in people's lives. Through it people can grow in perseverance and in the maturity that leads to wisdom and obedience to God (James 1:2-8; cf. Heb. 5:7-9). One can learn a contentment that does not depend on the circumstances of life and even experience the joy of victory over suffering when suffering loses its power to direct one's life (Phil. 4:11-12; cf. Rom. 8:35-37). The more people recognize that life and ethics are about character and virtue as well as right decision making, the more they will appreciate the significance of the contributions suffering can make to their lives.

It is no coincidence that much of the most profound writing, biblical and otherwise, has been done out of an experience of suffering. In such circumstances people can gain a new perspective on the significance of life and fresh insight into life's meaning and the human condition. They can discover God-given capacities in themselves that they never knew were there. At the same time, their weaknesses and self-centeredness are exposed in the refining process of suffering, and God can use suffering to restore their faithfulness (Prov. 3:11-12; Isa. 48:10; Heb. 12:5-11; Rev. 3:19). They can receive God's assurance that "my grace is sufficient for you, for my power is made perfect in weakness" and learn that dependence can be something good (2 Cor. 12:9).[10]

With so much to gain, it might seem worthwhile to promote suffering in one's life. However, just as people find life only by losing it, so people gain the value of suffering only when they oppose suffering as a genuine evil (albeit helplessly) and yet experience the goodness of God in its midst.[11] The experience of suffering is fundamentally different for people who intentionally seek it out, for they have an inescapable knowledge that they are merely undergoing what they have chosen. They lack the sense of being afflicted with something difficult that they must somehow overcome or endure.

There is a problem, though, with locating the value of suffering exclusively in the benefit that it brings to the sufferer. From a Christian perspective, the fact that God and other people also benefit is a crucial consideration. Much is indeed at stake for God in human suffering. The glory and power of God were demonstrated when the man born blind was healed (John 9) and when Paul received the grace to endure (2 Cor. 12). Suffering provides us with an occasion to trust and praise God for more than just the good gifts God has given us.

The suffering of Job is very instructive on this point. In the opening chapter of the book of Job, Satan claims that Job worships God merely out of self-interest. God considers the matter important enough to allow Satan to inflict great suffering on Job (God apparently refuses Satan's suggestion that God be the one to inflict the suffering — see Job 1:11-12). God is glorified both by Job's faithfulness and by his limitations, through which he learns more about God and himself. By contrast, God expresses anger toward Eliphaz and Job's two other "comforters" "because you have not spoken of me what is right, as my servant Job has" (42:7). "Speaking right" of God during and following suffering — trusting in God's promised faithfulness — brings great glory to God.[12]

One's suffering can also have substantial value for others. For example, a caregiver may learn valuable lessons from the manner in which a patient deals with his or her suffering. Alternatively, caregiving itself can be a heavy burden, particularly if it involves efforts to help the patient bear the burdens of suffering. As in the case of all suffering, the personal and vicarious suffering of the caregiver may well prove valuable only after an extended period of uncertainty or even despair.

Another way remains in which one's suffering may be of value to others. Suffering creates in some people the capacity to comfort others. "Praise be to the God . . . of all comfort, who comforts us in all our troubles, so that we can comfort those in any trouble with the comfort we ourselves have received from God" (2 Cor. 1:3-4).[13]

Suffering, then, has the potential to be very valuable. But of course it can also prove quite destructive. There are no guarantees that it will do anything more than reveal one's utter inability to cope with hardship — another reason for not bringing suffering upon oneself.[14] A consideration of the potential value of suffering will serve us not by pointing the way to a justification for all suffering but rather by revealing redemptive possibilities in the midst of what would otherwise be an unqualified evil. Those who can recognize this sort of value in suffering will be less inclined to do whatever it takes to be rid of the ostensibly meaningless experience.

Thus we come to the second common assumption about suffering — the belief that it should be removed at all costs. Western culture is profoundly influenced by a utilitarian outlook committed to maximizing happiness, an outlook that often degenerates into a personal hedonism, a commitment to maximizing one's own happiness. If happiness is what life is all about, then suffering must indeed be avoided at all costs. In particular, people must avoid the cross. Its crushing load on Jesus' back and the nails driven through his hands and feet epitomize the burden of the fallenness of the world that Jesus had to bear — in fact, chose to bear. Those who follow Jesus are called to suffer this fallenness with him, to take up crosses of their own.

The basic question, then, is whether God or suffering is going to set the agenda of one's life — and death. God's people will not find God's way by trying to avoid all suffering. They will find God's way as they strive to live God-centered, reality-bounded, and love-impelled lives — especially in the midst of suffering. In fact, the ultimate test of what is setting the agenda of our lives may well be how we deal with suffering in the face of death.

Such was the case for Jesus in the garden of Gethsemane. He was "overwhelmed with sorrow to the point of death" (Mark 14:34) and zealously prayed to be spared from the suffering that he knew would only get worse. Yet he affirmed that his primary commitment was to the larger purposes of God, whatever suffering they might entail. Needless to say, this encounter with suffering was not his first. He had learned obedience through other experiences of suffering as well (cf. Heb. 5:8). Admittedly, the absence of suffering is, generally speaking, something good — which is why Jesus prayed for it. But it is not the highest good — which is why he was willing to forgo it.

Believers are called upon to take up their crosses and follow Jesus — to be servants of Christ. Far from enjoying a life free of suffering, servants of Jesus in a fallen world will necessarily suffer. That is why, after claiming to be more a servant of Christ than some other self-proclaimed leaders, Paul justified his claim by cataloging his suffering (2 Cor. 11:23ff.). If the epistle to the Colossians is any indication, he understood his sufferings as intimately related to those of Christ (Col. 1:24ff.). Although Paul's sufferings were directly tied to his spreading the gospel, suffering endured out of faithfulness to God, whatever the circumstances, involves identifying with Jesus (and Jesus identifying with the sufferer) in a mysterious way.[15] In this sense suffering can be seen to have a kind of sacramental aspect.

Recognizing the nature of suffering is particularly important because of the reality-bounded nature of ethics. Only in light of such recognition does the notion of rejoicing in sufferings make sense. Past realities pave the way, good things are happening now in the midst of faithful suffering, and great joys lie ahead.[16] "Therefore we do not lose heart. Though outwardly we are wasting away, yet inwardly we are being renewed day by day. For our light and momentary troubles are achieving for us an eternal glory that far outweighs them all. So we fix our eyes not on what is seen, but on what is unseen" (2 Cor. 4:16-18).

If people fix their eyes only on what is seen, then the demands they place on suffering will rarely be satisfied. People insist, for example, that their suffering be meaningful and fair. But when people find meaning only in those things that they experience as meaningful, they have made themselves God. At that point their experience rather than God's will becomes authoritative, in line with the utilitarian spirit of the age. Their perception needs to be enlarged to include the unseen.

Our present experience of happiness simply does not provide us with an adequate basis for evaluating our suffering or making decisions about how we should live or die in the face of it. Even self-interest dictates that our decisions should be reality-bounded, that we should take all aspects of reality into account. Our decisions should also be love-impelled, made with reference to the implications of those decisions for the lives of others as well as ourselves.[17] Most importantly, decisions should be God-centered, in the recognition that only God — no individual, even oneself — is worthy of absolute devotion. "If we live, we live to the Lord; and if we die, we die to the Lord" (Rom. 14:7-8). Our commitment is to God, even when that entails suffering and death.

Ending It All

These reflections on death and suffering have major implications for well-motivated decisions to cause one's own death or the death of another in the face of illness or disability (so-called active euthanasia). So do the analyses of the God-centered, reality-bounded, and love-impelled dimensions of life in Part I. Some of these implications and related considerations suggest that taking a patient's life is inherently wrong.

Other implications and considerations suggest that this action inflicts unacceptable damage on human community. Let us first consider the inherent wrongness of "ending it all" when medicine cannot do enough.

As we have seen, life has special significance that goes far beyond the notion of "value," according to the described perspective. It is not something that can simply be traded off against anything else of value in utilitarian fashion. Rather, "life" entails a way of living, a basic orientation, an alignment with the nature and purposes of God. So the choice between life and death is a profound one, encompassing all dimensions of life and all dimensions of death. To kill someone, including oneself, even with the best motivations, is to realign oneself radically with death and disobedience instead of God, who works for the good and for life even in the midst of suffering and death. It is to admit defeat and to decide self-servingly to assist the enemy.

On the face of it, there is something odd about endeavoring to eliminate suffering by eliminating the sufferer. Those who do so apparently fail to distinguish between the person involved and the suffering that person is undergoing; they would appear to assume that people are nothing more than the suffering or happiness they are experiencing at the moment and that suffering is an unqualified evil that must be removed at all costs. Such assumptions need to be exposed for the fallacies that they are. Relief of suffering, by its very nature, belongs in the service of life rather than the service of death. That profound pain in some ways eclipses the person is a tragedy to mourn, not a pattern to emulate.[18]

Furthermore, people are under an illusion when they think that they can understand death and know exactly when it is appropriate. God has the power to spare anyone from death and suffering. That God does not always do so when people think it would be appropriate shows that God has a different perspective than they do on such situations. " 'My thoughts are not your thoughts, neither are your ways my ways,' declares the LORD" (Isa. 55:8). Apparently there is more at stake sometimes than people realize.

The desire to control death becomes more suspicious when we recall that death is a means God has used to keep in check the rebellious human attempt to become God. The original temptation to eat the special fruit was a temptation to "be like God" (Gen. 3:5). The people ate, and they began to become like God (v. 22). So God decided to thwart this aspiration by limiting the length of their life through death (v. 22). People today do not like that limitation any more than the earliest people liked the limitation of the forbidden fruit. Just as people ate the fruit because doing so promised desirable results (Gen. 3:6), so people today continue to try to usurp control over God's next limitation, death, by deciding when it should occur based on expected desirable results. From this perspective, deciding when someone should die is a striking but not surprising manifestation of pride and, ultimately, rebelliousness. The insult to God is compounded in that they thereby reject the gift/loan of life as worthless.

People may not be aware of any bad motivations in their aspiration to control death. Like Eve in Genesis, they may simply want to achieve something desirable. Moral motivations, though, are only part of what is important, as we have already seen. Intentions and actions are also crucial. Both the act and the intent of ending someone's life are wrong, though people who do so may well be evaluated more or less harshly depending on their motivations.[19]

The inherent wrongness of causing the death of a "relatively innocent"[20] person brings into question two slogans commonly used to justify ending someone's life. One is the so-called "right to die." As explained earlier from the described perspective, people should exercise great caution in claiming rights for themselves, since people have rights, but they have no right to rights. Rather, they have a duty to treat others with the respect due those whom God has made and for whom Christ has died. If one person is to have a right to something, others must have a duty to provide it. The problem with invoking the concept of a right to die to justify ending someone's life is that there is no duty on the part of others to bring about that death; it is in fact so far from being a duty as to be a morally unacceptable option. The concept of a right to die, employed in this way, is based on a misunderstanding of freedom as autonomy. Rightly conceived, freedom does not give people the authority to make their own moral law but rather enables them to live as God has created and intended them to live (see Chapter 3).[21]

The other questionable slogan is "death with dignity." In this case the problem is not with the term itself but with how it is used. Dignity is as important in death as in life. However, the assumption that dignity is incompatible with great suffering, or that suffering inflicts an indignity so grievous as to warrant killing the sufferer, is mistaken according to the described perspective. Human dignity is centered in God, something that people become most aware of when they reach the limits of their own strength and ability. Suffering itself is not the enemy of dignity — a bad response to suffering is. Choosing (and causing) death is one such bad response, for it rejects life and the One who is the source of life and dignity. This is the indignity of "death with dignity."[22]

As suggested earlier, ending one's life is not only inherently wrong but also destructive of human community. The damage is most apparent when medical professionals become involved in the killing. The medical profession has traditionally been guided by the Hippocratic Oath, which includes a commitment not to kill a patient even if the patient asks to be killed. As we have seen, this commitment is in harmony with the described Christian outlook.[23] People trust their very lives to medical professionals on the assumption that they have devoted themselves to life, health, and caring. Involving the profession in killing represents a radical change in its place within the community. It undermines its status as a profession that can unequivocally be counted on to support life in the ongoing struggle between life and death.

The potential damage to the important caregiver-patient relationship is great. Trust is absolutely critical in this relationship. Without it, patients will not provide essential information about how bad their condition is, and caregivers will not be able to provide effective care. A newspaper cartoon succinctly tells the story. It pictures a terrified hospital patient — newspaper headlines in front of him reading "Euthanasia Being Pushed" — gripping not the bed adjuster controls or the TV remote control unit but the hotline button to the police. If it is perceived that the medical profession has entered the life-ending arena, some patients will begin to wonder if every injection, pill, or new IV bag is designed to cure or to kill — to end the pain or the patient. The problem will be particularly acute when, as is increasingly the case, patients do not have long-standing relationships with their caregivers. Even where there is such a relationship, the weakness of illness can be expected to produce groundless fears.[24]

The damage to human community is not merely a result of the caregiver's involvement in causing the deaths of patients, however. Society's endorsement of this practice is destructive irrespective of who implements it. It constitutes an admission that it is acceptable to give up on life. The willingness of individuals to hold onto life in the midst of ambiguity and destructiveness has long served as an eloquent testimony to others that they too can continue to trust and hope.[25] The converse is equally true: those who quietly give up on life send the message to others that it is acceptable for them to consider doing so as well.

This undermining of community occurs even if patients make the decisions on their own and take their own lives. The problem is still greater if others participate in the decision or killing. Nonpatients are called upon to shift their basic orientation from life to death — not for themselves (which would be tragic enough) but for others. Accordingly, they are called upon to bear ultimate responsibility for another's life in a way never intended by God. Killing involves getting rid of people, not keeping and sustaining them as well as circumstances permit. We are all called to be our brothers' and sisters' keepers. One who keeps looks toward life, while one who kills looks toward death, though both keepers and killers may be standing in the same place as caregivers.

Involving people other than the patients themselves in decisions and actions to end life not only reorients more people from life to death but also introduces a temptation to self-centeredness. When killing patients becomes an acceptable option alongside caring for them in the midst of their suffering and dying, caregivers (especially family members) suddenly have a major vested interest in which option is selected. Among the many considerations involved in making such a decision, the fact that killing the patient would remove the burden of caregiving (and perhaps preserve and make available an inheritance) will not be insignificant for some people.

The statements of so-called "mercy killers" in the past have often been telling in this regard. "I killed her because I could not bear to see her suffer" may literally mean what it says — that first and foremost the action reflected the killer's need to be free from his or her own discomfort. Barriers to killing patients not only protect society in general and the patient in particular but also protect caregivers from their own weaknesses — from subtly self-centered decisions that may well haunt them for the rest of their lives.

It is quite possible for patients as well as caregivers to make flawed decisions to end life when they are experiencing emotional and physical duress. We will look further at the meaning of a patient's request to die in Chapter 6, but it is

important to note here that decisions to give up on life often
do not reflect the patient's true wishes.[26] The problem is not
simply the patient's capacity to decide, though there is much
in serious illness and suffering that can compromise this
capacity. The problem also involves the voluntariness of the
decision. If choosing death becomes a socially accepted alternative, then patients needing much care may begin to consider
themselves selfish merely for choosing to live. The pressure
on the elderly and those with disabilities would be particularly great if death came to be seen as a "solution" to disability
and old age. The escalating costs of health care would only
increase this pressure.

Although historical parallels are never exact, many
people have observed certain similarities between the
developing openness toward so-called "active euthanasia"
today and the favorable attitude toward ending the *lebens-
unwertes Leben* ("life not worthy to be lived") that developed
in Nazi Germany.[27] Those making this comparison are not
necessarily passing judgment on the motives or moral character of people today; nor are they necessarily oblivious to the
current respect for patients' wishes. In many cases they are
pointing out the parallel primarily in order to underscore a
similarity in the way of thinking involved. People in pre-Nazi
and Nazi Germany gradually began to think of life more in
terms of its value than its sanctity. Having crossed this bridge,
they found it easier to consider the benefits of eliminating life
of lesser value in order to preserve and promote life of greater
value. Decisions made on the basis of what was most valuable
— rather than on the basis of the God-centered, reality-
bounded, and love-impelled outlook found in the Bible —
became more dangerous as the government obtained the
power to carry this way of thinking to its logical social extreme.

We have already noted some of the ample evidence that
this sort of utilitarian approach to life is becoming more wide-

spread today.[28] Some people are even reinterpreting the moral mandate to love to include ending life in order to end great suffering.[29] But as we have seen, this reinterpretation lifts love of neighbor out of its reality-bounded context and severs it from love of God. The utilitarian "love" that results is not truly love (in a biblical sense) but a counterfeit that should be called by another name. Such "love" is not shaped and guided by God's created reality (including the life guide and the nature of death); rather, an idolatrous devotion to the removal of suffering motivates this "love" to contradict and deny that reality. Removal of suffering is indeed good, but not at all costs. To reject the ending of life impaired by illness (or age or some other disabling condition) is not to accord erroneously high value to that life; it is to place it outside the realm of valuing.[30]

In light of this perspective, the challenge to suffer not for worldly reasons but "as a Christian" (1 Pet. 4:15ff.) takes on a new significance not intended in the original context. Anyone can suffer because of committing crimes and being punished — or even because of being ill. To determine, however, out of faithfulness to God, not to end one's life despite the temptation to do so, brings a new meaning to continued suffering. It is a special opportunity to glorify God. "So then, those who suffer according to God's will should commit themselves to their faithful Creator and continue to do good" (v. 19).

It does not fall to the patient alone to pay the price of faithfulness, however. It is relatively easy to challenge others to be faithful, but it is immoral and heartless to do so if we fail to provide them with what they need from us in order to be so. After all, society's technological expertise is sometimes responsible for prolonging and even intensifying the suffering of the dying process.[31] Suffering and dying persons need an extensive amount of support: pain control, bodily care, and personal presence. Anyone can give the last of these and at least be vigilant to ensure that the first two are provided. The strength of the temptation to end some patients' lives today may ultimately be as much an evidence of the breakdown of our communal faithfulness to one another as it is an indication of deteriorating personal faithfulness to God (or deteriorating understanding of what faithfulness requires). A God-centered ethics must not merely be reality-bounded; it must be love-impelled as well.

CHAPTER 6

Deciding against Treatment

Nancy Cruzan lay unconscious for years in a rehabilitation hospital while her parents sought court permission to discontinue all life supports including the feeding tube. The hospital refused to follow the family's wishes. Helga Wanglie's predicament was just the opposite. The hospital considered further treatment of her futile and wanted to stop, but the family insisted that treatment be continued.[1] In other situations, such as Bill's (see the Introduction), the family and hospital agree with each other but not necessarily with the patient.

As we have already noted, the issue of who has responsibility for treatment decisions is very important. However, more is at stake according to the described perspective. The available choices will not necessarily all be equally moral, and there is a pressing need to distinguish between better and worse decisions when people's lives are at stake.

One distinction sometimes made is that between so-called "active" and "passive" euthanasia — often with a view to condemning the former and commending the latter. This terminology is confusing, though, not only because of the negative connotations of the word *euthanasia* but also because the active-passive distinction obscures the important ethical issue at stake here. Ethically the key question is not whether any action taken by the patient or another person is the medical cause of death (as in "active euthanasia") but whether anything is done *or left undone* with the intention of causing the patient's death. Intention is the issue.

So-called active euthanasia is unethical for a host of reasons ultimately rooted in the intention to cause death. However, so-called passive euthanasia — letting an illness or injury take its fatal course without attempting to stop it — may equally be rooted in the intention to cause death. When such is the case, it, too, is unethical for similar reasons.[2]

Suicide

Just as actively causing death in the face of illness or injury is morally analogous to intending death by withholding or withdrawing treatment, so is suicide. Admittedly, suicide tends to have darker moral connotations than the treatment decisions we have been considering because we tend to have a harder time accepting the validity of the reasons people have for attempting to commit suicide. Yet a decision to refuse treatment is quite similar ethically to a resolve to commit suicide whenever the decision has the intention of bringing about death. For that reason, a brief review of some of the moral problems associated with suicide may contribute to a better understanding of why choosing death in the face of illness is so problematic.[3]

One difficulty with suicide is that it constitutes an abdication of moral responsibility. It represents a refusal to take on the often difficult conditions of human existence. Moreover, it manifests an unwillingness to bear, in love, with the weaknesses of the person for whom one has a unique and special responsibility: oneself.

Suicide is similarly problematic in the context of human

community. We are all diminished when any one of us commits suicide. For one thing, even in the case of someone whose life presently seems worthless, we have lost the unpredictable contributions that this individual might have made directly or indirectly to the lives of others had he or she chosen life instead of death. But quite apart from such potential contributions, one person's suicide also has the effect of discouraging others in their own struggles. Even a suicide committed out of a motivation to relieve caregivers from suffering cuts a tie that binds all of us together and supports us all in our task of living.

Particularly problematic is the attitude toward God implicit in most suicides. Suicide is a statement that there is no hope for an acceptable future, that such a future is not within God's ability and will. It constitutes an attempt on the part of people to determine the end of their lives, as if they know fully the goal for which God has sustained them to this point. However, it is God's prerogative to determine when there is no purpose for a life to continue. To assume *ultimate* responsibility for one's life is to reject God, no matter when in the course of life one elects to do so.

For these and other reasons, then, suicide is morally objectionable. But suicide is unlike many other morally objectionable actions in that it rules out any subsequent actions: one cannot feel remorse for having committed suicide, nor seek forgiveness, nor take any action to undo the damage that has been done. There is no possibility of retracting fatal decisions that appear in hindsight to have been misguided. Suicide leaves no room for human fallibility.

The discussion of suffering and death in Chapter 5 is relevant to a consideration of the moral implications of suicide as well. Submitting to the dictates of suffering and death when life can go on is far from a dignified dying. Changing sides and joining the enemy (death) at the end of life is hardly a reliable way to please God and be assured a place in God's eternal kingdom, if that is our aspiration. On the other hand, those who try to escape from God and the difficult lot that God has given them in life will find that death only hastens the point at which they must face God.

Admittedly, a perspective that is not informed by theological considerations may support the assertion that suicide can be a rational, desirable, and legitimate expression of one's freedom. However, within the God-centered, reality-bounded, and love-impelled perspective described here, suicide has none of these virtues. Most importantly, it overlooks and contradicts the way God has created the world to be, including the way human freedom is to be exercised (see Chapter 3). This aspect of the problem is not addressed by historical observations about what originally prompted the church to become so concerned about suicide. Some have claimed that strong prohibitions against suicide developed in Christian circles either because of the overly lax attitudes inside or outside the church toward suicide or on the basis of mistaken or presently irrelevant religious arguments. Whether or not such claims are valid, the numerous moral problems with intending death remain.[4]

The Bible does indeed record various examples of suicide that it neither commends nor condemns explicitly.[5] Since the Bible communicates its message through both the failures and triumphs of people, this silence says nothing about the moral legitimacy of suicide. A broader analysis of the biblical materials is necessary to determine into which category or categories suicide falls.

The death of Jesus is particularly instructive at this point because of his role as example. While Jesus did not resist his death in the sense of trying to escape from his captors, he did not seek death in the way that a person committing suicide does. The Garden of Gethsemane scene (Matt. 26:36-46; Mark 14:32-42; Luke 22:39-46) graphically suggests that Jesus did not want to die — that he was prepared to do so only if it was

God's will to use his death to accomplish some particular purpose. God uses evil as well as good, and the speeches of Peter in Acts 2 and 3, the prayer of the disciples in Acts 4, and the speech of Stephen in Acts 7 all characterize Jesus' death as an evil — as an immoral killing. The key point is made in advance by Jesus himself: he must die in accordance with God's purpose, but woe to the one who is instrumental in his death (Matt. 26:24; Mark 14:21; Luke 22:22). As we have already noted, we cannot assume merely because an action has good results and God works through it that it is inherently good or that we ought to seek to do it.

When an individual rejects medical treatment with the intention of bringing about death, the action is morally similar to suicide and is immoral for many of the same reasons that suicide is immoral. Which of these reasons are applicable in any given case will vary depending on the particulars of the situation. But we should note that not every decision to withhold or withdraw medical treatment is rooted in an intention to bring about the death of the patient, and in such cases, analogies with suicide and actively ending a patient's life are not applicable. Before we turn to a consideration of this latter category of decisions, however, I would like to take a brief look at one more line of argument that seeks to justify forgoing treatment with the intent of bringing on the death of the patient.

Quality of Life

Decisions to withhold or withdraw treatment are sometimes made on the grounds that the patient's quality of life is (or will soon be) too low and there is no significant prospect of improvement. Death is judged to be better than continued living. We will take a closer look at certain particularly troublesome instances of this predicament in Chapter 7, but at this point we should consider the general matter of seeking death in order to avoid a low quality of life.

One problem with seeking death under such circumstances is that death entails much more loss than gain. Although such actions prevent or bring to an end a bad situation, they do so at the price of abandoning God and embracing the enemy, death. People may fall into this betrayal almost unawares by proceeding from the mistaken assumption that what matters in life is the quality of one's life and that some lives are not worth living. Such views reflect utilitarian and hedonistic presuppositions that people's lives must be justified by what they contribute to others or at least by the pleasure they provide to themselves.

According to the perspective developed from the Bible in Part I, however, life draws its significance from the fact that it is created and sustained by God. It requires no other justification: it is a trust from God. Paul's outlook in 1 Corinthians 4 is therefore instructive in the present context, even though he is not specifically addressing the issues being discussed here. "It is required that those who have been given a trust must prove faithful," he writes. "I care very little if I am judged by you or by any human court; indeed, I do not even judge myself" (vv. 2-3).

What matters is not how others value the quality of a person's life — or even how that person values it — but whether one is living faithfully in accordance with God's purposes. Remaining life-oriented in the face of suffering and death is an important part of that faithfulness. This stance is not an idolatrous "vitalism" that justifies absolutely anything that will extend life even the least amount of time, as will soon become evident. Rather, it is a rejection of using judgments about quality of life as the basis for deciding who lives and who dies.

Such decision making is not only inherently mistaken but can also be quite destructive. It undermines care and trust in caregiver-patient relationships by shifting the focus away from the kind of total support for the patient that provides special care in response to special weakness. Instead, at some point not always clear to all concerned, the focus becomes whether or not the patient is worth saving — a qualitative criterion that can mean different things to different people. This way of thinking serves as an ever-present temptation to caregivers, including family, to be free from the burden of care that may well be detracting (sometimes markedly) from their own quality of life.

Patients themselves are often sensitive to the burdens their illness imposes on others. If patients feel that their lives must be of sufficient quality to justify these burdens, then they are put in a difficult position. Since caregivers are bearing the burden of care, patients may understandably feel that caregivers should have some say in whether or not the patients are worth it. Some patients, disinclined to ask awkward direct questions, will test caregivers' views on this matter by offering to refrain from present or prospective treatment, so that death will ensue. In some cases they make the offer by presenting it as a decision they have already made. A ready acceptance of the offer by family, physicians, or other caregivers may unintentionally confirm such patients' worst fears. The message they get from the caregivers is that their lives are not worthwhile. Quality-of-life thinking thus confuses critical communication and greatly complicates the crucial assessment of the patient's true wishes.[6]

Despite the difficulty of making quality-of-life judgments about others, there are some extreme situations in which most people would agree that the patient's quality of life is essentially nonexistent. One such situation involves patients who are permanently unconscious and have lost the capacity to perceive anything from their environment — for example, patients in a "persistent vegetative state" or an unrelenting coma. Some people have argued for withholding or withdrawing treatment from such patients on the basis of their low quality of life. However, to do so on this basis would be to embark on the approach to decision making just criticized, albeit starting with patients at the low end of the spectrum. It is the way of thinking itself, not how far down the scale one is looking, that is the problem here.

The reason that it seems so completely useless to continue to treat certain patients, such as those who are permanently unconscious, may be that they have died (i.e., they have moved beyond the possibility of experiencing life in this world). Determining when death occurs is an important and complex issue in its own right, but it lies beyond the scope of this book. The Bible only identifies various signs of death; it does not present a technical, scientific definition of it. Suffice it to say here that distinguishing between living and dead patients is an ethically sounder and safer enterprise than attempting to draw distinctions between various degrees of quality of life.[7]

Distinguishing the dead from the living is also important because different actions and even language are appropriate in relation to each. If a patient has died, then treatment is stopped as a matter of course (unless the body must be sustained temporarily for some purpose such as organ transplantation). Permission to stop treatment need not be obtained from the family, and it is inaccurate to talk in terms of the patient "completely dying" once treatment has been stopped. Death has already (completely) occurred, and continued treatment is a waste of resources as well as abusive to the body.

A related language issue concerns "vegetable" terminology. Regardless of whether or not it is suitable to liken dead bodies to vegetables, referring to living human beings as "vegetables" (or saying that they exist "in a vegetative state") is an inappropriate characterization of something created and living in the image of God. The terminology has demeaning connotations and invites inadequate treatment, in violation of the life and justice guides as well as the mandate to love.[8]

Employing permanent unconsciousness as a criterion either for death or for an unacceptable quality of life is, in any case, unwise until this condition can be diagnosed with certainty. There are a number of well-documented cases in which patients who had been diagnosed as existing in a "persistent vegetative state" by neurologists experienced in the diagnosis of this condition nevertheless regained consciousness.[9] Regardless of the criteria being used for determining death, though, the ethical outlook described in Part I suggests that the death of a living person should not be intended even if that person's quality of life is low. What if treatment is withheld or withdrawn without intending the patient's death? We will address that question in the remainder of this chapter.

Inappropriate Treatment

Just as withholding or withdrawing treatment can be wrong, so initiating or continuing treatment can also be wrong. For example, if a person is going to die soon whether or not treatment is provided, then the life guide is not at issue in any significant sense. The justice guide may be equally irrelevant if the person is not being devalued because of any particular attribute such as a (perceived) low quality of life. We should distinguish between burdensome treatment and burdensome life at this point. Judging a treatment to be too burdensome when it provides no significant benefit is different from judging life itself to be too burdensome. Unlike the latter judgment, the former may involve no assessment of the worth or value of the person per se but rather a recognition that treatment does not contribute anything to the patient's well-being.

In fact, treatment may on balance be harmful. When death is drawing near and can no longer be avoided, continued treatment may inflict terrible pain and suffering on a

patient that never would have occurred apart from the treatment. Such a misuse of technology is not surprising, for the
history of technology is filled with morally ambiguous technological developments and applications. Sometimes medical
technology is misused from the best of motivations, due to
insufficient understanding of what the technology is actually
accomplishing. At other times the misuse of medical technology reflects the self-centeredness of fallen human nature.
Caregivers may yield to the temptation to employ or forgo
medical technology in order to ease their own pain or guilt
rather than basing their decision on a genuine commitment
to do what is right for the patient. A God-centered, reality-
bounded, love-impelled outlook provides ways to distinguish
the proper and improper use of medical technology.

The God-centered dimension, first of all, has much to
say about the moral character of those making treatment decisions, caregivers and patients alike. God-centered people
have turned from self to God, allowing God to begin to re-
shape their character, including their motivations and intentions. Without this reshaping, the imposition of external ethical principles in an attempt to control actions is inherently
doomed to failure. Such an attempt overlooks the influence
of who people are on how they live and underestimates the
importance to God not merely of what people do but also of
why they do it.

A God-centered approach also emphasizes the importance of seeking God's purposes for the world and living in
accordance with them. In the context of treatment decisions,
this includes recognizing that disobedience may lie in doing
too much as well as in doing too little. There is no virtue in
over-treating "just to be sure." One can become so zealous in
trying to sustain biological life that one ceases to attend to the
God who created it.

The charge of "vitalism" is warranted at this point. A
form of vitalism does indeed underlie the unwillingness ever

to withhold or withdraw treatment. This never-say-die attitude is particularly problematic in the caregiver, but it may
characterize the patient as well. It is radically at odds with a
God-centered perspective. God has allowed death to limit
physical life — a reality that we must take into account. If we
fail to do so, we rebel against God by making an idol of life.
Idolatry is subtle: it takes something that is good and treats it
as if it were God. As important as life is, we must remember
that it is a gift from God, not a god itself.[10]

Accordingly, under certain circumstances withholding
or withdrawing treatment can be obeying God, not playing
God. We play God if we ascribe absolute significance to life
and, derivatively, to the medical technology that sustains it.
We play God if we assume the right to make judgments about
which lives are *worth* continuing — if we choose to become
the medical cause of death rather than accept another cause
that can no longer be stopped. However, truly recognizing
that beyond a certain point physical life must end is far from
playing God. It is instead resisting the temptation to claim
God's ultimate responsibility over life and death, acknowledging that extending the suffering of dying by employing
every possible technology to the bitter end is hardly admirable.

As we noted in Part I, this God-centered perspective is
integrally related to a reality-bounded perspective. We are
called to respect and live in accordance with the world God
has made. Whereas so-called mercy killing is wrong from this
perspective because it is based on a mistaken view of life and
death, the status of forgoing treatment is not so unambiguous.
A decision to forgo treatment may in fact respect the realities
of life and death, at least when the intention is not to bring
on death. The individual making such a decision may understand that physical life is extremely important but that it is
not the only aspect of the person. When nothing can be done
to maintain physical life to any significant degree, the person

as a whole can be cared for by not extending the suffering of the actual dying process. To prolong such suffering unnecessarily is not only to make an idol of physical life but also to remove physical life from its integral relation with the rest of the human person created in the image of God.

Moreover, Christians believe that "to die is gain" (cf. Phil. 1:21). The reality of life as God has created it extends beyond the temporal limitations of physical life. Believers can look forward to a resurrection into a new dimension of life beyond physical death — actually a continuation of the eternal life they have already begun to enjoy. There is a sense in which they will not be "home with the Lord" until after they have physically died (2 Cor. 5:8). So there is little incentive to hold on desperately to every last minute of physical life, at any cost, as if there were nothing more to life, as if death could be defeated in this way. Christians instead hold on steadfastly to Christ, with and through whom they can overcome death.[11]

That there may come a time when further treatment is inappropriate is particularly evident from the third aspect of the described ethics, its love-impelled dimension. In its broad sense, as we have seen, the ethical mandate to love encompasses the other two dimensions. In its narrower sense, however, the call to love is specifically a call to promote the well-being of people, as far as that can be done within the bounds of God-created reality. Since the situation in view here is one in which no such bounds are being violated by withholding or withdrawing treatment, the question is whether or not the well-being of patients in such a situation is always best served by further treatment. Experience shows that it is not.

Further treatment may produce nothing more than a prolongation of the dying process, thereby extending the suffering of patients. Their final hours might be better spent in composing themselves for death and drawing to a close important relationships than in a vain struggle against dying. Love, like the practice of medicine, is more fundamentally a matter of caring than of curing. Accordingly, the responsibility and privilege of caring remains even when curing is no longer possible. In fact, under such circumstances, caring may well require that treatment designed to cure be withheld or withdrawn.[12]

The tentativeness of this conclusion is important. As long as one is living within the bounds of God-created reality, it is difficult to generalize about what love-impelled moral actions will look like. So much depends on the unique experiences of the particular patients (and caregivers) involved — their stories and the stories of the communities of which they are members. Caregivers must pay attention to these stories, with discernment and understanding, if they want to give patients the care they need. Nevertheless there are some distinctions and perspectives that can prove helpful to patients and caregivers as together they confront the challenge of living in the face of death. It is to these distinctions and perspectives that we turn in Chapter 7.

CHAPTER 7

Important Distinctions

Many years ago Karen Ann Quinlan became the symbol of what many people did *not* want from health care — being kept alive in a permanently unconscious state. Reports frequently chronicled a loving father coming again and again to his daughter's bedside to provide whatever care was possible. Only after she had spent a long period of time on a ventilator and there had been a protracted court battle was the ventilator disconnected and this father's child allowed the possibility of death. More recently another father chose not to risk such a prolonged struggle. His child had been unconscious for four months and the future looked bleak. So Rudy Linares came to the child's bedside, gun in hand, ordered everyone out of the room, disconnected the ventilator, and tearfully held his son until the child died.

As we noted in Chapter 6, the question of whether death is intended in decisions to withhold or withdraw treatment is crucial. Nevertheless, it is far from obvious how to answer this question in many situations. In what sense, if any, did these two fathers intend the death of their children? Both loved their children. Perhaps the more appropriate question, then, is how love can best be expressed in such trying situations. A response must grapple with four important distinctions according to the described perspective. Each distinction involves an ethically significant aspect of the patient's medical condition or treatment.

Terminal vs. Imminent

The first distinction has to do with the seriousness of the patient's condition. When a particular illness or other medical condition is expected to result in the patient's death eventually, no matter what medical interventions are undertaken, the patient's condition is commonly referred to as "terminal." If treatment will likely prevent death from the medical condition at issue, then the condition is not considered terminal. In nonterminal situations, to withhold or withdraw lifesaving treatment is to intend death, in that death would not have resulted from that condition had treatment been given. Such a failure to provide treatment is morally problematic for all of the reasons we examined in Chapters 5 and 6.

What about terminal situations? To answer this question we need a more careful definition of terms. In a very real sense we are all terminal cases in that we will all die. Even if the term is tied to a particular medical condition, it covers situations that must be distinguished ethically. Patients who can live for a decade with their terminal condition fall in a different category than those who cannot survive more than a few more moments. The former still have substantial lives to live, whereas the latter do not.

Whether or not the life guide is relevant, then, is a matter of judgment. At some point fairly close to the time of death, when there is no reasonable likelihood of life continuing to a significant degree (with or without treatment), the mandate to sustain life loses its force. When treatment cannot truly sustain life, one is not necessarily intending death by forgoing treatment. Treatment may simply not have any worthwhile benefit; it may, in fact, serve only to add to the burden of the dying process.

A person who can live for years with a terminal condition is in a different situation. There is a significant period of life ahead. The fact that this person is dying should not obscure the fact that he or she is *living* — and will continue to do so, perhaps for a very long time. Moreover, the longer a patient is expected to live, the greater the possibility that means will be discovered to allow the patient to live even longer or with a better quality of life. Forgoing treatment when life can continue in this way involves some sort of assessment that life is "not worth it," whatever that means. In such a case, the issue is not the likelihood of life continuing beyond the present but rather the quality or significance of the life that can continue, and we have already noted the problems with choosing death on the basis of this type of consideration.

So it would seem that we need some category more focused than "terminal" to characterize the medical condition of those who only forgo treatment when death can no longer be significantly delayed by treatment. Traditionally, the term "imminent death" has served this purpose well. It is a flexible term, applicable to patients expected to die within several hours, days, or weeks (occasionally months) according to competent medical judgment. Accordingly, it has been able to accommodate a variety of medical conditions in which the length of the final dying process may vary somewhat. Yet it is distinct enough to have been widely employed in legal and medical contexts alike to distinguish those dying now from those who will die later.[1] Unfortunately, in the minds of some it has recently come to be associated only with those within hours of death — thereby becoming too restrictive. While the term will be retained here in its traditional, flexible sense, another similar term may have to be substituted eventually if the traditional flexibility of "imminent death" cannot be preserved.

When death is not necessarily imminent (i.e., imminent regardless of treatment), the life guide and the associated refusal to align oneself with death support the provision of treatment.[2] But the two basic ethical questions raised earlier remain: Is death intended? and Is the patient willing?

The issue of whether death is intended underscores the importance of closely monitoring the patient's condition. Treatment is warranted only as long as it serves to forestall death or at least provide a significant medical benefit. When it no longer does so, then the reason for starting treatment in the first place is no longer present, and treatment may be withdrawn.

The issue of the willingness of the patient underscores the importance of maintaining open communication in the patient-caregiver relationship. If a patient decides that treatment (or life itself) is too burdensome and so rejects treatment, the caregiver should acknowledge the seriousness of the decision. After the caregiver takes due care to ascertain that the ethical criteria of capacity, voluntariness, information, and understanding have been met (see Chapter 4), then the patient's wishes should be honored. But the caregiver must be very careful in such a situation to be certain that the patient's request is a genuine request to forgo treatment and not a disguised plea for affirmation. Open communication is essential to such a determination. Caregivers who respect a patient's genuine decision in this matter do not thereby affirm the morality of the decision; they merely acknowledge the patient's God-given freedom. People must be accorded the freedom even to make objectionable choices.[3]

On the other hand, when death is imminent even if treatment is provided, the reality-bounded dimension of ethics does not provide any guidance either mandating or opposing treatment. In such situations, as in so much of life, the love-impelled dimension of ethics (in its narrower sense of neighbor love) becomes definitive. Every situation must be attended to carefully and individually. Treatment does not automatically have to be withheld or withdrawn once death is imminent. It may be the case, for example, that family members feel the need to spend more time with the patient. Or the counsel or mere presence of the patient may temporarily make a critical difference to a relative or friend in a particular situation. Patients living for others and not merely for themselves will take such considerations seriously.

Other factors that may influence patients to continue treatment in the face of imminent death, however, are not so benign. Caregivers operating out of the war model may strongly (sometimes coercively) urge continued treatment out of an idolatry of life and a misunderstanding of their caregiving responsibility. Patients may seek maximum treatment to the very end because they are not confident that there is a middle ground between such efforts and merely being left to die. In the face of death, the loving support of others is critical for patients and families. Patients cannot make informed choices about treatment without knowing from day-to-day experience that everything possible will be done to care for their needs — even if a formerly (but no longer) life-sustaining treatment is discontinued. Caring must supersede curing as the more basic purpose of medicine, even when curing is a form that caring can take. If this principle is firmly in place, then caring will continue when curing is no longer possible.

Caring for a person includes caring for the entire person. According to the described perspective, people have non-material as well as material dimensions that together constitute an indivisible whole. This being the case, genuine caregiving must extend to matters of the spirit such as the patient's relationship with God. Problems in that relationship are not only important in their own right but may also constitute a source of the patient's illness. God, in any case, is the ultimate source of healing. Accordingly, the command to love — first to love God and then, similarly, to love people — calls caregivers to address this aspect of human need and source of illness alongside all others.

This recognition does not legitimate insensitive evangelistic bullying, but it does underscore the importance of being alert and attentive to more than merely physical needs. If the gospel of Jesus Christ is literally "good news" for the patient — if it can in some fashion help to address the patient's health needs — then the described perspective would indicate that it should be made accessible to the patient like other treatments. Any caregivers (family members, friends, chaplains, health care professionals, etc.) may be involved. They have to be sensitive to the patient's vulnerability whether or not death is imminent and take care not to impose their own values or outlook on the patient. Yet that very concern to make certain that the patient is allowed to make the choices requires that the patient who wishes to experience a deeper relationship with God, as well as the healing and peace that can result, be enabled to do so.[4]

While patients may choose to continue treatment even in the face of imminent death in order to deal with such matters, patients lacking decision-making capacity cannot so choose. They have lost the ability to make treatment choices and to deal with matters of faith on a communicative, cognitive level. If their only hope of establishing a relationship with God were to hinge on a virtually nonexistent chance of regaining communicative, cognitive ability, an argument could be made that special efforts to continue even burdensome life-sustaining treatment in the face of imminent death might be warranted. The patient's predicament has not caught God by surprise, however, and one may assume that God has provided appropriate opportunities for the patient to respond before this incapacitation. Moreover, a response in faith to God involves more than mere rational calculation. Who is to say that a patient without apparent decision-making capacity is not approached by God at a level of spirit that does not, under the circumstances, depend on the sort of capacity we typically assume to be necessary? In other words, patients need not be treated differently on the basis of speculations about the status of their relationship with God.

To this point I have been using the term "imminent death" as if it defines a distinct category into which all patients either do or do not fall. Actually, though, there is a gray zone. Whereas death is almost certainly imminent for some patients and just as clearly not so for others, it is difficult to say with any precision how long any given patient with a terminal disease has to live. The presence of this uncertainty does not invalidate the imminent/not-imminent distinction, however, any more than the existence of gray invalidates the distinction between black and white. The point here is that uncertain cases require special attention. The greater the likelihood that death is imminent and the greater the harm done if treatment is continued in vain, the stronger the rationale for treating the situation morally as if death is imminent. For instance, a patient who strongly prefers to die at home rather than attached to machines in a hospital has a valid justification for declining hospital care as long as there is a reasonable likelihood that death is imminent. Others may prefer to err on the side of continuing hospitalization as long as there is a significant chance that death is not necessarily imminent.

Withholding vs. Withdrawing Treatment

The second helpful distinction involving an aspect of the patient's medical condition or treatment is that between withholding and withdrawing treatment. In determining when it is morally acceptable to forgo treatment, it is sometimes thought that withdrawing (as opposed to withholding) life-sustaining treatment is tantamount to killing the patient and is just as wrong. Again the key question of whether death is intended can clarify what is at stake ethically.

Experientially, the withdrawal of life-sustaining treatment may indeed seem like killing the patient. Treatment is withdrawn and the patient's death follows soon thereafter. However, from a medical and ethical perspective the situation looks different. Withdrawing treatment is medically different from actively killing a patient (e.g., by administering a lethal injection of a poisonous drug) in that the medical cause of death is different. When treatment is withdrawn, the medical cause of death is the illness or injury itself. When the patient is killed, the medical cause of death is the action of the killer.

In pointing out this distinction between the medical causes of death I am not suggesting that withdrawing treatment is always morally different from active killing, however. It may not be different if its intention, like the intention of active killing, is the death of the patient.[5] On the other hand, if a patient is in such a deteriorated condition that death is imminent even with continued treatment, then a failure to withdraw treatment may only serve to prolong or even increase agony pointlessly. Treatment already begun should then be withdrawn for the same reason that treatment not yet begun would be withheld: there is no medical justification for it, and it may even be harming the patient.

The difficulty here, therefore, is not really medical or ethical; it is more a matter of how the situation is perceived. Before initiating treatment, caregivers must have a medical justification for the treatment. Their focus at this point is on the patient. But once treatment has been initiated, the focus sometimes expands beyond the patient to include the technology involved. Consciously or not, caregivers may come to view life-supporting machinery as a part of the patient. As a result, they may calculate the harm involved in "cutting off" a well-functioning respirator in the same way they calculate the harm involved in cutting off a perfectly good arm. But this is to misconstrue the situation. It is imperative that the patient (as opposed to the treatment) remain the focus, and that considerations regarding the use of life-supporting technology — whether initiating it or continuing it — be medically and ethically justified. Otherwise, we grant to technology the unique ethical significance that God has given to human life alone.

While withdrawing treatment is not necessarily any more problematic ethically than withholding it, it may nevertheless not be the preferred approach in some situations. Despite the logical distinctions, some caregivers cannot help but feel that to withdraw treatment is to cause the patient's death. Such is particularly the case when caregivers are asked to withdraw treatment that had been initiated much earlier by a different caregiver. If the treatment has served to hold death at bay for some time, it may be difficult to accept the idea that death can no longer be effectively resisted, especially for caregivers and patients operating out of the war model.

Nevertheless, these considerations may serve more to justify the need for a better understanding of what is involved in the treatment decisions at issue than they do to justify a preference for withholding treatment over withdrawing it. In fact, in many situations there are strong reasons to prefer withdrawing over withholding. It is often difficult to know whether a particular treatment will prove medically effective or acceptable to a patient unless it is tried for a while.[6] In other words, a trial period may be necessary to determine whether the treatment can satisfy the criteria that it provide an important medical benefit and that the patient is willing to accept it. In any case, patients are likely to be able to make a much more informed decision — one based on genuine understanding — if they have actually experienced the treatment under consideration.

Relieving Pain vs. Ending Life

A third important distinction requiring careful attention involves efforts to relieve a patient's pain, which may hasten the moment of death by relaxing the body. Is relieving pain in such circumstances tantamount to killing the patient, or do the two acts need to be distinguished ethically? Again, as with the previous distinction, the answer to both questions is sometimes Yes and sometimes No.

Our earlier discussion of suffering is relevant here. As we noted in Chapter 5, suffering is not an unqualified evil to be removed at all costs; it does have value. However, we can gain the value of suffering only when we oppose it — albeit helplessly — as an evil and yet experience the goodness of God in its midst. But if we reach a point at which we are no longer able to cope with suffering, if it overwhelms our capacity to experience God's goodness, then it loses its value and becomes merely destructive.

So we ought not to seek out or condone pain and suffering as if they were good in themselves. To the contrary, we can rightly seek to avoid them when that is morally possible. This outlook is reflected, for example, in Jesus' counsel to his disciples that when they were persecuted in one city they should flee to another (Matt. 10:23). Although Jesus did not spell out the reasons for this counsel, it appears that he wanted to spare his disciples from the suffering of persecution and free them to attend to other important matters. A similar perspective is instructive with respect to the medication of pain. It is morally acceptable — even desirable — to relieve pain in order to spare patients from suffering and thereby free them for a variety of pursuits, such as relating better to other people and to God.

Yet there are moral limits to this good enterprise from the perspective of the described approach. Contrary to popular and hedonistic utilitarian assertions, it is not ethically justifiable to end a God-given life — one's own or another's — merely in order to avoid suffering. This is not to diminish the difficulty of living out such a conviction. The agony Jesus experienced in wrestling with the issue of whether suffering or God would have the greater authority in his life was so great that "his sweat was like drops of blood falling to the ground" (Luke 22:44). Yet he chose faithfulness to God. Patients and caregivers are similarly tempted to avoid suffering by taking or administering pain medication in amounts calculated to cause death. Such intentional ending of life is morally wrong according to the described perspective.

It may also be misguided. One of the greatest contributions of the hospice movement is its demonstration that pain can be controlled much more effectively than was commonly believed before. In numerous hospices devoted to the care of those who are terminally ill (especially those with cancer), caregivers have learned that treating patients with love and understanding — as persons rather than cases — can make a profound difference. Physical pain can often be relieved with relatively small doses of medication when caregivers also take time to let patients express their anxieties and fears. If small doses prove insufficient, larger doses and more powerful drugs can be effectively used.

It is not always easy to identify precisely what type of medication and other forms of care will relieve a patient's pain. Caregivers sometimes lack the time or expertise to discover a particular patient's needs. However, compassionate, interdisciplinary hospice teams have demonstrated that such problems can be addressed. If physicians are unable to devote an optimal amount of time to understanding the complete range of their patients' needs, other team members (e.g., chaplains, social workers, nurses) can do so. In any event, it is not necessary to eliminate the patient in order to eliminate (or at least sufficiently control) the pain.[7]

As noted earlier, pain medication can do more than

merely relieve pain: it can also relax the body in such a way that it succumbs to a disease more quickly than it might otherwise. Should a caregiver necessarily hesitate to administer pain medication when this is a possible outcome? If death is imminent regardless of any further medical care, the answer is No. When there is no hope that medical treatment will add substantially to life, there remains only the obligation to care for the dying person as best one can, and relieving the person's pain is an important part of that care. A supporting ethical consideration is the intent behind the provision of the pain medication. The administration of such medication is not morally objectionable so long as it is given not with the intent to cause or hasten the death of the patient but out of a concern to relieve the patient's pain. Another supporting factor is that appropriately administered pain medication does not itself become the medical cause of death; it merely restores the body as much as possible to a pain-free state, and the terminal medical condition continues to worsen until death ensues.

If death is not imminent regardless of any further medical care, the situation is somewhat different with regard to pain medication. If it is possible that a patient might live a long time with proper treatment, then care must be taken not to undermine that potential.[8] Pain medication, though, is merely one part of the overall treatment. Most treatments have risks as well as possible benefits, and the patient must assess the contribution that pain medication can make to the effectiveness of the overall treatment. Evidence has long suggested that pain medication can actually contribute to a lengthened life, in that pain interferes with nutrition and rest, and generally weakens the body.[9] Pain medication is ethically problematic only if it is likely to render the rest of the treatment ineffective, thereby ending life well before it would end otherwise. Such is rarely the case.

While pain medication itself is generally not wrong, however, it should not be given in a dosage larger than necessary to achieve the desired goal. Caregivers should do what they can to preserve the patient's capacity to do such things as make treatment decisions and relate to other people and to God. Since overmedication can seriously impair these capacities, caregivers should avoid it.

Extraordinary vs. Burdensome Treatment

The fourth important distinction is actually a contrast between two pairs of distinctions. The issue here is whether treatment is best judged to be problematic when it is "extraordinary" (as opposed to ordinary) or when it is "burdensome" (as opposed to beneficial). The traditional distinction between extraordinary and ordinary treatment originated during the early days of surgery. At that time, surgery could be extremely painful because anesthesia was not available. Moreover, the effectiveness of surgery was often jeopardized by postoperative infections because of the lack of antiseptics. Accordingly, surgery was deemed an "extraordinary" treatment, and the implication was that people were not morally obligated to undergo it. The likely burdens of the treatment were just too great in comparison with the likely benefits.[10]

The problem with this distinction is that it commonly overgeneralizes. The distinction implicitly suggests that any given treatment can be understood to be either extraordinary or ordinary, and this in turn implies that the burden or benefit of the treatment is experienced similarly by all patients. Such is not the case, however. A treatment that seems quite ordinary to one may be experienced as extraordinary by another. Such experiential differences may be rooted in numerous other differences, such as contrasting spiritual outlooks or varying levels of family support. Even general perceptions of the status of a given treatment shift over time as a consequence of constant developments in the field of medicine. What seems

extraordinary today may soon seem ordinary, and people dis-
agree as to when a treatment switches categories.

Relying on a caregiver's categorization of a treatment is
further problematic because it subjects the patient to the
caregiver's judgment about what is normal (ordinary) treatment. A caregiver who has adopted the war model, for example, and who thus views death as the ultimate defeat to be
avoided at all costs, may present a given treatment (e.g., a
particular form of chemotherapy) to a patient as quite ordinary. Meanwhile, caregivers committed to other models might
characterize the same treatment as extraordinary because of
its limited prospect of benefit. The extraordinary/ordinary
distinction then becomes a device that caregivers use (often
unconsciously) to impose their own judgment about the appropriateness of treatment on patients. This problem is particularly acute when a patient is encouraged to employ the
distinction in a living will. By simply rejecting all "extraordinary" measures in certain situations, the patient may be con-
ceding critical treatment judgments to the caregiver in a document designed precisely to avoid such caregiver discretion.
Patients may especially want to retain more control (for themselves or their surrogate decision makers) over judgments
about controversial treatments such as artificial nutrition and
hydration.[11]

The problem here is not with the concerns underlying
the extraordinary/ordinary distinction as much as it is with
the form that the distinction takes. In this form, the distinction
implicitly places the emphasis on the nature of the treatment
itself and how it is to be classified rather than on the way it
is experienced uniquely by each patient. Because it is so important that the patient be willing to receive whatever treatment is provided, the patient's own assessment of what constitutes benefit and burden should play the most prominent
role. Admittedly, the extraordinary/ordinary distinction
could be construed so as to place the emphasis on the benefits

and burdens as experienced by the patient. If that is the point of the distinction, however, it might better be stated in terms of burden and benefit. The patient's explicit task then becomes to distinguish between burdensome and beneficial treatment.

What role should the burden/benefit distinction play in ethical decisions concerning treatment? It can play a decisive role when death is imminent regardless of treatment. As we have already noted, in such situations the love-impelled dimension of ethics (in the narrow sense of promoting the well-being of all affected) is definitive. In burden/benefit language, this means that patients should consider the burdens and benefits of continued treatment for themselves but also be sensitive to the implications of their decisions for family members as well as any other affected individuals and groups.

When death is not imminent if treatment is provided, however, other reality-bounded considerations take priority. The issue of whether death is intended becomes key. According to the described perspective, what matters most is not whether people are satisfied with how much benefit treatment will yield. The crucial question is whether they are being faithful to God by continuing to sustain the life that God has entrusted to them. A decision that life is "not worth it" is fundamentally off the mark.

It must be emphasized, however, that an obligation to sustain life entails an obligation to receive a given treatment only if that treatment is likely to be life-sustaining in a significant sense — only, that is to say, if it offers a reasonable likelihood of adding significantly to a patient's life. Every treatment has its risks and costs, and so a given treatment will virtually never be justified if it provides insignificant benefits such as an added minute or two of life. In fact, the chance that a treatment may directly or indirectly lead to an earlier death — or to an equally early death that is more painful — must be considered when deciding whether treatment is warranted.

Patients can often legitimately decline treatment on the basis of such possible outcomes, particularly when the treatment is experimental and the risks not fully understood.

What if a patient is offered a treatment that would likely be life-sustaining but would seriously affect the lives of others in an unwanted fashion? Might it be possible for patients to be "life-intending" by caring more for the lives of others than for their own lives, even to the point of forgoing life-sustaining treatment that could prolong life for a significant length of time? The death of Jesus is instructive on this point. Like a patient for whom a death-forestalling treatment is available, Jesus could have avoided (capture and) death. However, he chose not to do so because something of greater significance than his life was at stake. He chose instead to lay down his life for others.

It is morally commendable to risk one's life to pursue something as important as, or more important than, that life. In a "fallen" world, we experience conflicts between even the most significant moral mandates. The task of patients, then, is to discern any considerations in their situations that may outweigh the God-centered, reality-bounded, and love-impelled mandate to sustain their own lives. One such consideration would appear to be the lives of others.

The lives of others could be at stake in various ways. If the life-sustaining resource that a patient needs is scarce, such as a donor heart for a transplant, then by forgoing treatment the patient may make it possible for another to receive treatment and live. Paying for treatment may involve an analogous situation. If the resources so spent could instead be used to save the lives of others, then forgoing treatment might be warranted in order to save others' lives. The "other" in view, for example, might be a family member with a desperate need.

Alternatively, there are places around the world where even a relatively small amount of money could sustain numerous lives by providing food or lifesaving vaccines. The words of 1 John 3:16-17 are striking in this regard: "this is how we know what love is: Jesus Christ laid down his life for us. And we ought to lay down our lives" for others as well. The passage goes on to suggest that anyone who has material possessions and sees his brothers or sisters in need but has no pity on them must be devoid of the love of God. This passage is commonly understood as a call to a figurative laying down (i.e., opening up) of our lives to meet the life-threatening financial needs of others. And yet Jesus quite literally gave up his life — suggesting that this sort of self-sacrifice may be appropriate for others as well. Admittedly, a patient's decision not to consume scarce resources will not usually have the effect of freeing up resources that actually get provided to others who desperately need them — at least not if the patient is acting as an individual. However, if the patient is acting as part of a community, then self-giving can serve as a sign of faithfulness pointing to the possibility that communal action can enable and ultimately call forth a new set of priorities for resource allocation (as explained further in the Conclusion).

Self-sacrifice, then, is most clearly justified if one can be certain that it will serve to sustain the lives of others by meeting a vital need. But it is not often easy to be certain that this will be the outcome. How can we know, for example, that the life-threatening needs of family members will go unmet without self-sacrifice on our part? In the face of such uncertainty, we have to rely prayerfully on the best discernment we can muster concerning what is required to meet these needs. Intention is crucial in this matter. To be drawn to the prospect of self-sacrifice out of a sense that life is not worth continuing is to demean God-given life and to intend death — and this, as we have seen, is morally objectionable. Self-sacrifice is justifiable only if it provides a better way to affirm life than one's own treatment would — namely, by supporting the lives of others. Needless to say, it is also crucial that only those people contemplating self-sacrifice be allowed to make this decision;

it would be ethically unacceptable if it were imposed on them against their will (even subtly) by others.

The implications of this perspective for family members and others financing a patient's life-sustaining care are also worth noting here. We all have a responsibility to care for those who are seriously ill, especially for our biological family and brothers and sisters in the faith. The basis of this responsibility is the reality that God has created us to live not merely individually but also in community with others. The responsibility is distinctly love-impelled as well.[12]

However, the responsibility to give, while warranting substantial sacrifice, does not entail a moral requirement to subject oneself or one's family to life-threatening harm in the process, lest the jeopardy to one person's life merely be spread to others. Accordingly, the apostle Paul explains to the Corinthians that, in giving to meet the desperate needs of other believers in Jerusalem, they are expected only to give according to their means. "Our desire is not that others might be relieved while you are hard pressed" (2 Cor. 8:13).[13] Families, church congregations, and others, then, must engage in the same discerning process as patients in order to assess when the cost of funding a patient's life-sustaining treatment is too great for those who must go without those funds as a result. Nevertheless, in particular situations love may call forth a sacrifice that goes even beyond normal expectations. As the Macedonians (who gave "beyond their ability" — 2 Cor. 8:3) serve as the example Paul uses to prompt the self-centered Corinthians, so such examples can serve to prod people today from self-centeredness toward an equal regard for others.

While general ethical guides can help us in making decisions, there is no escape from the crucial role that discernment must play for patient and caregiver alike. To recognize this is to gain new appreciation for Paul's prayer for the Philippians as a model of how people should pray for those

touched by serious illness or disability: "this is my prayer:
that your love may abound more and more in knowledge and
depth of insight, so that you may be able to discern what is
best . . ." (Phil. 1:9-10). Discernment is influenced by many
factors, such as the circumstances one is in and the information one has.[14] However, three other key factors should also
be noted.

First, as Paul's prayer implies, God can nourish the love
within people and expand their capacity for discernment.
There is no substitute for the encouraging Spirit of God, especially when one is prone to despair as the vitality of life ebbs
away. Human admonitions for patients and caregivers to act
or not act in certain ways at such a time typically fall on deaf
ears.

Second, the moral character that we develop profoundly
influences our ability to discern well. The extent to which a
patient will characterize a given treatment as unacceptably
burdensome is in no small measure determined by virtues of
character such as humility and love. The same is true for
others contemplating giving up personal funds so that a
patient might be treated. In other words, ethics understood
as the study of what ought to be done is rather impotent if it
is not joined with personal formation. Personal formation
(sometimes referred to as Christian discipleship) involves the
cultivation of the moral character necessary in order for
people to be what they ought to be, in part so that they may
do what they ought to do.

Third, discernment is more than an individual matter; it
is profoundly shaped by one's community. The significance
of community resides not merely in the way people tend to
be influenced by the values of those around them. It also (and
perhaps more importantly) involves the fact that what one
experiences as an unacceptable burden is greatly dependent
on who is available to help shoulder it. A patient's bad decisions may be as much the result of the failure of the patient's

community to love as they are the result of any moral short-comings on the patient's part. Admittedly, we have an obligation to protect the patient's God-given freedom to accept or reject any treatment. However, there are better and worse decisions, and the better ones are rarely reached alone.

PART III

ALLOCATING VITAL RESOURCES

CHAPTER 8

Medical Assessments and the Elderly

Who should live when not all can live? Who should receive a donated organ when five candidates need it? Who should get a bed in the intensive care unit when space runs short? Who should be given any expensive treatment at all? The answers to these questions are deeply touching the lives of countless people in the United States and around the world today, such as Bill and his caregivers (see the Introduction). In the past this problem has received only limited public attention, but that is rapidly changing. What does the described approach have to say as people struggle to decide who should live and who should die?

The Allocation Problem

It is not possible for me to provide anything more than a brief overview of the problem here.[1] In essence, medical scarcity in the more developed countries of the world can broadly be described in terms of two phases. First, there was a low-tech

153

phase in which basic lifesaving drugs and other medical services were not available in sufficient quantity to meet the
needs of all. As most of these scarcities were overcome, however, there developed a general perception in some countries
that lifesaving care could be provided for all in need. Now
these countries have entered a second, high-tech phase of
scarcity in which more advanced technologies such as kidney
dialysis, organ transplantation, intensive care, and other expensive treatments are not available to all in need.[2]

Many less developed countries are still in the low-tech
phase. Large numbers of children there die for lack of vaccines, antibiotics, oral rehydration therapy, or the health care
personnel to administer them. Some countries not only continue to struggle with these low-tech scarcities but also face
the high-tech allocation dilemmas accompanying the introduction of expensive medical technologies.[3]

The future does not promise a solution to medical scarcity. Hopefully the magnitude of the scarcity in the less developed countries will be lowered through worldwide
cooperative efforts, but economic, social, and political constraints will likely hamper such efforts. Even in the more
developed countries scarcity will persist for several reasons.
First, new technologies are so expensive that the costs of
making them available to all has become prohibitive in some
cases. Second, the scarcity of some treatments (e.g., organ
transplantation) is not a function of money but of the limited
supply of other resources (e.g., available organs). Third, technological advancement will continue to yield new lifesaving
treatments that will be available only to a minority until they
can be developed and produced on a sufficiently large scale
to meet everyone's need (if that ever occurs).[4]

In the face of such a predicament, how are the recipients
of scarce lifesaving medical resources being selected? Numerous criteria are currently being employed. Sometimes those
judged most valuable to society are preferred; sometimes it is

those with stable home environments or the ability to pay. On the other hand, those thought to be living lives of insufficient quality may receive lowest priority. For an indication of how a large group of health-care professionals weigh such criteria in making decisions about the allocation of vital resources, see Table 8.1 (on pp. 156-57). Similar considerations are employed in less developed countries such as Kenya.[5] Which of the various criteria are morally acceptable? Does a theological perspective on the world provide any guidance in these life-or-death decisions?

Age Criteria

We will take a closer look at the full range of criteria in Chapters 10 and 11, but at this point the age criterion warrants special attention because it is coming to exercise such a powerful influence over decisions about the allocation of vital resources. At a time when some treatment choices of "the elderly"[6] are being better protected through such means as advance directives (see Chapter 4), others are being curtailed. In an era of limited resources, a greater degree of choice is desirable. From an economic standpoint, for example, it is preferable that the elderly have the option to refuse costly treatments in favor of less expensive treatments or no treatment at all. In the end, however, when people want more treatment than a society can provide, some individuals' choices must be denied. The elderly appear to be prime candidates.

Age criteria already direct many patient selection decisions in the United States.[7] National and state surveys have confirmed some sizable support for such criteria.[8] Lifesaving treatments such as heart transplantation, intensive care, and kidney dialysis and transplantation have long been allocated on the basis of the age of the patient.[9] Medical studies con-

Table 8.1. Patient Selection Criteria

Criteria for Patient Selection	Relative Importance	Percentage Considering Criterion
Medical Benefit. Will the health of the prospective recipient be better with the treatment than without it?	4.2	95%
Likelihood of Benefit. How likely is it that the desired medical outcome will in fact occur?	4.0	96
Quality of Benefit. What quality of life can the prospective recipient expect if accepted for treatment?	3.8	97
Willingness. Has the prospective recipient explicitly or implicitly registered a desire to undergo treatment?	3.7	89
Length of Benefit. How much longer can the prospective recipient expect to survive with treatment?	3.6	96
Psychological Ability. How able will the prospective recipient be to cope emotionally and intellectually with the treatment regimen?	3.2	97
Age. How many years has the prospective recipient lived?	2.7	88
Vital Responsibilities. Does the physical life of at least one other person — or something equally important — depend on whether or not the prospective recipient lives?	2.5	69
Resources Required. Will the prospective recipient be likely to require particularly long or expensive treatment?	2.2	66
Supportive Environment. How supportive (financially, emotionally, etc.) will the prospective recipient's family, friends, and community be?	2.0	61
Progress of Science. Will significant scientific knowledge be gained from treating the prospective recipient?	2.0	58

Criteria for Patient Selection	Relative Importance	Percentage Considering Criterion
Social Value. How much will society, including people individually, benefit if the prospective recipient is treated?	2.0	56
Ability to Pay. Does the prospective recipient have enough money or insurance to pay for the required services?	1.8	43
Impartial Selection. Should prospective recipients be treated as fundamentally similar and, therefore, selected impartially by lottery or on a first-come, first-served basis?	1.7	31
Favored Group. Is the prospective recipient a member of a certain group, identified by geographical location, veteran status, or the like?	1.4	27
Sex. What is the gender of the prospective recipient?	1.0	1

The figures in this table come from a study in which 453 medical directors of kidney dialysis and transplantation facilities in the United States were asked to assess the degree to which a variety of criteria affect their determination of who should receive vital medical treatment. They were asked to rank each of the criteria listed above on a scale of increasing importance from 1 (= Unimportant) to 5 (= Very Important). The numbers in the first column ("Relative Importance") indicate the average response of those surveyed. The numbers in the second column ("Percentage Considering Criterion") indicate the percentage of the respondents who give the criteria any weight at all in their determinations.

I offer a more complete statistical analysis and discussion of this study in an article entitled "Selecting Patients When Resources Are Limited: A Study of U.S. Medical Directors of Kidney Dialysis and Transplantation Facilities" (*American Journal of Public Health* 78 [February 1988]: 144-47).

trolling for physiological differences among patients indicate that even nonscarce resources tend to be provided on the basis of age.[10] Outside the United States, age criteria are also widely employed.[11] The denial of lifesaving dialysis to some patients in Great Britain is only the most publicized of many such situations worldwide.[12]

The prevalence of an age criterion, particularly in Great Britain, suggests that the criterion may well become more prominent in the United States during the next few decades. If resources devoted to dialysis are restricted, then the British parallel will be particularly influential.[13] In fact, whereas only 10 percent of dialysis directors that participated in the U.S. study referred to in Table 8.1 employ an age criterion today, 85 percent indicate that they would do so under conditions of greater resource limitations.[14]

unfair

Beyond the realm of dialysis, too, the elderly are likely to fare less well than others in U.S. patient selection decisions for a variety of reasons. Because the elderly require a disproportionately large amount of medical resources, a relatively great potential savings lies in excluding them from treatment. The lack of assertiveness on the part of many elderly (at least the very old) plus the cultural value placed on youth also make an increasing emphasis on an age criterion likely.[15]

What does this situation look like from the God-centered, reality-bounded, and love-impelled perspective developed in Part I? A God-centered perspective, first of all, suggests that human observation, values, and reasoning are all limited. Rather than trusting in human perceptions of who the elderly are and how worthy they are of lifesaving health care, people would do well to learn as much as possible about God's perspective from the Bible, among other sources. People should also resist the temptation to base treatment of the elderly on "the good of society" as that standard is commonly understood (i.e., in a simple utilitarian fashion).

Since the lives of the elderly are at stake, a reality-bounded perspective is similarly going to be interested in who the elderly are and how they compare to other potential recipients of health care resources. Moreover, it will be concerned about the implications of basic ethical guides such as life and justice. A love-impelled perspective, in turn, will be committed to improving the well-being of all in society, including the elderly, within the bounds of the governing realities. A good place to begin a more detailed analysis, then, is with a look at the nature of the elderly and of human life itself, as far as the Bible can shed light on these matters.

The Elderly

Who are the elderly? Two characteristics stand out at various points in the biblical writings. First, they often have a special perspective that comes with age. "Is not wisdom found among the aged?" asks Job. "Does not long life bring understanding?" (Job 12:12; cf. 15:10; 32:7). The elders (normally elderly) are therefore in the best position to give good counsel (Deut. 32:7; 1 Kings 12:6ff.), and a family that has lost all of its elderly is said to have been severely punished (1 Sam. 2:31). Wisdom is frequently presented as a function of the life experience that only the elderly have. However, because it is also a product of righteousness and God's Spirit, it is possible for the young to have it (Job 32:8-9; Eccles. 4:13) and the old to lack it (Prov. 16:31; Job 12:20).[16]

A second characteristic of many elderly — at least at some point — is weakness. Old age is acknowledged in the Bible as a time of suffering and vulnerability (e.g., in Eccles. 12:2-5; 2 Sam. 19:35). Knowing that insensitive people take advantage of the weakness of the elderly, the psalmist prays, "do not cast me away when I am old; do not forsake me when my strength is gone" (Ps. 71:9; cf. v. 18).

Both the wisdom and the weakness of the elderly call for appropriate responses. An appropriate response to wisdom is respect. Evil nations are sometimes characterized by their lack of respect for the elderly (Deut. 28:50; 2 Chron. 36:17; Isa. 47:6). It is a dark day when "the young will rise up against the old" (Isa. 3:5), when "elders are shown no respect" (Lam. 5:12). We are instructed instead to "rise in the presence of the aged, show respect for the elderly and [so] revere your

God" (Lev. 19:32). Such texts recognize that the economic value of the young is greater than that of the old (Lev. 27:1-7 is explicit on the point) but that the way people are to be valued and treated has to do with more than economic worth. The elderly are to be respected for their wisdom — but also simply for who they are as elderly persons (Prov. 20:29). The point of valuing the elderly for their wisdom is not ultimately to accord them greater significance than the young but to counterbalance the utilitarian tendency of some societies (such as the United States) to overvalue the productivity of the young.

An appropriate response to the relative weakness of the elderly, on the other hand, is protection. God is frequently portrayed in the biblical writings as the protector of the weak (Exod. 22:22-27; Ps. 10:14; 35:10; 140:12; Acts 20:35; 1 Cor. 8:9-12; 2 Cor. 12:9-10), and God's people are challenged to be the same (Prov. 31:8-9; 1 Thess. 5:14). So it is not at all surprising to find God affirming, "even to your old age and gray hairs I am [the One] who will sustain you" (Isa. 46:4). God's identification with the plight of the helpless has understandably been heralded as a theological cornerstone for treatment of today's elderly.[17]

From this perspective the elderly are as worthy of lifesaving care as anyone else. In fact, whether a particular culture values the wisdom of the elderly or not is ultimately beside the point. All persons are God's creation in God's own image and the objects of God's sacrificial love in Christ (Gen. 1:27; John 3:16). It is this basic equal worth of all that demands that all be respected and that the weak accordingly receive special protection.

If anything, the tendency of the elderly to be physically weak and separated from the power that accompanies culturally recognized economic productivity makes them especially worthy of Christian concern. Their equal claim upon society's lifesaving resources needs to be protected. Even if theoretical justifications for excluding the elderly were not flawed in their own right, they would engage people in the practice of abandoning the elderly and in that sense excluding them from communal care — a destructive precedent.[18] If an elderly individual volunteers to let someone younger have priority over her or him in the distribution of limited lifesaving resources, this act may be an admirable expression of sacrificial love. To require such sacrifice, however, is to demean the elderly as a group and to take from them the opportunity to give.

Life

Just as the biblical materials cast light on who the elderly are, they also illumine the nature of human life itself in a way relevant to the assessment of age criteria in health care. We have already examined in some detail the concept of life as a moral guide. Two additional characteristics of life, especially relevant in the present context, stand out in opposition to nontheological views of life. The first is that *life is spiritual.* The second is that *life is eternal.*

Linked to God, life includes but transcends the material sphere. The spirituality of life contrasts with common views of life at two important points. First, people tend to live by what they see — by appearances rather than by faith — and the elderly may appear to be relatively unproductive and insignificant. However, if what matters is not economic achievement but, for example, righteous character and relationship with God, then the elderly can be as fruitful as anyone (Ps. 92:14; cf. 1 Cor. 4:16).[19] Second, we tend to categorize people in ways that elevate ourselves and put others down. A spiritual perspective looks beyond such worldly classifications as Jew versus Greek or slave versus free and views all people as loved and sought by God (Matt. 28:19; cf. Jonah 4:11) and potentially one in Christ (1 Cor. 12:13; Gal. 3:28; Col. 3:11). From this perspective, efforts to classify certain people by age in order to exclude them from access to health care should at least be suspect. Moreover, those steeped in the youth-oriented values of North America need to be challenged by alternative values in other cultures. No culture is gospel.

More specifically, the fixation on youth and the productivity orientation of Western culture need to be assessed critically by those from other cultures who have a much greater appreciation for persons per se and the elderly in particular. Research has shown that many cultures view the elderly differently than they are viewed in North America.[20] The described perspective calls us to value persons for more than just their productivity. It is possible for North Americans to move significantly in this direction without swinging completely over to an indifference toward productivity, which could also be destructive in its extreme form.

The other additional characteristic of life often acknowledged in the Bible — the fact that *life is eternal* — also contrasts with common views of life at more than one important point.

First, when people view temporal life as all that there is, maximizing the length of that life becomes a matter of ultimate importance. Among those who do profess belief in an "afterlife," many view it as something subsequent to "this life" and thoroughly different from it in nature. The perspective of some biblical writers, however, challenges this view. While some writers do focus upon the future dimension of eternal life, others add the conviction that eternal life begins not later but now. A person who believes in God "has eternal life" already and "has crossed over from death to life" (John 5:24; cf. 1 John 3:14). From this perspective, physical death is not nearly so significant a transition as it is commonly considered to be. As sleep is merely a transition from one day to the next, so death may be simply referred to as "being asleep" (1 Cor. 15:6, 18, 20, 51). To be able to sleep and so go to be with Christ is actually "better by far" than living long (Phil.

1:23). In other words, for those truly concerned with the ultimate good of a person, access to a long life pales in significance compared with access to an eternal life. (The lives of
those who do not choose life with God also continue eternally
— albeit separated from God in accordance with their choice
[Matt. 8:11-12; 25:46; Luke 14:15-24; 16:26, 31].)

There is a second way in which an eternal perspective
on life minimizes the significance of attempts to lengthen life
(through age criteria in health care or otherwise). In the face
of eternity, a lifetime is but a few hours (Ps. 90:4; cf. 2 Pet. 3:8),
a momentary breath (Ps. 39:5; cf. James 4:14), a fleeting
shadow (Job 14:1-2; Ps. 144:4; Eccles. 6:12). Even to extend life
by years is in the greater scheme of things to extend it by only
a few seconds.

These aspects of the eternal perspective do not provide
direct arguments against the use of age criteria in health care,
but they do argue against the strong tendency to idolize length
of life, and they provide a better frame of reference for considering the many other arguments against age criteria.

One final implication of an eternal perspective is closely
related to the second but is somewhat more directive. Necessarily brief in the face of eternity, temporal life may end at
any moment. When one least expects it, the end may be at
hand (Luke 12:16-20; 1 Thess. 5:1-4). Accordingly, ethical
living in the present is crucial (Rom. 13:8-12). The point here
is not that planning for the future is unnecessary but that we
should treat with special seriousness immediate needs that
can in fact be met. Health care has traditionally reflected this
perspective by directing the major portion of available resources (preventively and therapeutically) to present needs
that can demonstrably be met, while at the same time devoting significant resources to research for the future.

In this light it may well be appropriate to emphasize
diseases of the young when allocating research funds, for we
can appropriately pursue a variety of future-oriented ends

through research. But it is quite a different matter to exclude the elderly from receiving specified health care resources in order to improve the life prospects of the young. Such a course of action morally compromises the meeting of definite medical needs by making decisions about who receives care subordinate to the pursuit of other goods such as long life. In the biblical writings, a full life span may be understood as something good given by God, along with good food and water (Exod. 23:25-26). Using patient selection as a means to pursue any such goods rather than to respond to medical need is fundamentally a utilitarian (or misplaced egalitarian) endeavor that dilutes the commitment that health caregivers have to all persons.

Deciding to treat patients on the basis of strictly medical considerations may seem a straightforward way to exclude inappropriate influences, but such is not the case. Many so-called medical justifications for excluding the elderly from lifesaving health care are actually driven by nonmedical considerations. We would do well, then, to distinguish the various medical justifications and to assess their legitimacy individually. With a clearer grasp of the medical issues, it will be much easier to address the nonmedical bases for excluding the elderly in the next chapter.

We should distinguish four types of medical justifications, since they constitute significantly different arguments for age criteria in health care. Three of these — length of medical benefit, quality of medical benefit, and likelihood of medical benefit — involve comparisons of patients. The fourth, medical benefit, involves determining in the case of each patient whether a significant benefit is likely to result from treatment. The first three justifications are dubious according to the described perspective.[21] In some instances the problems are pragmatic, but there are also deeper substantive difficulties inherent in the justifications. The fourth justification is sound, but it justifies a medical rather than an age criterion when applied to the elderly.

Length of Medical Benefit

Some people favor age criteria because they believe that scarce resources should be given to those who will receive the greatest (i.e., longest) benefit if treated. The elderly, as a rule, will not live as long as younger patients and so will not receive as great a benefit. There are a number of difficulties with this rationale.

One difficulty with a length-of-benefit justification is the uncertainty of the prognoses involved. It is impossible to predict with precision how long a person will live. When a patient is suffering from multiple illnesses, predictions are especially problematic.[22] Because of the high probability of major errors in prediction, it may simply be too risky to rely on length of benefit as a basis for patient selection.

Another problem with this justification is that it does not take into account the significance of personhood per se. It is mistaken to try to distinguish lives on the basis of quantifiable factors such as the length of time that patients are expected to live. As we have already noted, such considerations are secondary when life itself is at stake. This outlook has been voiced particularly strongly in Italy, among other countries. Italians have tended historically not to exclude from scarce dialysis even those patients who are suffering from terminal illnesses (beyond their kidney disease) that dialysis will not affect. Why, the Italians have reasoned, should those with a shorter life expectancy receive lower priority than those whose expectancy is longer through no merit of their own?[23]

Subjectively it is also difficult to claim that a longer life is more important to preserve than a shorter one. Each person's life is uniquely important to that person. The objective counterpart to this argument is that each person should have an equal right to life. The right to life (i.e., the duty of others to respect it) does not expire after a certain number of years or gradually diminish; we all ought to have access to life (within limits) irrespective of our circumstances.

A final difficulty arises with regard to reusable resources such as hemodialysis and, to a lesser degree, intensive care. In this context, employing length-of-benefit considerations can ironically end up saving fewer lives. Given a limited medical resource such as hemodialysis, for example, one can either treat a small number of people for long periods of time or a larger number of people for shorter periods of time. Since younger people are more likely to need longer periods of treatment than older people, an inclination to treat the young rather than the elderly will mean that for a fixed amount of treatment time, however measured, fewer people overall will be treated. If persons (and not just unqualified longevity) matter, this is an unattractive by-product of the length-of-benefit rationale.

Quality of Medical Benefit

Some people believe that the elderly will usually not have as high a quality of life following treatment as will younger patients, and they support giving priority in patient selection to younger patients on this basis. There are several important problems with this view.

First of all, there are practical difficulties. Quantifying qualitative considerations in order to be able to compare patients is extremely difficult. Identifying precise trade-offs between relative likelihood, quantity, and quality of benefits can be even more complex.

A more fundamental difficulty is that not only is it impossible for one person to determine what another person's quality of life will be after a given treatment, but it is inappropriate even to attempt to do so. When people do try to make quality-of-life judgments about other people's lives, they typically judge on the basis of various objective, observable indicators of quality of life. But there is significant evidence suggesting that such objective indicators do not correlate well with patients' subjective experience of their own lives.[24] The fact that it appears to someone else that I am experiencing a low quality of life does not mean that I necessarily share that view.

There is an important difference between observing and experiencing. Well people (observing patients' quality of life) and sick people (experiencing it) view issues of quality differently.[25] What is unacceptable to the well may be quite acceptable to the sick. In fact, studies document that physicians differ from patients (and from nursing assistants as well) in their assessments of those patients' quality of life.[26] The validity of some people making qualitative judgments about the lives of others, then, is open to serious question. It may be that one simply cannot make qualitative judgments without personally experiencing that which is being qualitatively evaluated.

Furthermore, different people have different standards by which they subjectively judge quality of life.[27] This point is graphically illustrated by a British debate that centered largely on quality-of-benefit considerations. A British hospital decided to remove a patient by the name of Derek Sage from dialysis treatment on the grounds that his quality of life was quite low. The warden at Simon House, a center for homeless men where Sage was living, argued that Sage had been doing well while receiving dialysis and was eating and sleeping well. Hospital staff, on the other hand, described Sage as a demented, intermittently violent, dirty, and doubly incontinent man with a tendency to expose himself and masturbate while being examined. The warden countered that Sage did not typically behave in this way and that he did so at the hospital because the place frightened him.[28] It is admittedly difficult to be certain of all the factors that entered into this particular treatment decision. All too often, though, a judgment that a patient's quality of life is too low is really a statement that the person making the judgment would rather not have to continue to deal with the patient in the patient's current condition.[29]

What may really be going on in such instances is a veiled form of social-value assessment — the sort of human-centered reasoning we considered in Chapter 1. Some people are being excluded because their quality of life following treatment will be so low that they will provide little benefit to society in exchange for the precious resources they are receiving. Benefiting society is a worthy aspiration in line with the love-impelled dimension of ethics, but love operates within the bounds of God-established realities such as life and justice. Social-value assessments violate those bounds by claiming priority over life itself — that is to say, over who will be enabled to live. Moreover, they fail to account for the spiritual and eternal dimensions of life.

Empowering some to judge the social value (i.e., quality of life) of others is particularly dangerous for the very patients who already constitute the most disadvantaged segment of society and are the least productive as a result. Certain social groups predictably bear the brunt of this discrimination — most notably the poor and the elderly. They are reduced to their functional dimension as if there were nothing else in personhood worth respecting.[30] While we will take a more detailed look at social-value selection in Chapter 10, it is important to note here that we would do better to view successful treatment in terms of sustaining a quality of life that is significant in the eyes of the patient.

The ethical demands of freedom and justice also come directly into play here.[31] Age criteria based on imposed judgments about quality of life deny people the freedom to determine the sufficiency of their quality of life *for them*. In terms of justice, if persons are fundamentally equal, then they should have equal access to lifesaving resources. The relative quality of their lives should be irrelevant when life itself is at stake. There may be a price to pay for the protection of freedom, justice, and life in terms of the overall quality of benefit produced by a limited supply of resources — but things of great value are rarely obtained cheaply. Sometimes the anticipated quality of life following treatment depends on the efforts of persons other than the patient, such as family members. Particularly in these instances, imposing requirements of quality on a patient's life seems unjustified. If a low quality of life is expected after treatment, that should serve as a reason to provide special help where possible in addition to life-sustaining treatment, not a rationale for withholding both. Medicine rightly devotes many of its resources to enabling people to live lives of the highest quality possible. These efforts at their best, though, in line with the ethical priorities of the described approach, involve trying to make low-quality lives high-quality rather than letting low-quality lives perish in order to preserve higher-quality lives.

Likelihood of Medical Benefit

A third form of medical justification for an age criterion involves the likelihood that patients will benefit medically from treatment. Knowing that elderly patients are less likely to benefit from certain treatments than are younger patients, some physicians support age criteria on these grounds. However, this justification is flawed in important ways.

To begin with, this justification denies any chance of treatment to some patients who would probably benefit from it. Treatment goes first to those individuals who are most likely to benefit from it and then, as resources permit, it goes to those who are less likely to benefit from it. If resources are limited, treatment may well have to be denied to individuals who would probably benefit from it in an absolute sense even if they would not be as likely to benefit as other candidates. In a sense this justification does promise to ensure a productive use of resources, but it does so at too great a cost according to the described perspective. It does not adequately respect the significance of the lives of all those involved, for the life of each person who has a reasonable likelihood of benefiting from treatment depends on having an opportunity to obtain treatment. This problem would exist even if the justification could guarantee the best results in every case. In fact, no such guarantees are possible. Caregivers can determine the relative likelihood that a patient will benefit from treatment on a rough statistical basis only, and this leaves considerable room for error. In any given case, the preferred patient might die even with treatment, while the patient denied treatment might have survived if treated.

There are other serious problems with this likelihood justification as well. For one thing, its preoccupation with efficiency makes it dehumanizing. Like social-value considerations, it tends to favor efficiency over equal regard for persons (especially equal regard for the significance each person attaches to his or her own life). There is more to the health of a society, however, than physical well-being. The fairness and humaneness with which people are treated, among other things, are also critical. A society that ignores such concerns in its pursuit of efficient medical care may stave off the effects of illness for a while only to end up incapacitated in a more significant way by inhumanity and insensitivity. Such is the eventual result of ignoring God-established bounds.

A likelihood-of-benefit justification is also weak in that it depends on a clear determination of the relative likelihood that an individual will benefit from treatment, and such determinations are difficult to make. Theoretically, for this justification to be valid, caregivers would have to be able to dis-

tinguish a patient with, say, a 10 percent likelihood of benefiting from a patient with a 12 percent likelihood. But under
normal circumstances, nothing like that sort of accuracy is
possible. The clinical data necessary to make more than edu-
cated guesses are usually not available.[32] Even those who
favor likelihood justifications in general tend to base their
support on the stipulation that it is possible to make prognoses with some exactness.[33]

Detailed comparisons of all candidates for treatment are
also problematic because they interfere with medicine's basic
responsibility to the patient. Rather than directing physicians
to pursue treatment for any patient who will benefit medically
from it, a likelihood justification requires them to compare
the candidates so that some can be favored over others. The
trust that patients have in their physicians and medical institutions — so essential to effective medicine — may be seriously undermined as a result. Patients will know that any
information they supply indicating that their recovery might
be difficult will lessen their chances of receiving any treatment
at all.

Sometimes the elderly as a group rather than individual
older patients are excluded from treatment on the basis of
their statistically lower likelihood of benefit with treatment.
The problem with this approach is that it withholds resources
from some individuals on grounds that do not apply to them.
Grouping people together under a single label, such as "the
elderly" is a relevant basis for medical treatment decisions
only if all the people in that group share the same relevant
medical characteristics. While it is true that most elderly
patients are not able to tolerate certain medical treatments
well, for example, the assertion that *most* are not implies that
some are, and it is unfair to exclude individuals who are likely
to benefit simply because they belong to a given class. The
described approach suggests that medicine should keep the
needs of the individual patient clearly in view, as does God.

Medical Benefit

There is a fourth form of medical justification for an age criterion that, unlike the other three, does not compare individual patients or groups of patients. It is a yes-or-no assessment. Those who use this criterion seek to allocate treatment to all (and only) those who will likely receive significant benefit as a result of the treatment. Implicit in this justification are minimum levels of likelihood, quality, and length of benefit necessary to justify the allocation of medical resources to patients.

Many factors are a part of the medical evaluations needed to apply a medical-benefit standard, and the results will not always be clear-cut or uniform among physicians. Sometimes a trial use of a resource will be the only way to determine if a patient will benefit from it. Nevertheless, the point of the standard is straightforward: to try to benefit all and only those who can benefit.

This form of medical justification is much better grounded than the other three according to the described perspective. It is rooted squarely in the notion of responding to human need in whatever medical form it exists. The notion of need includes the idea that some disease or injury condition is present and that a patient's life is thereby undesirably altered. Determining what constitutes an undesirable alteration is a value judgment that requires careful examination with respect to each resource. A need for a life-sustaining resource implies that a patient's life is in jeopardy without it.[34] As we have already seen, need and equality work together as basic components of distributive justice in the biblical writings. We are called to meet life-sustaining needs with equal regard for all persons.

Sufficient clinical data must be collected to establish limits regarding how much of a particular resource is genuinely needed by patients in various medical circumstances. For instance, the sickest patients may ironically not need a particular resource at all, if they have deteriorated to the point where the resource would no longer be of benefit to them or if their death is imminent from other unalterable causes. Furthermore, caregivers have to determine what constitutes minimum levels of likelihood, quality, and length of benefit with as much specificity as the circumstances will allow (such that no one who can reasonably be expected to benefit significantly from treatment is excluded). Even with such limitations, though, the requirement of need has long proven to be a helpful guide in selecting patients.[35]

The critical question for us in this context, however, is whether the legitimate treatment rationale of medical benefit can rightly be used to justify an age criterion. In the final analysis, it cannot. Once again, the essential problem is that the characteristics of the elderly as a class simply do not apply to every elderly individual. Some elderly patients may indeed be so sick that they do not "need" a particular life-sustaining resource (in the sense explained above), but others will have a genuine need for that resource. A given elderly person may be in better physical condition to undergo treatment than a younger person. Certain elderly patients also have a strength of mind and heart that make them better candidates for treatment than some patients half their age.[36] So finding a simple cut-off age beyond which people do not warrant a particular life-sustaining treatment on medical grounds is necessarily problematic. Any such cut-off will be arbitrary, unfair, and disrespectful of the elderly as persons. Such determinations violate God-established bounds in their pursuit of convenience and efficiency.

In fact, should the elderly have some particular difficulty making use of needed resources, then need itself can be seen to dictate that special efforts should be made to overcome these difficulties (especially if the need is in some measure society's fault). Special need — if it can reasonably be met —

scarcely justifies offering less care; to the contrary, it supports an argument for providing greater care. When the elderly have found it difficult to withstand the immunosuppressive regimen employed in kidney transplants, for example, the response of some caregivers has been to try different immuno-suppressive regimens until they have found a treatment that does work, rather than simply excluding them from consideration for treatment altogether.[37]

In the end, it may be appropriate to exclude certain elderly patients from certain treatments, but such exclusions should be made on the basis of their inability to benefit medically from these treatments rather than on account of their age as such. We have to be careful about how we use language; we should take care to identify as "medical" only those matters and criteria that are in fact medical. Age per se is not a medically relevant factor in determinations about individual patients, since medical problems that make one elderly person a bad candidate for a given treatment may not affect another. We generally cannot even assume that a given elderly person has a short life expectancy.[38] It is preferable according to the described approach, then, not to use age as a medical criterion. The focus should be on the medical liabilities commonly associated with old age, and not age itself, as potential reasons for excluding a patient from treatment. It is certainly true that many elderly patients are so physically weakened that they make poor candidates for organ transplantation or intensive care; but others bear up fairly well in these circumstances.[39] In fact, studies show that although the elderly have often been excluded from dialysis treatment, many of those who have received it have done well.[40]

Accordingly, age is best not identified as a separate patient selection criterion at all. Rather, its most appropriate role is probably as one of many "symptoms" to be looked for by the physician making the medical assessment required by a medical-benefit criterion. Like any observed symptom, age can be an indicator of a possible medical problem. It serves best as a tool the physician uses in applying a medical criterion, not as a criterion in its own right. From this perspective it is inappropriate to single out age during a discussion of selection criteria in a way that implies that it is more than just one among many symptoms considered in a medical assessment. It is more a rule of thumb for medical assessment than for patient selection in general.

Even in such a restricted role, age considerations must be carefully handled to ensure that they are not accorded more influence than is warranted medically. It is easy enough to underestimate the ability of some elderly patients to endure treatment when life is at stake; and technological developments consistently make treatments more endurable. In the end, the only way to know with confidence how the elderly will bear up under a given treatment may well be to treat them in large numbers, as was done during the early days of dialysis in Italy.[41] Whenever possible, a therapeutic trial can be employed to facilitate more individualized assessments.

All these considerations combine to suggest that the growing U.S. support for age criteria in health care does not have a sound medical basis. In fact, this support more likely reflects certain social, economic, or even philosophical attitudes and values understandably not shared by the whole society or by various other cultures. It is to these nonmedical, social justifications of age criteria that we turn in Chapter 9.

CHAPTER 9

Nonmedical Exclusion of the Elderly

Age criteria in medicine are widespread even though they lack a satisfactory medical basis. One explanation for this state of affairs is that many of the most influential justifications for age criteria are nonmedical in nature. Indeed, age considerations are sometimes hidden within more general "social" and "economic" justifications, as may have been the case in Bill's situation (see the Introduction). What are the nonmedical justifications for age criteria, and how legitimate are they from a God-centered, reality-bounded, and love-impelled perspective?

The Justifications

Many believe that age criteria are legitimate because they encourage the productive use of medical resources.[1] There are several types of explicitly productivity-oriented justifications.

One type involves the contention that age criteria will help to ensure the best possible return on the investment of resources: the young are more likely to contribute more to society for a longer time than the elderly.[2] Another type of productivity-oriented justification focuses on the convenience of an age criterion. Unlike uncertain and somewhat subjective medical judgments, a patient's age is a comparatively objective and precise basis for selection.[3] Moreover, some proponents argue that it can often be applied without major resistance from the elderly, who as individuals (if not collectively) can be relatively unassertive.

A final productivity-oriented justification has to do with the financial savings that can be achieved if the elderly are denied lifesaving resources. For example, if those over 55 years of age were excluded from treatment for renal disease in the United States, 45 percent of the costs of the renal disease program would be saved.[4] In other areas such as intensive care, the elderly use such a disproportionate amount of resources that there is also a great financial gain where they are excluded. After all — though it is tragically stark to acknowledge — death is the ultimate economy in health care expenditures.[5]

An age criterion might also seem appealing from a perspective such as the described approach, which respects such moral guides as life and justice. Interestingly, part of its appeal stems from what it is not: in the face of some lifesaving medical care today that is prone to dehumanize people by trying desperately to forestall death at all costs, an age criterion recognizes that it is appropriate to accept death when old age arrives.[6] Furthermore, although "ageism" is sometimes asserted to be as discriminatory as racism and sexism, the criterion actually avoids much of the criticism directed against racism and sexism. Racism and sexism are considered evil primarily because only certain people are penalized because of their race or sex. But *everyone* is subject to old age (if death does not intervene first).[7]

It can be argued that rather than promoting inequality, an age criterion promotes equality — specifically, an equal opportunity to live to the same age as others.[8] Some base this argument on a right to a minimum number of life-years.[9] Others focus on the value of each year of life rather than each person per se, arguing that we should employ an age criterion in order to maximize the total number of life-years saved by medical efforts.[10]

A variation of the equal-opportunity justification has to do with the concept of life span. Some people contend that there is a natural life span (perhaps seventy or eighty years) that is normative for human beings rather than merely a statistical average at the present moment in history. Once people have reached this age, they argue, medicine should generally no longer be concerned with saving (extending) their lives. They have lived full lives, and resources should be devoted instead to those who still have important life projects ahead of them.[11]

One further egalitarian proposal is that people should be treated equally not so much in the present moment as over a lifetime. Health care should be provided in such a way as to enable all people to live as long as possible.[12] To achieve this end, the resources available must be distributed throughout each person's lifetime so as to protect against early death. Expensive lifesaving resources, then, might be made available only to the young, with personal care services enhanced for the elderly (and preventive as well as other basic care perhaps provided to all).[13] Some argue more radically along these lines that all resources should be channeled to the young to increase their prospects and the elderly should be encouraged to commit assisted suicide.[14] Unlike a more utilitarian concern to maximize the total number of life-years saved — which would often entail helping some at the expense of others — this outlook adopts the perspective of the typical individual and appeals to the notion of "prudence." If each person had a fixed amount of health care resources to spend over a lifetime, it is reasoned, it might be prudent to confine expensive lifesaving care to the earlier years of life.

An Assessment

While these justifications have a certain intuitive appeal, they do not hold up well under careful scrutiny. Consider first the productivity-oriented justifications. Excluding the elderly would indeed ensure a better return on the investment of health care resources, but in the process it would demean people. Such justifications proceed as if the only relevant moral concern is to get the most productivity out of a group of machines, and this analogy is simply not appropriate. To the contrary, persons of any age are intrinsically valuable apart from their productivity according to the described approach, because of God's love for them. Those who adopt a utilitarian, human-centered approach improperly allow a concern for good consequences — whether love-impelled or not — to operate beyond the bounds of the ethical guides of life and justice (see Part I).

An age criterion is also attractive because it is convenient. It provides an objective standard for making difficult decisions about the allocation of vital resources. And yet the mere fact that a standard is objective does not mean that it is appropriate. The patient's height would constitute an equally objective — though obviously irrelevant — standard.

An age criterion is also convenient in that the elderly may well be the weakest and easiest to exclude from treatment, but they ought to receive more care for that reason, not less. In the biblical materials, the reality-bounded guide of justice upholds not only the fundamental equality of all persons but also the importance of special support for those most in need.

Admittedly, using an age criterion would provide a disproportionate savings in the cost of health care. But spending a disproportionate sum on a given age group is not necessarily inappropriate if that age group has a disproportionate amount of legitimate needs. For example, a disproportionate amount of educational dollars has appropriately been spent on children in the past.

The other arguments on which we have touched may at first glance appear to be more in line with the described approach, but they too are deficient. For instance, the need to accept death when it cannot be avoided can be seen as a good reason to adopt a medical-benefit criterion. However, this justification is not relevant when applied across the board to the elderly, since individual cases will vary from the average. A given elderly patient may receive additional decades of life if treated. On the other hand, the argument that an age criterion is less morally objectionable than selection on the basis of race or sex because it applies to everyone equally (at least all those who live long enough) may simply be admitted. However, the evils of racism and sexism do not stem solely from the fact that they single out certain groups in society for different treatment; they are evil more fundamentally because they involve disadvantaging people for illegitimate reasons. So unless it can be demonstrated on other grounds that age in itself constitutes a legitimate reason for excluding the elderly from medical treatment, society must guard as fastidiously against ageism as against racism and sexism.

The three remaining justifications for excluding the oldest patients from treatment — arguments from equal opportunity, life span, and prudence — require somewhat more detailed attention.

Equal Opportunity

An equal-opportunity justification supports giving people an equal opportunity to live a long time, thereby maximizing the life-years saved. The most dubious aspect of this justification from the perspective of the described approach is the way it values life-years rather than lives (persons). People are more than sums of life-years that are accumulated like property.

Accordingly, murderers are typically not punished less for killing sixty-five-year-olds than for killing twenty-five-year-olds. Life is equally precious at any age. Although it is indeed better to preserve someone's life for a longer rather than a shorter time, it is another thing to suggest that we should seek to preserve one person's life for a long time at the price of denying any chance of living to another.

As we have already seen, an age criterion directed at seeking a maximum savings in life-years can have the curious effect of saving fewer lives overall. Since younger patients who are treated for chronic complaints will typically live longer than elderly patients who receive treatment for similar complaints, they will use up more resources in their lifetime, leaving less for others. For example, a young person might require dialysis treatment for years — a period of time during which many elderly patients nearing the end of their lives might be treated. By directing the benefits of treatment to a few young people rather than distributing them to more people of various ages, an age criterion will reduce the number of people helped.

Two problems unrelated to maximizing life-years are also involved in attempting, by means of an age criterion, to equalize the opportunity people have to live a long life. The first of these involves the manner in which we calculate the patient's opportunity to experience life. Say two women need the same scarce lifesaving resource. One of them is thirty-five years old; the other is thirty-six years old but has recently emerged from more than a year spent in a coma. If we are making decisions on the basis of an age criterion, whom do we choose? Usually the younger woman would be the preferable candidate on the grounds that her shorter life has given her less opportunity to experience life. However, in this case the older woman has had the lesser opportunity. If we concede that it is valid to consider issues like these in making a decision in the matter, we open the door to any number of imprecise qualitative considerations in the assessment of who has had the least opportunity to experience life. One person who supports this approach admits that such assessments would be "an overwhelmingly complicated task," calling it "procedurally and administratively a nightmare."[15] And yet how would we justify excluding such factors? A patient's socioeconomic or spiritual condition may have much more to do with her or his lifetime experience of well-being than does age. Age provides too rough an approximation of lifetime well-being (or present physical health for that matter) to be determinative when something as important as life is at stake.

The other problem related to equalizing the opportunity to live long concerns the past access of patients to resources. Should a younger person who has already received years of life-extending medical care be automatically preferred to an older person who has received very little? A strictly employed age criterion would say so, although it seems less than accurate to suggest that the younger person has not been given as great an opportunity to live as the older person.

Life Span

No more attractive from the described perspective is a variation of the equal-opportunity justification that limits lifesaving care to those who have not yet reached their natural life span. The very notion of a normative life span is debatable.[16] Even if a theoretical biological limit to the human life span is granted, the actual life span has grown through the years as life-extending care for the elderly has improved. An age criterion of the sort envisioned here would hinder medicine from extending even good-quality years at the end of life.

Furthermore, such an age criterion would demean those living beyond the natural life span. One supporter candidly admits this problem, given the world as it presently exists.[17] However, the problem is also intrinsic to the justification. Those who support this justification assume that extending medical care to those beyond the natural life span is not warranted because these people have already "accomplished" and "achieved" everything of significance that they can.[18] An implicit productivity orientation is revealed here: what matters is what one succeeds in doing. According to the described perspective, however, the significance of life is to be found as much in "being" as in "doing" — as much in relating to others as in completing tasks. Moreover, our life goals change as we grow older. We have different values at different ages. Those who argue that the elderly no longer have any goals left to reach are probably thinking only in terms of their own (often productivity-oriented) life goals.

While those who support the life-span justification are generally not aware of their productivity bias, they do typically acknowledge a commitment to maximizing quality of life. In fact, this commitment may in the end provide more support for a quality-of-life criterion than for an age criterion. One supporter admits that an age criterion excluding elderly patients from care is not warranted unless their quality of life is low.[19] In any event, a quality-of-life criterion can be as problematic as an age criterion. It is no easier to assess another person's quality of life accurately than it is to determine if people have essentially completed their life goals — at least without relying on the statements of the patients themselves. There is little reason to assume that all older persons will value their continued life less than younger persons value theirs. Moreover, neither group is likely to be forthright about the degree to which they no longer value their lives if what they say could cost them their lives. The alternative is to withhold resources only from those who voluntarily forgo treatment — but that is to impose neither an age nor a quality-of-life criterion.

Prudence

The final justification of an age criterion also raises a debatable issue. Is it truly prudent to distribute health care resources throughout life so that only certain resources are available at each stage of life? If the concern is to make more personal care services available to the elderly, an age criterion for acute care is not necessary. All that is needed is to place a greater priority on personal care services when the larger allocation decisions are being made. If an age criterion does have any warrant on prudential grounds, it would not sanction comparing individuals in order to favor the younger. At best it would sanction the exclusion of entire age groups from consideration for a scarce resource, but even this is questionable because of its overly idealistic and harmful nature.

In an ideal world this proposal might be appealing, but even proponents admit that it would be wrong to introduce age criteria in one health care setting and not in another. They also admit that age criteria may be politically unacceptable in any setting.[20] The potential strength of the proposal lies in its vision of distributing vital resources equitably throughout an individual's lifetime, but in the end the elderly will likely experience the reality of exclusion from treatment more keenly than they will appreciate the theory that lies behind it. The politics of the issue centers on which groups will gain greatest access to the most resources. Moreover, were the proposal applied throughout a nation such as the United States, existing social and economic injustices could cause the application of an age criterion to make things worse.[21] As we have already seen, the justice guide demands that we address present injustices as part of identifying what a just alternative might look like. The issue of health care for the elderly is no exception.[22] The potential injustice of an age criterion is so compelling that even those who in theory support age-based rationing may be forced to admit that their proposal "is in no way a recommendation for the introduction of such practices in our present world."[23]

Regardless of how attractive a proposal might be in theory, the question is how it would affect us if it were put into effect in the world as it is. So we have to ask ourselves some tough questions. How likely is it that injustice will persist in the world? Will the basic goodness of people triumph, or will we have to take injustice into account in our deliberations about the allocation of vital resources? A God-centered and reality-bounded perspective speaks directly to such questions. People as well as the policies and institutions they establish are less than God intends them to be because people are fundamentally self-oriented rather than God-and-other-oriented (Ps. 14:2-3; Jer. 17:9; Rom. 3:10-12, 23). While it is possible to turn from self-centeredness to God and others, experience and the biblical materials alike testify that the majority of people will never do so (Matt. 7:13-14; Luke 13:23-24).

Accordingly, there is a pressing need for social strategies that take this reality into account and seek to promote the best possible policies in light of it. Good intentions and commitment to laudable concerns such as equal opportunity, a natural life span, and prudence are not enough. It is misleading and perhaps even dangerous to propose age criteria that would be immoral if implemented "in our present world."

The potential harm of a prudentially based age criterion, though, extends far beyond its excessive idealism. For example, while it might not be as thoroughly discriminatory as racism or sexism, it is subtly discriminatory. It assumes that all persons move through all age categories, but the fact is that many people are born with congenital, genetic, or environmental handicaps that will prevent them from living as long as others. Moreover, a prudentially based age criterion would generate conflict between elderly persons who had never required health care but were now being denied needed lifesaving treatment on the one hand and younger persons now preferred as candidates for scarce lifesaving treatment regardless of how many medical resources they had used in the past. The proposal would also impose constraints on the liberty and welfare of elderly individuals that would often seem unbearably harsh to them, even if these constraints were objectively prudent.[24] In a sense the scheme is very paternalistic in that it adopts one understanding of what prudence entails and imposes it on all. No personal discretion is allowed regarding whether or not to pursue lifesaving therapies in later stages of life.

An additional drawback of such a proposal is that it would produce a serious injustice during the first generation it was adopted. The elderly of that generation would be denied lifesaving resources without having previously received the special benefits that the program would accord to younger people. Moreover, these elderly would be denied resources that they had paid for throughout their youth. In effect, some elderly would be forced to give up their lives for the good of all generations. Such well-intended oppression is the sort of classic utilitarian injustice described in Chapters 1 and 2. To try to rectify such injustice during the first generation of transition to the new system would entail shifting considerable resources that belong elsewhere, thereby creating new injustices. This problem is not merely theoretical. When Social Security legislation was first passed, the idea of giving that first generation of elderly less income support than subsequent generations was soundly rejected — even though those elderly had not paid into the system from which they would be receiving.[25]

A similar problem would occur every time a new lifesaving technology was introduced. The elderly would be given no access to it — even though the justification for this exclusion would ostensibly be that they had had priority access to it when they were young. In the end, the prudential approach assumes a level of stability in the health care system over a person's (actually, every person's) lifetime that is unrealistic.

The prudential approach may be still less attractive if it entails assisting the elderly to die. The specter of doctors, not to mention society in general, encouraging people to die so that health care resources can be saved is ominous indeed, and yet there are those who favor such an approach. Proponents admit that such suicidal decisions could not be considered truly voluntary unless some of the savings generated by those who chose to end their lives were made available to provide decent supportive health care for the elderly who chose not to be killed.[26] But in that case the approach would become increasingly self-defeating as savings financed better health care for the elderly, thereby lessening the impetus to end life. Nor is it obvious that most people would opt for death over illness, even if supportive services were limited.

Overarching Critiques

Implicit in these evaluations of the various justifications for an age criterion — and going beyond them — are two basic critiques. One has to do with values and the other concerns the matter of rights.

Values

The age criterion in most of its forms reflects certain nonmedical values. Among these, the value of youth is prominent. In some countries, such as the United States, such a high value is placed on youth that it affects the practice of medicine generally. Research indicates that the older patients are, the less likely they are to be treated — even resuscitated — under the same medical circumstances.[27] So it is not surprising to learn that some people originally supported funding dialysis for all who needed it because it looked as if primarily young adults would be the beneficiaries.[28] No more surprising is the enthusiasm for allocating health care resources generally on the basis of maximizing the quality-adjusted life years to be saved. This approach commends, as an objective ethical criterion, making whatever decisions save the most life (calculated by multiplying the number of life-years saved by a factor reflecting the quality of those years). The approach is inherently biased toward funding treatments that are mainly beneficial to the young.[29]

Youthfulness is attractive for various reasons, but especially for the productivity that normally accompanies it. Economic productivity is highly prized in many countries — so much so that the elderly and others like them who are on the whole less economically productive are looked down on and stereotyped.[30] The decision to exclude them from lifesaving health care is merely a particularly serious instance of this devaluation. As we have already seen, it is rooted in the failure to give sufficient moral weight to the value that God attaches to every life irrespective of age.

The diminished value accorded to the elderly and their corresponding limited access to certain lifesaving medical resources are ultimately the product of various cultural values which themselves need to be evaluated in the light of the Bible, according to the described approach. It is sometimes difficult, however, for one immersed in those values to recognize where they are at odds with biblical perspectives. As suggested in Chapter 1, people are blinded by the cultural values of a fallen world and tend to overlook certain emphases found in the Bible. They are convinced that their own way is obviously right, so they feel no need to look at the world through another culture's eyes. Sometimes there is no other way for people to recognize their blindness, though, than to discover what others can see that they cannot.

The common view taken of the elderly in a country like

the United States, for example, is rather different from the one characteristic of the Akamba people of Kenya (though Western influences are now altering the Akamba view somewhat). The Akamba view persons as much more than economic beings. They accord an elderly poor person as much respect as a rich or otherwise socially important person. In fact, old age calls forth a unique veneration.[31]

The high level of respect accorded to older people in Akamba society is intimately bound up with that culture's view of the relationship between the individual and the community. Whereas the utilitarian view common in the United States conceives of the social good atomistically in terms of individual (mainly job-related) contributions summed over the breadth of society, the Akamba view presupposes a social network of interpersonal relations within which one becomes more and more an essential part the older one becomes. The more personally interwoven a person becomes with others through time, the greater the damage done to the social fabric when that person is torn away by death. This extended-kinship social system commands a sort of spiritual loyalty and is ceremonially celebrated in various practices and rituals.[32]

The cultural values regarding old age lead many Akamba to make decisions about age-related resource allocation that are very different from those generally supported in the United States. When asked in one study whether an older or a younger man should be saved when there are resources enough to save only one, many Akamba medical personnel argued that even a very old man should be preferred because he "has more responsibilities" and "is a father to many people."[33] The latter expression, though often literally true in the traditionally polygamous Akamba society, here evokes a broader thought. The older man is a leader, a wise counselor, and an inspiring figure worthy of respect within his community.

There are viable alternatives, then, to the economic, individualistic, youth-oriented outlook adopted by many in countries such as the United States. Other countries — Sweden, for instance — could also be cited as examples of places where greater respect for the elderly leads to age criteria (when they exist at all) that are much less restrictive than those in the United States.[34] Alternative attitudes toward the elderly are indeed possible.

Different views of the elderly arise at least in part from different views of productivity. Even in a culture that places a high value on economic productivity, it could be argued that the elderly are more deserving of reward than anyone, since they have made a productive contribution to society throughout their lifetime. From this perspective there may be a special moral obligation to provide the elderly with the various kinds of care that they need.[35] Older people may still have major lifetime achievements before them. Moreover, the value of the elderly to society is more than economic in nature. They often have special virtues cultivated over a lifetime, such as wisdom to share and patient love to bestow, as well as various (though perhaps unspectacular) services to provide. Those who assume that the elderly do not contribute much to society may make that assumption in part because they do not expect much of them and do not hold them accountable to be all that they can be. Claims about their diminished mental abilities have in fact been challenged by multiple studies. Should the elderly be penalized simply because their society overlooks, perhaps inadvertently, the true value of their contribution?[36]

It is important to realize, then, that the notion of people's value is more complex than it first appears. But beyond this, it is even more important from the described perspective to insist that the very attempt to justify the continued existence of the elderly in terms of their social contributions is misplaced. We have already examined the problem with thinking of people in terms of value, since that subjects human life to utilitarian trade-offs (see Chapter 3). People have different *worths* in a social sense, but their worth as persons is intrinsic to who they are by God's design.[37] From this perspective the version of the prudential argument that encourages the elderly to end their lives for the benefit of society at large is particularly distressing. It would involve engineering such intrinsic valuing out of society by systematically cultivating in people a sense of obligation to die when they are first thought to be terminally ill.[38]

Rights

The notion of intrinsic worth is foundational to the second overall critique of an age criterion mentioned earlier: an age criterion is weak not only because of the dubious values that undergird it but also because it constitutes a direct violation of basic human rights. The right to life — or, more precisely, the right to lifesaving resources — is an acceptable notion from the described perspective as long as it is properly understood. As explained in Chapter 1, people have rights, but they have no right to rights. Rather, they have primarily a duty to treat others with the respect due those whom God has made and for whom Christ has died.

From this perspective, a person's life should be preserved simply because it is a human life. The age attached to that life is irrelevant. One's right to life does not diminish a little every day that one lives. Basic human rights rooted in God's intentions for humanity are not so variable. They are attached to personhood per se. A year of life at any stage of life can be equally precious. It has been suggested that the elderly have a right to humane termination procedures rather than a right to continue living.[39] Such a point of view, though, conserves society's resources without sufficient attention to how persons per se are treated.

Since an age criterion is often applied by excluding all

patients above a certain age, it also can be seen as violating basic rights in discriminating between patients when there is no just basis for doing so. At this point the argument presented in Chapter 8 becomes particularly relevant. On average, elderly patients may not fare well with certain treatments, and yet a given elderly person may be better able physically and emotionally to endure treatment than many younger individuals. While some may end up with a low quality of life, others will not.[40] Fixed age cutoffs are arbitrary and a violation of the ethical guide of justice, which would have us regard each person's need with equal care.

Overall, "rights" language may be helpful. However, it may be misleading where the resources necessary to honor those rights fully do not exist or have not been made available. Under such circumstances the related language of equal *respect* may be more helpful (especially in the context of equal needs). According to this language, an age criterion is disrespectful of the elderly as persons not only because it excludes them from treatment as a class but also because it fails to recognize individual differences that would make some individuals better candidates for treatment than others. In the process of showing such disrespect to an entire group of people, society itself can become brutalized — rendered insensitive to the immediate needs of some of its members. The love-impelled dimension of ethics requires that the frame of reference remain communal. We must not seek to meet the needs of some in ways that entail the neglect or exclusion of others.

Even in the case of schemes in which the concern is not age per se but some other goal such as distributing limited resources prudently throughout people's lifetimes, an important symbol may be at stake. When the elderly are left to die with no access to lifesaving treatments that are available to others, people actually do abandon the elderly and in that sense exclude them from communal care. Although philosophical justifications for such action might be offered, the damage to society's sense of responsibility for all of its members would be done. What is needed instead in some societies such as the United States is a thorough welcoming back of the elderly as full members of the community.[41]

There are many reasons, then, for resisting the nonmedical justifications being advanced for excluding the elderly from lifesaving health care. In particular, the propensity of Westerners to value youth and productivity so highly needs to be critiqued by those from other cultures such as the Akamba, who have a much greater appreciation for persons generally, especially the elderly. Seeing the elderly with new eyes, we might well discover that they are as important to the human race as the young. We might also find a corrective for the propensity to value everything (and everyone) in terms of its achievement and come to value people irrespective of what they can contribute.

CHAPTER 10

The Pursuit of Social Benefit

The debate over age criteria is merely a microcosm of the much broader debate over patient selection criteria. In situations like Bill's (see the Introduction), people pick and choose from a considerable variety of medical, economic, and social criteria as they make their decisions. In the debates that such predicaments generate, a God-centered, reality-bounded, and love-impelled approach contrasts significantly with an outlook more congenial to certain widely held contemporary values. In this chapter, we will take a close look at criteria associated with the latter approach — specifically, criteria reflecting the unbounded pursuit of social benefit.

Criteria oriented to the unbounded pursuit of social benefit are human-centered rather than God-centered in the sense outlined in Chapter 1. If ethics is not centered in God and God's intentions for the world, people tend to shape their lives around what looks good or beneficial to them. If they are sensitive to the interests of others as well as themselves, they tend to approach decisions about patient selection on the basis of what will produce the greatest overall benefit in light of the diversity of interests present in society.

To achieve this end in the context of patient selection,

people employ a variety of social-benefit and sociomedical-benefit criteria. Each has an affinity with the love-impelled dimension of ethics in its concern to benefit people. However, each has numerous flaws rooted ultimately in its neglect of the God-centered and reality-bounded dimensions of ethics. In particular, each elevates the love-impelled dimension above the reality-bounded dimension rather than allowing reality-based ethical guides to define the limits within which neighbor love properly operates.

Social-Benefit Criteria

Social Value

The most generic attempt to base patient selection on what will produce the greatest overall social benefit involves the use of a social-value criterion. This criterion entails a commitment to produce as much social benefit as possible through patient selection without the constraint of basic ethical guides such as freedom, justice, and life. The patients given preference are those judged most valuable to society. In light of the utilitarian spirit of the age, it is not surprising to find studies documenting that this criterion has been employed frequently.[1] Use of this criterion involves doing what God has reserved exclusively for the Final Judgment: making overall judgments concerning the value of individual human lives and contributions. Only God is able to make such judgments, because God alone is omniscient.

After all, the task is enormous. A decision must first be made about the sort of potential contributions to society that should be considered when patients are assessed. The contributions that people value in many countries, such as the United States, are so diverse and intangible that they simply cannot be quantified and precisely compared. Studies in countries such as Switzerland and Great Britain document that physicians considering the same pool of cases make different selection decisions based on a variety of social considerations.[2] So there appears to be little likelihood that those making the decision would be able to agree on, much less rank, the contributions that are valuable to society. Even supporters of the criterion at the level of theory tend to despair over this issue.[3]

The problem of calculating a patient's social value becomes still greater when we look to the future. Any assessments we make are necessarily based on today's values. How can we know what skills, attributes, or wisdom might be of greatest value tomorrow? And yet if our goal is to maximize social benefit by allocating vital resources to the most valuable individuals, we really need some way to know what the society of the future will consider important. Since we have no access to precise foreknowledge, we may well end up saving the wrong people.

If the identification of accurate social-value standards is problematic, applying them is no easier. In order to determine what sorts of contributions people are likely to make, we would have to know everything about them. In many life-threatening situations there would not be anything like the amount of time that would be required for the detailed research that would be necessary to make such determinations. Even if we did have an abundance of time, the sheer quantity and cost of the research would probably outweigh the benefits that the social-value selection would provide.

Furthermore, there are several other complicating factors. For instance, how would we go about assessing the relative value of such intangible personal characteristics as generosity, charisma, humor, and the like? In any determinations of this sort the door would be wide open for the personal biases of the people doing the selecting to intrude. Social-value selection during the early days of dialysis in the United

States generated particularly graphic examples of the ways that patient selection can be skewed by such biases.[4] Probably the most publicized of these examples occurred at the Seattle Artificial Kidney Center, where life-sustaining dialysis reportedly went to people involved in the community activities valued most by members of the selection committee.

Another complicating factor is that it is not really possible to gauge the contribution that people will make to their time until after they have died. At any earlier point in life, experience tells us that it is very hard to predict with confidence exactly how well people will end up fulfilling their potential. The difficulty of knowing in advance the precise degree of rehabilitation that patients will achieve following rigorous operations or treatments only makes matters worse. And even if we did have the knowledge and skill to use the right social-value standards and select the right people for treatment, the outcome might still be far from optimal in terms of social value produced. In order to maximize social value, society must achieve an optimal mix of different (e.g., vocationally different) types of people rather than a concentration of whatever type of person would be ranked highest on the social-value scale.

In other words, nothing short of divine omniscience, unavailable to human beings, is needed to employ a social-value criterion accurately. Even with comprehensive knowledge, people would lack the wisdom to judge which persons would best be kept alive in view of God's eternal purposes. No wonder social-value selection has been widely criticized as "playing God."[5] Members of the selection committee at the Seattle Artificial Kidney Center during the early days of dialysis felt such guilt for their attempts to play God that they eventually disbanded the committee.[6]

From the very beginning of human history, according to the described perspective people have tried to go their own way — to take God's place, to play God. As it was in the beginning, though, the temptation to play God is usually subtle enough that the violation of God's purposes is not very evident to the violator. To avoid making this mistake, we need a sense of the differences between people and God, as well as the differences between God's intentions for the world and our own ideas of what is best. With such perspective we can wisely and creatively be people rather than foolishly and destructively playing God.

The harmful effects of employing a social-value criterion illustrate well the destructiveness of playing God. First of all, the criterion unfairly discriminates against those groups that cannot contribute as much to society as others. It is bad enough when such groups are in effect punished for a lack of ability that is no fault of their own — when disabilities are a circumstance of birth, for example. But it is even worse when empowered people deny adequate medical care — deny life itself — to those who have not been able to produce equal achievements because they have been systematically discriminated against in the past. In such cases, a social-value criterion only serves to multiply the destructiveness.

A number of groups in society are especially victimized by such compounded discrimination. As we saw in Chapter 3, they are the very people for whom God has a special concern. One such group is people living in poverty. Simply because they have been born without wealth, class privilege, or opportunities to develop their natural abilities, some poor persons find themselves unable to contribute much of value to society, and for that reason a social-value criterion dictates that they should be denied life-sustaining medical resources. Those denied a good education or unable to find a job fare similarly. Where social services have been made available, some people have been able to overcome such disadvantages. Those who have not had the benefit of social services in the past are precisely those most likely to be denied life-sustaining resources in the present.

Other groups that would likely rank low on most social-value scales include people who are mentally and physically disabled as well as members of traditionally disadvantaged racial groups and foreign citizens — perhaps women also if society (or the group deciding) does not value them as much as men. Those with little political power might well lose out when social-value standards are designed, perhaps unconsciously, to benefit those with control over designing them. Other losers would be the creative nonconformists such as Socrates and Thoreau (whom society, to its eventual detriment, is always eager to be rid of) and criminals, even when they have fully paid the penalty for their crimes. A particularly troublesome form of double jeopardy is involved in the case of such criminals: the social-value criterion convicts and punishes them twice for the same crime, the second time handing down a death penalty.

The very nature of the social-value criterion demeans human dignity. It robs people of their unconditional worth as creatures of God and defines them purely in terms of their value (especially usefulness) to others. It reduces the unique significance of human life to the interchangeable value of things. People are treated as if they are mere objects for barter, mere machines that are best left unrepaired when it is no longer efficient to fix them. In cases in which this criterion has been applied, observers have been appalled at the callous way patients have been handled.[7] Others have noticed that once social value is considered in the context of allocating scarce lifesaving resources, it begins to influence who receives health care in other situations where resources are not scarce.[8]

The destructiveness of the social-value criterion touches even the important relationship between the caregiver and the patient. Over the years a great reservoir of trust has built up in patients toward the health care professions because patients have seen that physicians and other health care professionals have consistently made decisions on a medical basis in the patient's best interests. This trust has enabled the professions to provide health care much more effectively, since patients have provided the private information (embarrassing symptoms, life-style habits, etc.) needed for caregivers to make accurate diagnoses. However, when a social-value criterion is applied, the health care professions seek to ensure the good of society before the good of the patient. A breakdown of trust is inevitable.

A social-value criterion, then, is destructive in a variety of ways, all flowing from a misguided attempt to play God. According to the described perspective, this de facto rejection of God not only ignores who God is and what God has done but also ignores the future reality of Christ's return, which may occur at any moment. The decision to allocate vital resources to patients on the basis of their long-term value to society is obviously based on the assumption that there will be a "long term." It adopts an open-ended view of human history rather than one in which the world as we know it will be brought to an end by God. The biblical materials give us reason to question whether there will be time enough for the benefits sought through social-value calculations to be realized. Rather than sanctioning an approach that depends on consequences that may not occur, in a future that may never happen, the described ethical approach counsels living in accordance with God's lasting intentions right now. It challenges people to be God's rather than gods.

Progress of Science

The medical conditions of patients vary considerably, and they are not equally interesting from a scientific perspective. One patient's treatment may yield only limited knowledge about the effectiveness of the treatment, perhaps because of other complicating medical conditions, while another's may reveal more useful information regarding the effectiveness of the treatment in curing a particular disorder or perhaps a variety of disorders. A progress-of-science criterion would favor the latter patient on the grounds that treatment would then contribute more to the advancement of science. In other words, this criterion is really just a particular type of social-value criterion.

Although various people have advocated a progress-of-science criterion, its use has gone virtually undocumented. There is some evidence, however, that it was employed in the United States during the days of dialysis scarcity before federal funding relieved the scarcity.[9] A more recent study indicates that support for the criterion persists in the arena of kidney transplantation and would resurface should dialysis resources again become scarce in the United States.[10] That the degree of support reported in this study is almost identical to the support expressed for a social-value criterion again suggests that the two criteria are fundamentally the same in terms of their ethical basis.

Accordingly, a progress-of-science criterion shares nearly all of the weaknesses we have noted with regard to a social-value criterion. A few of the particularly relevant considerations are worth highlighting here, beginning with the way that the progress-of-science criterion involves "playing" (and hence rejecting) God. To employ the criterion accurately, one would need a divine foreknowledge regarding which patients would yield the most useful information if given preferential treatment. It is rarely possible to anticipate with sufficient precision the relative likelihood and significance of information to be gained in this way. Comparing the value of such information in a particular case with the other social values at stake is similarly problematic.

A progress-of-science criterion also directly violates the important freedom guide that is part of the reality-boundedness of ethics according to the described perspective. Employing this criterion involves patients in an experimental process as well as a medical treatment. Patients are no longer selected primarily because they need treatment; rather, the patient's suitability to participate in the experiment also plays a central role. It is probably not possible to obtain ethical consent under such conditions. Those who lack scientifically interesting disorders are not eligible to participate in the experiment, so they are never asked to consent. Those who have such disorders might consent, but it is doubtful that in doing so they would satisfy one of the four elements of ethical consent — voluntariness (see Chapter 4). These patients would in effect be told that they may either consent to special gathering of information — and perhaps added tests and procedures — or probably be denied a treatment essential to saving their lives. The threat of death is profoundly coercive.

Such problems would be bad enough if a progress-of-science criterion were the only way to obtain the desired scientific information. However, there are ways to obtain the same information without resorting to this criterion. Even if patients of greatest interest to researchers were not specifically chosen on the grounds of this criterion, it is likely that they would be chosen for the treatment on other grounds over time. Eventually a sufficiently large group of these cases would provide the body of evidence that researchers were looking for. The only drawbacks would be that it might take longer to gather the information and it would have to be gathered from all over the country rather than a single test site. These would scarcely constitute insurmountable problems, however: the information on the cases could be centrally collected, and sample cases could be examined at particular locations. If an impartial-selection criterion (described in Chapter 11) were employed, this approach would somewhat resemble a typical randomized clinical trial.

If a more controlled study were necessary, a large cooperative effort with standardized procedures could be undertaken involving patients of the required type who had been selected at various centers without reference to a progress-of-science criterion; or such patients could all be flown to the same medical center, assuming that the prospective value of the research justified the expense. Both approaches have been employed in the past as part of experimental protocols. In other words, the use of a progress-of-science criterion may truly be justified only by convenience — quite a weak rationale for violating the justice and freedom guides, among other important ethical considerations.

Favored Group

In deciding who will receive scarce lifesaving resources, medical facilities may also take a patient's group identity into account. This is most commonly done by considering the geographical location of one's residence (specified areas closest to the facility are given priority) or the social group into which one falls (e.g., children or veterans). This criterion in general does not appear to be widely supported. Certain forms of it, however, such as prioritizing local or national residents for organ transplantation and giving veterans special access to a variety of resources, have more proponents.[11]

In its reliance on considerations of social benefit, this criterion shares some of the weaknesses already identified in relation to social-value and progress-of-science criteria. These weaknesses will become apparent as we examine the three major justifications of a favored-group criterion.

The first justification is fundamentally the same as the last one examined in relation to a progress-of-science criterion: convenience. Health care (along with many other services) is commonly provided to particular groups of people by particular facilities — by community hospitals to members of the surrounding community, for example — and it is convenient to continue this practice when scarce lifesaving resources are in view. However, what is morally acceptable in much of health care is not necessarily acceptable when treatment is lifesaving and scarce. Lifesaving care is analogous to treatment in an emergency room, where caregivers have traditionally saved lives without reference to the patients' social group or place of residence. When treatment is scarce, patients rejected at one facility cannot necessarily obtain treatment at another, just as emergency patients cannot always survive transfer to a second facility if rejected at the one to which they first go.

To make people's lives depend on where they happen to live or what social group they happen to be a part of is more than arbitrary — it is unjustly discriminatory. Poor communities often end up with relatively less access to vital resources. The reasons for their poverty and inferior health care resources may have little to do with their own merit and much to do with public decision making, which can be insensitive to those who are politically weak. As we have seen, such insensitivity to poor and weak persons is a serious affront to God.

The second major justification for favored-group criteria has to do with medical considerations. It is true, for example, that some transplantable organs will perish if they must be transported long distances. However, others (e.g., kidneys) can survive long enough to be transported throughout the country and beyond. Treatment is also not as likely to be effective when patients must travel long distances for treatment or follow-up care. The problem here, however, may be more a matter of the patient's finances than anything else. Given adequate financial resources, the patient might be willing and able to live near the treatment center for the required time. When such is the case, the criterion at issue is really a form of ability-to-pay criterion, which we will consider shortly.

Even if favored-group considerations were to have a

genuine medical justification, a favored-group criterion per se is not justified. Such a circumstance would warrant a medical-benefit criterion (see Chapter 11) instead. Favored-group considerations may have a certain legitimacy when they serve to inform medical assessments, but even then it is important to keep in view the general undesirability of such considerations. Otherwise we will probably not make sufficient effort to meet the needs they seek to address. Rather than deny patients treatment on the grounds that they would have to travel too far to receive it, for example, we may be able to provide transportation assistance or financial support to make relocation possible during the treatment period.

One further medical consideration has to do with the supply of organs for transplantation. Some have argued that organ donation might decrease if organs are made available to foreign nationals or nonlocal recipients. Yet, it is far from clear that people's willingness to donate hinges on this consideration. In fact, the evidence suggests that donations from resident ethnic communities increase when nonresidents of similar ethnicity are allowed to receive transplants.[12] Moreover, local organ donation may be hurt more by a requirement that organs be transplanted locally in a mediocre facility than by a policy that allows them to be transplanted with greater success elsewhere.

The third major justification for a favored-group criterion involves exceptional situations in which no one is disadvantaged when the criterion is employed. The theory behind this justification sounds plausible: people should have the freedom to purchase their own scarce lifesaving medical resources as long as the freedom of others is not thereby restricted (i.e., the supply available to other persons is not reduced). For example, the supply for others may not be affected if individual patients privately pay for the use of a piece of equipment made exclusively to accommodate such private demand (we will consider the matter of the patient's ability to pay at a later point). A group of people — even an entire state or country — could similarly produce special resources available only to its own members as long as the resources available to nonmembers were not thereby limited.

What sounds good in theory, however, does not fit most actual situations. For example, special access to scarce lifesaving resources by veterans for disorders not related to their term of service would not seem to be justified by this exception. In this case, the national government would be devoting resources to a particular group of people rather than to others without the compelling kind of special rationale that is arguably present in relation to service-related disorders. But the described perspective suggests that people instead have a higher obligation to respect the lives of all patients equally, regardless of the positions these patients have held in society or the contributions they have made to it. The fact that service in the armed forces and subsequent veteran status have not traditionally been open to all social groups, such as women, only further undermines the legitimacy of giving veterans special access to treatment when life itself is at stake.

The issue of organ transplantation in a country such as the United States presents another example. Even though some states provide special funding for treatment, their efforts to restrict access to organ transplantation exclusively to their own residents are problematic in that millions of federal tax dollars were spent to develop the technology involved.

An analogous problem exists with restricting transplantation to residents of a given nation. Advanced technology today is virtually always the product of international cooperation, at least to some degree. A relatively developed country such as the United States, moreover, has benefited extensively from the inexpensive raw material and labor obtained from other countries. In fact, U.S. nationals frequently obtain medical care while abroad, sometimes traveling abroad specifically for the purpose of such care. These considerations would seem to justify some sort of quota system that would ensure at least limited access to transplantation for people from other countries.[13] The ethical problems with such a provisional favored-group criterion, however, should prod countries to move as quickly as possible toward an international network of transplantation technology and organ sharing in which favored-group criteria are unnecessary.

Sociomedical-Benefit Criteria

Likelihood, Length, and Quality of Benefit

There are six other selection criteria that, like the three criteria just examined, are fundamentally flawed in their human-centered elevation of benefit over other more important ethical considerations. Three of these remaining criteria — likelihood of benefit, length of benefit, and quality of benefit — purport to be medical rather than social in nature. However, as we noted in Chapter 8 in the context of treatment of the elderly, these justifications are not concerned merely with sustaining the lives of people in need. Unlike a straightforward medical-benefit justification, they seek to maximize other benefits at the expense of providing each patient in need with an equal opportunity to obtain vitally needed treatment. For this reason and the others we considered in Chapter 8, the described approach suggests that these three criteria should be resisted.

Admittedly, a likelihood-of-benefit criterion may have some appeal if it is understood merely as a means of saving as many lives as possible. However, it operates differently from other criteria designed to maximize the saving of lives. The practice of selecting one patient for treatment rather than another because that patient is more likely to benefit from the treatment founders on our inability to predict accurately who

will in fact benefit. We may be able to make good predictions
in a significant number of cases, but there will always be some
in which the patients who are selected for treatment will not
live and the patients passed over for treatment might have
lived had treatment been administered. In such cases, the
likelihood-of-benefit criterion promotes the violation of both
the life guide (i.e., more lives are lost) and the justice guide
(i.e., not all in need are given equal opportunity to be selected).
There is an echo of this way of thinking in Romans 3:8, "let
us do evil that good may result" — an approach to life Paul
rejects as unacceptably human-centered for all of the reasons
we noted in Chapter 1.

Psychological Ability

In addition to age, which we have already considered at
length, there are three other criteria that present themselves
as largely medical when in fact they are better classified as
social-benefit criteria. The first of these is psychological ability.
This criterion favors those with the willingness as well as the
intellectual and emotional capacity to cope with treatment or
with life in general. In light of the potentially close relationship between the adoption of this criterion and the likelihood
that treatment will be effective, the significant support for the
criterion in medical circles is not surprising.[14]

Nevertheless the criterion is seriously flawed. Like some
of the other criteria we have considered, it involves "playing
God." Its legitimacy depends on a foreknowledge and omniscience that people simply do not have. For example, to
apply the criterion, one would need to know exactly what
stresses a patient would have to endure with a particular
treatment. Some stresses may be anticipated, but others vary
from case to case.

Moreover, even if certain stresses could be anticipated,
one would need to understand what psychological charac-

teristics would render a patient unable to cope. Yet the human ability to cope with adversity has persistently defied exhaustive analysis. Many a patient has responded well to treatment despite psychological assessments that predicted the contrary.[15] Psychological testing is often helpful in revealing a patient's present condition, but it is less accurate in predicting how that patient will respond to future stresses.[16] It would be arrogant to presume to be able to make consistently accurate comparative assessments involving two or more patients. Moreover, this arrogance would threaten the lives of those whose psychological ability was even slightly underestimated.

A psychological-ability criterion is further problematic because it so often serves as a cover for other considerations that are more clearly objectionable, such as the convenience of the medical staff. For example, a medical staff may use the criterion (consciously or unconsciously) to screen out the sort of unruly, noncompliant patients that make the treatment of other patients more difficult. The staff may also prefer not to have to expend the greater effort necessary to care for patients whose psychological stability is impaired. As we have already seen, though, convenience is a weak rationale for violating the moral guide of justice.

Similarly, the criterion may merely serve to cloak personal bias. Physicians' judgments about the coping abilities and cooperativeness of patients are much more subjective than the physiological assessments they engage in. Like everyone else, physicians find that they can work best with those most like themselves. Some believe that virtually all forms of psychological impairment limit the patient's quality of life and hence make it inappropriate to grant that patient equal access to treatment. Even specialists in psychological assessment are subject to personal bias, as evidenced by the degree to which assessments of a given patient can vary from one specialist to another.[17]

It is not surprising, then, that psychological-ability criteria can serve as a hidden form of social-value criteria to exclude socially undesirable persons from lifesaving treatments. Patients who are limited in their abilities to interact with others, perhaps due to some disability or other perceived deviation from the social norm, are particularly vulnerable to such exclusion. It is telling that when social-value assessments of candidates for dialysis were ended in favor of strictly medical criteria at Seattle's Swedish Hospital, for example, psychological testing was also ended.[18] We have already noted the many ethical problems associated with social-value criteria. Ironically, even on social-value grounds a psychological-ability criterion may not be as warranted as it appears to be at first glance. History is replete with evidence that very unstable individuals have made major social contributions.

Admittedly, there are some cases in which the psychological inability of patients is so great that in all probability they would not benefit medically from treatment. Strictly speaking, though, in such cases the reason such patients are excluded from treatment is purely medical. Those who would invoke a psychological-ability criterion in these cases mistakenly assume that they involve considerations other than medical benefit. Psychological ability, like age, should be considered as merely one of several factors to be assessed in determining whether a patient meets the medical-benefit criterion.

Even understood in this limited way, psychological considerations would rarely prove definitive in excluding patients from treatment. Seldom are psychological problems so severe and hopeless that they cannot be treated in a way that renders a life-sustaining treatment workable. The treatment itself may alleviate the problems, as in the case of dialysis. Or psychological difficulties may be the result of stress, which can often be relieved through counseling that addresses both the nature of the illness involved and the life-sustaining potential of the treatment.[19] When psychological instability persists, special treatment programs can sometimes be established to provide the care necessary to enable the treatment to be effective. Psychological assessments would then generally serve to identify patients needing special care rather than being used as a means of identifying patients to exclude from treatment.

To guard against inappropriate use of the criterion, the described approach implicitly commends several precautions. The burden of proof should fall on those who would exclude a candidate from further consideration, in light of the life-or-death nature of the selection decision. As when resources are in unlimited supply, medical benefit should be the governing standard. If the medical significance of a patient's psychological difficulties is uncertain, all available steps should be taken to gain better understanding. It is sometimes possible to give patients an experience similar to the treatment needed in order to test their ability to cope with it. For example, candidates for dialysis are often placed on the strict diet necessary for the treatment months before dialysis is begun, and this can give an indication of whether they would be able to understand and handle the discipline. When a reusable resource such as intensive care space or dialysis is at issue, patients can also undergo a trial period of treatment to test their ability and willingness to cope with it. If, after such a trial period, reasonable doubt about their psychological ability remains, then there are insufficient grounds for excluding them from treatment on the basis of a psychological-ability criterion.

Supportive Environment

A supportive-environment criterion favors those patients who will have the most supportive living environment during and following treatment. The environment at issue here includes the care provided by family, friends, and health care personnel as well as the facilities and other material resources available to patients. Both in the United States and in other countries this criterion has frequently been advocated.[20] Nevertheless, it shares many of the weaknesses of the criteria we have already examined.

First of all, to employ this criterion effectively, one would need a level of knowledge that God alone possesses. Little is agreed on — or in many cases, even known — regarding the relation between a variety of environmental factors and the medical benefit that a patient receives from treatment. One study, in fact, has discovered that certain types of strong families may be a hindrance to effective treatment because of the high level of stress they experience when a family member is threatened by serious illness.[21]

The vagueness of the link between environmental and medical considerations is troublesome for an additional reason. Although some connection may exist, to overgeneralize it would lead to the exclusion of certain people from treatment unfairly for reasons that do not apply to them individually. Children from a two-parent home may automatically be considered more suitable candidates for treatment than children from a one-parent home, even though some of the former settings are more unstable and unsupportive than some of the latter. Some caregivers might assume that a household containing a reformed alcoholic would be relatively unstable, whereas in reality the opposite may be true. Experience shows that many individuals who appeared to be poor candidates for treatment according to a supportive-environment criterion have fared quite well with treatment.[22]

The supportive-environment criterion has also been used to cloak such objectionable criteria as social value and quality of benefit. It can be used, for example, to screen out those patients whose life circumstances make it more likely that they will be a burden to society and will have to endure a relatively low quality of life — uneducated persons, for instance. The very fact that the correlation between the environmental support available to patients and the medical effectiveness of their treatment is difficult to gauge and largely subjective invites such misuse. Indeed, the criterion readily cloaks discrimination on the basis of the patient's ability to pay, in that certain types of supportive care are too expensive for poor people to provide.

Like social-value and psychological-ability criteria, an environmental-support criterion can also be used to disguise personal bias. People show a propensity to consider others with life-styles radically different from their own, as well as those with less intellectual ability, to be inferior and relatively unsupportive.[23] Specifically, patients belonging to racial and ethnic groups with living patterns that vary considerably from those of the individuals who are allocating vital resources may be disproportionately excluded from access to treatment.

Another injustice of the criterion is even more blatant. It can deny treatment to patients for reasons over which they have no control. For example, it might endorse withholding treatment from a child on the grounds of an inadequate home environment even though it is the child's parents who are responsible for this poor environment, not the child. Patients in this predicament ought not to be denied treatment on environmental grounds. If possible, they should either be provided with the support they need as part of their treatment or an alternative treatment should be found in which the lack of environmental support would not be so critical. Admittedly, additional costs may be incurred by pursuing either of these alternative approaches, but such costs should not outweigh the patient's need for life-sustaining care. The ethical guide of justice dictates that special need calls for extra care, not less care.

If a situation were to arise in which the absence of a supportive environment — and the inability to provide one

— truly rendered treatment medically futile, then treatment should not be provided. However, the basis for reaching this conclusion would not be a supportive-environment criterion per se; rather, it would be a medical-benefit criterion, which we will examine at some length in Chapter 11. A patient's environment is simply one of a variety of factors that have to be assessed before it can be determined whether a patient will benefit medically from treatment.

Even as a component of establishing medical benefit, environmental assessment should remain subject to several guidelines implicit in the described perspective. First, the existence of a general correlation between any environmental factor to be considered and the medical effectiveness of the treatment in view must be clearly established. Next, the unique features of each situation must be carefully identified, since the level of personal support necessary varies significantly from individual to individual. According to one study of transplant recipients, the time and energy required of their families ranged from "a lot" to "a little," with at least 25 percent of the recipients at each end of this spectrum.[24] Finally, if there is serious doubt about the medical significance of the environmental factors involved in a particular case, these factors should not be allowed to influence the selection decision.

Ability to Pay

The last problematic selection criterion, ability to pay, favors those with the money, insurance, or other resources necessary to pay for treatment. In the United States, health care has never been available to meet every need irrespective of one's ability to pay. Many millions of people have inadequate private or government health care insurance, and many millions more have none at all. The consequences are predictable: the uninsured use health services only about half as much as the insured and are more likely to die from treatable conditions as a result.[25] Such a situation must necessarily concern anyone sensitive to the mandates of the justice guide and God's commitment to the poor. Ability to pay has played a major role in controlling access to such resources as dialysis, organ transplantation, intensive care, and even emergency care in the United States.[26] Other countries have demonstrated a still greater reliance on this criterion.[27]

Because an ability-to-pay criterion is closely related to a free-market approach to health care, one might think that there would be extensive support for the criterion in largely capitalist countries. However, there is great opposition both in the United States and elsewhere.[28] The primary reason is that an ability-to-pay criterion does not protect the freedom of all so much as it protects the freedom of those with resources to obtain treatment while ensuring that those without resources will have no such freedom.

For a market to function morally as a vehicle through which people can exercise their freedom of choice, all must have sufficient knowledge about their options and the resources to pursue at least their top-priority choices. That way, all can obtain what is most important to them by devoting a sufficiently large share of their resources to it. The problem with health care is that people do not have similar knowledge or sufficient resources. Accordingly, the disadvantaged are reduced to desperation bidding, to paying virtually any percentage of their resources for care. The idea of fair prices seems out of place in such a context. A person's level of desire for a lifesaving resource is simply not reflected accurately. Poor people lack what is minimally necessary to bargain for expensive items through the market, and rich people need devote no more than an insignificant portion of their resources to obtain life-sustaining care.

Moreover, an ability-to-pay criterion not only fails to protect people's freedom but is also harmful in its own right. For instance, the spectacle of desperate patients bidding against each other in a free market system of distributing lifesaving resources — in fact, the mere knowledge that life is being bought and sold — undermines the commitment to the incomparable and intrinsic significance of human life.

The criterion also unfairly discriminates against a variety of people. Those who are weak from illness are particularly vulnerable to exploitation under a free market system. Elderly persons are denied treatment disproportionately often, because many are poor and less able to obtain long-term loans due to their age. Whatever their age, poor people as a group are consistent losers when an ability-to-pay criterion is employed. Such predictable discrimination for reasons sometimes beyond the victims' control is most odious when people's lives are at stake, and it constitutes a direct violation of the justice guide, which calls for a special concern for the basic needs of the poor. It is particularly unfair to deny people access to technologies the development of which they have helped pay for through taxes and to deny poor people organ transplants when they as a group contribute to the supply of available organs.[29]

An ability-to-pay criterion also benefits whoever can marshal extraordinary influence. Those with the best access to the media have sometimes been able to elicit sufficient financial contributions from the community to satisfy a monetary ability-to-pay criterion, for example. Communities have sometimes been able to pressure a government or insurance company into funding treatment for a particular person. In order to obtain major community support, though, a patient's family often must have the sizable amount of money necessary to finance a massive publicity effort. If patients can get a famous personality or an influential politician to support their cases, they too may have a particularly good chance of being treated.[30]

Distributing vital resources according to one's access to media or political influence (and the associated ability to pay) is morally troublesome. Not all people are attractive enough to gain major media coverage. Not all people have the necessary connections with individuals in the publicity arena. Not all people have privileged relationships with key political figures or the kinds of skills to persuade insurance companies or others to provide needed funding. In fact, there is evidence that people have been unable to obtain the necessary funding because of their skin color, the interest level of their physician, and other irrelevant factors.[31] Life is too precious to depend on such considerations. The ethical guides of justice as well as life are blatantly violated by this approach to patient selection.

As is often the case when the reality-bounded dimension of ethics is disregarded, this approach tends to be counterproductive in the long run. It is demeaning to patients because it reduces them to begging for the privilege of remaining alive. It also proves terribly disruptive to the lives of the families involved. Ultimately, society as a whole is the loser as patients are pitted against patients, physicians against physicians, and politicians against politicians — all clamoring for attention every time individuals need lifesaving resources. People may eventually become desensitized to all appeals for financial help — perhaps even to the urgent need for organ donation.

Since ability-to-pay criteria in their various forms are so objectionable, it is best to avoid them whenever possible. The best way to do this is to render them unnecessary by making wise budgetary decisions at the macroallocation level. For instance, a society could decide to develop only those lifesaving technologies that it is willing to fund for all. Soon after a technology is invented, its ultimate costs (i.e., costs after significant cost-reducing refinements) would need to be projected and a decision made as to whether or not a nation could afford to devote public funds to develop it and provide it to all in need. Alternatively, facilities that profit from the provision of scarce lifesaving treatments could be taxed to generate part of the funds required to make these treatments accessible to all. Leaving this matter solely up to the charitable inclinations of health care institutions is not likely to prove sufficient, if past experience is a valid indicator (although there are admirable examples of generosity).[32]

Although the ability-to-pay criterion is generally undesirable, the described approach may sanction the use of an indirect form of it. If people have the money to obtain or even create a medical resource that is otherwise scarce because limited funds are available (e.g., a new dialysis machine or intensive care bed), then they should be permitted to finance their own treatment. The freedom guide requires as much, as long as their actions do not compromise the freedom of others to obtain treatment. Admittedly, the inequity of wealth that makes these special purchases possible only for some may not be just. However, a health policy cannot be held responsible for eradicating all social evils. Any health system would be more just if such prior injustice were eliminated, and major efforts should be directed to that end.

On the other hand, if a resource is scarce not because of limited funding but because of the limited availability of the health care resource itself — as in the case of organs for transplant — then it is not legitimate for people to purchase treatment. Were they to do so, they would undermine other selection criteria rooted in basic moral guides such as justice. Moreover, less wealthy patients needing the resource would almost certainly be fatally harmed by such private actions. Freedom is not honored when some flourish at the direct expense of others.

An analogous exception exists when patients can provide (i.e., obtain) the organ they need for transplant, as opposed to supplying the financing. Some people who would not otherwise donate an organ will elect to do so for the benefit of a child or close relative. There are also documented examples of individuals who would not have donated organs had they not been allowed to designate particular nonrelated recipients.[33] This exception can be considered morally acceptable only if it does not affect the supply of organs available to other patients. To ensure this, living donors could be required to sign affidavits testifying (1) that they would not have donated the organ in question without the appeal from, information about, or relationship with a particular recipient and (2) that they are unwilling to make the organ available to anyone other than the recipient. A donor advocate could also be assigned to ensure that no pressure from the potential recipient or others has improperly influenced the donor's decision. If such safeguards prove unworkable or insufficient, then it may be necessary to limit designated recipients to relatives of the donor. A unique sense of obligation on the part of living donors toward relatives is common.

Although barring ability-to-pay considerations in most health care situations entails a financial cost, it is not unusual in any sphere of life for it to cost something to adopt the most ethical policy. Nevertheless, if the cost is great enough, other more basic ethical factors such as the life guide may come into play. An ability-to-pay criterion could conceivably be required in exceptional situations, then, not for financial reasons per se but because of these more basic ethical factors.

For example, ability-to-pay considerations may occasionally be necessary if the only alternative is allowing people to die who otherwise could be treated. Such may be the case when facilities will have to close (or never open in the first place) if they do not employ an ability-to-pay criterion for at least some of their services. The life guide suggests that it is better to treat some (who can pay) than none at all — at least during the interim while those involved seek the financial means to treat all. Two conditions must be met, however, if an ability-to-pay criterion is to be justified in this way. First, there must be no possibility that the facility can operate without employing the criterion, and second, it must be the case that closing the facility would jeopardize patients' lives

— that is to say, it must be the case that no other medical facilities in the area could step in to provide the treatment normally provided at the facility in question. The situation that fulfills both of these conditions is rare.

A similar exceptional case may arise when a facility or locality has only limited funds. Difficult choices must be made about what forms of health care to subsidize. We cannot ethically subsidize a particular treatment (and thereby avoid an ability-to-pay criterion) if doing so in effect would restrict resources needed for preventive care or another treatment and result in a greater overall loss of life. It might be wonderful to fund liver transplants completely for three patients at a particular facility, but if such a program would dry up funds needed to supply prenatal care to many hundreds of women and hence lead to the deaths of more than three infants, it would not be ethically justifiable.

We should generally seek to avoid the use of an ability-to-pay criterion, then, though admittedly it may not always be morally possible to do so. When it cannot be avoided, it ought at least to be the last criterion applied. Only after a patient has been identified as the best candidate for the next available resource on the basis of medical and all other legitimate criteria should considerations of ability to pay be introduced. While it would be tragic if purely monetary considerations should lead to a denial of treatment at this point, this ordering of criteria would at least have the effect of focusing the kind of attention on the patient that might prompt the private donation of funds to pay for the treatment. At the same time, this approach would serve to prod those responsible for allocating limited resources to a greater awareness of the number of patients who were being left to die exclusively for lack of financial support. Such an awareness would challenge them to face the justice issues involved more squarely.

In the end, the pursuit of social benefit leads to a number of criteria that are fundamentally flawed because they are human-centered. It is not the concern for social benefit that is mistaken but the attempt to pursue such benefit outside of its proper ethical context.

CHAPTER 11

Determining Who Lives

The God-centered approach developed in Part I offers a positive alternative to the human-centered criteria examined in the previous chapter. It does not look to what people value at the moment but rather strives to root ethics in what God intends for the world, as best that can be known through the Bible, prayer, reason, and communal and individual experience. We should not be surprised that there are moral "givens," for there is a Giver who has created the world to thrive when it operates in particular ways. God's ways are not necessarily people's ways, nor are they necessarily intuitively obvious. They do involve people in promoting human well-being, in line with the utilitarian spirit of the age. In fact, the described approach places great emphasis on attending to the uniqueness of each patient and situation. At the same time, this love-impelled dimension is bounded by moral guides such as truth, freedom, justice, and life that are inherent in the reality of the world God has created. It may be far from obvious which of these guides, if any, is relevant in any particular situation. Careful attention to the individual patient and the social context is essential.

The Individual Patient

Attending to each patient in an appropriate manner entails giving due respect to each patient's particular wishes and values. As we have already noted, God takes human choices very seriously: love is genuine only if it is voluntary and uncoerced. Even when eternal destiny is at stake, people are free to choose for or against God. And just as people are granted the freedom to make eternal choices, so they should be granted the freedom to make critical decisions that may extend their lives here and now. They should ultimately be at liberty either to forgo scarce lifesaving medical treatments or to pursue treatment.

Willingness

In other words, a willingness criterion is warranted to ensure that only those who genuinely want treatment receive it. A willingness criterion has widespread support in medical practice.[1] It also corresponds to the first of the major ethical considerations we examined in Part II — the patient's wishes. Whether the issue is ending treatment or beginning it, the patient's wishes are extremely important. We have seen that determining the patient's true wishes is more complicated than the common notion of "informed consent" might suggest, although helpful guidelines are available.

While respect for freedom entails considering the patient's willingness to receive treatment, freedom in the biblical writings is not synonymous with license. Some choices are better than others; some, for example, are more in line with the ethical guides that God has provided. The significance of the life guide suggests that it is generally appropriate for people to want to receive resources they need in order to stay alive. Other people such as family members also may need the continued presence of their ill relatives for a variety of reasons. Yet the example of Jesus adds the admirable alternative of laying down one's life so that others might live — an affirmation of life in its own right. If such prioritizing of the lives of others is to be a genuine expression of freedom, though, the decision must be that of the person making the sacrifice. It must not be the forcibly imposed judgment of society or the subtly imposed suggestion of any other individual. Ultimately, then, a willingness criterion suggests that a patient's wishes regarding whether or not to receive a scarce lifesaving resource should be honored, although some wishes may be more morally commendable than others.

Attending to the individual patient in an appropriate manner also entails giving due attention to each patient's medical condition. Given the tremendous significance that God ascribes to the life of every person, we should seek to meet the vital needs of each to the fullest extent possible. This understanding of life and justice points to the importance of two other patient selection criteria: medical benefit and imminent death.

Medical Benefit

A medical-benefit criterion, first of all, dictates that resources should go to those who genuinely need them. As explained in Chapter 8, it includes for further consideration in the selection process all (and only) those who will likely receive a significant medical benefit as a result of treatment. In addition to serving as a criterion in its own right for the allocation of vital resources, the medical-benefit criterion serves as the basis for assessing the medical legitimacy of any other selection criterion. We have already seen how it can inform an ethical assessment of age, supportive-environment, and psychological-ability selection criteria. Not surprisingly, then, the medical-benefit criterion is commonly advocated and employed in the practice of medicine today.[2]

Admittedly, other medical considerations such as likelihood of benefit, length of benefit, and quality of benefit have a place in assessing medical benefit. Rather than using these considerations as criteria in their own right to compare and rank candidates for treatment, however, a medical-benefit criterion employs them in a noncomparative and minimal sense. Those who lack a reasonable likelihood of receiving a significant length and quality of benefit from treatment are excluded from treatment on medical grounds. "Significant" here means the smallest amount that can reasonably be considered important. If living a year longer, for instance, can reasonably be considered a significant benefit, then the minimal length-of-benefit requirement of the medical-benefit criterion should not be longer than a year. Candidates expected to receive borderline medical benefit from treatment should probably not be excluded from treatment on the basis of this criterion in view of the imprecision of the judgments involved.

Imminent Death

All who will die because they lack access to a particular resource need that resource, but those who will die *imminently* because they lack such access fall into a category of special need. They require the resource now, unlike others who can survive for a while without it. So if one is to attend to the particular medical need of each patient in an appropriate manner, an imminent-death criterion becomes an important vehicle. The criterion allots priority treatment to those whose death is expected within a few days or weeks (or perhaps slightly longer) according to competent medical judgment. Although this definition of imminent death is not precise, it is the best that the circumstances will allow, and it has been found workable by many in clinical practice.[3] In fact, some sort of imminent-death criterion has long played an important role in patient selection.[4] According to a national survey, it also enjoys a broad measure of public support in the United States.[5]

Because of serious problems with certain forms of the criterion, however, we need to look carefully at the way it is employed. For example, some forms of the criterion give priority to patients who have deteriorated to the extent that they can no longer benefit significantly from treatment. Such an application of the criterion neglects the important medical-benefit criterion. An imminent-death criterion should instead give priority to those candidates who are within, say, two weeks of being disqualified from treatment on the basis of the medical-benefit criterion. Such predictions are often difficult to make, especially when patients who do not seem to be very sick are nevertheless at significant risk of dying (e.g., those with rapidly deteriorating heart conditions). If a prediction cannot be made with reasonable accuracy, the imminent-death criterion should not be employed.

For those who are concerned that an imminent-death criterion aspires to an unrealistic degree of precision or is open to abuse, three remedies are available. First, we can avoid the attempts that some have made to break down the time period when death is imminent into subperiods. These smaller categories are more difficult to define precisely and place more emphasis on precise categorization than is necessary. Patients ought simply to be categorized as being in or out of the imminent-death period. Second, whenever caregivers have reason to question whether a patient is in the imminent-death period, they can err on the side of safety and include all such questionable cases in the higher priority category. Meanwhile, research can continue so that clinicians will become more adept at determining when the death of a particular patient is imminent. Third, all documentable evidence of the imminence of death can be documented and subject to later review. Sanctions could then be imposed on anyone invoking the criterion when it clearly is not applicable — which is to say, anyone manifestly violating standard medical practice.

The Social Context

Impartial Selection

While attending to individual patients — their wishes as well as their needs — it is also essential that we attend to their social context. There may be many other patients who want and need the same treatment. As we have seen, justice entails equal provision for all those in need. However, in situations of scarcity, when all alike cannot receive the needed resources, the best that can be done in the interests of equality is to provide each patient with an equal opportunity to obtain treatment. (Whether people responsible for their own illness should be denied access to scarce lifesaving resources is a justice issue of a different sort; but such a consideration is presently too difficult to apply in the practice of health care.)[6]

An impartial-selection criterion that selects patients randomly is the surest way to protect equal opportunity. Such impartial selection may strike some as irrational and unappealing because of its arbitrariness. However, this arbitrariness is its ethical strength according to the described perspective, for it guards against the intrusion of comparative evaluations of the worth or value of persons. In fact, this arbitrariness may even act as a subtle incentive for those who hold economic and political power to reduce the scarcity of resources, since impartial selection would preclude them from relying on their special position to obtain priority access for themselves, their family, or their friends should they need treatment. The arbitrariness of impartial selection would also serve to keep the tragedy of scarce resources clearly visible, unlike social-value selection, for example, which may give the appearance that a "solution" to the scarcity has been found. A clearer awareness of the scarcity will tend to stimulate greater efforts to reduce it.

The use of impartial (random) selection to prevent im-

proper human decision making has a long history. In the Bible
it is sometimes seen as a way to leave the decision to God
(Prov. 16:33; cf. Josh. 18:6-10; 1 Sam. 10:20-21; 14:42; 1 Chron.
26:13; Neh. 10:34; Esth. 3:7; Prov. 18:18; Jon. 1:7-8; Acts 1:24-26),
but it is also employed there simply to ensure that a decision
does not reflect the value judgments or preferences of the
decision-maker (Num. 26:55; Judg. 20:9-10; Job 6:27; Joel 3:3;
Obad. 1:11; Nah. 3:10; Matt. 27:35). This latter motivation has
been particularly influential in the practice of medicine, where
impartial selection has received significant support in situations such as determining access to organ transplantation,
kidney dialysis, and vital vaccines.[7]

Impartial selection generally takes one of two forms.
One is a traditional lottery in which names are randomly
selected from a list of all patients waiting for treatment. The
other is a first-come, first-served approach. Since the time that
each person is stricken with a medical condition and seeks
treatment is more or less random, the first-come, first-served
approach functions as a sort of natural lottery. The first-come,
first-served approach has more commonly been employed in
health care than has the lottery, perhaps because it does not
seem quite as starkly random as a lottery.

From the perspective of justice, however, randomness is
precisely what is being sought. In fact, one moral problem
with the first-come, first-served approach is that it is not truly
random or impartial. Patients with greater wealth (and those
with the greater power, information, and confidence associated with the wealthier classes) have better access to
health care generally and to referral networks in particular.
Accordingly, they tend to get on the waiting lists for scarce
medical resources sooner than those who are less wealthy and
empowered.[8]

The first-come, first-served approach may seem just on
grounds other than randomness, however. For instance, many
would find appealing its insistence that those who have

waited longest should be treated first. And yet, while such a priority may be justifiable in most situations, it must be disputed when life is at stake. No amount of waiting can make one person deserve life more than another. With a lottery, some might have to wait longer than others because of "the luck of the draw" — but that would be better than leaving some to wait longer just to get on the waiting list because they are victims of social inequities.

Moreover, the first-come, first-served approach to patient selection also has two bad side effects that a lottery avoids. One stems from the fact that the criterion favors the patients who have been waiting longest for treatment: it tends to select the sickest patients, the patients with the least likelihood of recovery. As a result, it produces limited results or even wastes vital resources altogether. The second bad side effect of the first-come, first-served approach stems from the fact that it creates legitimate expectations on the part of patients about the order in which they should be treated. Once such an order is established, patients will understandably be annoyed if it is interrupted to accord special priority to an individual — for example, when ethically mandated by the imminent-death criterion. The approach thus has the effect of promoting ill will among patients and caregivers. These two side effects are worth considering in our evaluation of the first-come, first-served approach, but they remain secondary considerations. The primary consideration here is the justice issue — that is, identifying the form of impartial selection that is most truly random and thus impartial. A lottery is usually the preferable form.[9]

Justice is not the only basic guide that undergirds an impartial-selection criterion, however. If equality were all we were interested in, then it could be argued that the best way to ensure it would be to deny treatment to everyone alike.[10] But other concerns are also important. As we saw in Part I, life has a unique significance rooted in God and is worthy of great care and respect. The life guide teaches us that the equality we seek should be life-affirming rather than life-denying, and so the guide supports a criterion like impartial selection which protects as many lives as possible while safeguarding equality.

Resources Required

Respect for life entails two additional criteria rooted not in an assessment of the patient as an individual but in larger social considerations. The first of these criteria dictates that patients needing less of a given resource should be treated before patients needing more of the same resource if a greater number of lives can be saved as a result. A resources-required criterion has not received as much attention as other selection criteria, partly because the possibility of a major disparity in the amount of resources required by various patients does not arise in relation to many treatments. Patients who need a kidney transplant, for instance, all alike need a kidney, and once a kidney has been received by one person it cannot be used by another.[11] In other circumstances, however, such as the early allocation of penicillin and the provision of dialysis, the criterion has played a significant role. Those needing less of the resource, or needing it only temporarily, have traditionally received priority.[12]

It is important to distinguish this criterion from a more general utilitarian endeavor to maximize the benefits resulting from the use of limited resources. A resources-required criterion recognizes that life has special significance and is not merely something of value that can be traded off against other things of value. Unlike utilitarian attempts to compare incommensurables, the criterion simply prefers more of that which is uniquely important, human life, over less of the same.

Because choosing some over others is never a light matter in view of the importance of equality, those employing the resources-required criterion should be relatively certain that they will in fact save additional lives by doing so. It would be wrong to grant one patient priority over another on the basis of a negligible difference in the amount of vital resources each is predicted to require for treatment, since such predictions are inherently imprecise. Only major disparities in the amount of resources required should be employed as a basis for patient selection, according to the described approach. Perhaps the clearest case is the choice between someone needing a vital scarce resource (e.g., an artificial organ) long-term and one needing it only temporarily. Such a choice involves using the same resource either to sustain the long-term patient or to save the lives of many patients with temporary needs, one after the other. If it is not clear whether a given patient falls into a priority group, it would be best here as elsewhere to err on the side of caution and include the patient when something as important as life is at stake.

Vital Responsibilities

The final criterion suggested by attending to the social context similarly affirms the special importance of life. Yet it differs from the resources-required criterion in that it broadens the scope of what the social context entails. Taking into consideration patients and nonpatients alike whose lives may be affected by selection decisions, a vital-responsibilities criterion favors patients on whom the lives of others literally depend. Classic illustrations of its use include providing antibiotics and other scarce treatments in wartime to those able to return most quickly to battle in order to prevent further killing — killing either of people on the patient's own side only or, more broadly considered, of people on both sides through a faster conclusion of the hostilities. Similarly, it has often been determined that those with medical expertise should be treated first so that they can regain the capacity to treat others.[13] At issue here is the importance of all human lives, patients and non-patients. Any selection decision resulting in more lives saved receives support from the life guide. Unlike a likelihood-of-benefit criterion, which sanctions some immoral selections along the way in order to save more lives in the long run, a vital-responsibilities criterion (like a resources-required criterion) saves additional lives every time it is applied.

Unless the goal of saving more lives remains clearly in view, this criterion can collapse into a mere social-value criterion designed to favor those who are considered to be more "important" or "valuable" than others. So it is essential that anyone being favored by this criterion be truly indispensable to the saving of others' lives — a condition that rarely applies — and that they not be so weakened following treatment that they would be unable to perform the service on which others' lives depend. Each case must be considered on its merits rather than automatically approved because of its type. Even top politicians, physicians, and military leaders would not usually qualify for special priority.

An Overall Approach

The vital-responsibilities and resources-required criteria illustrate particularly well the close relationship between the reality-bounded and love-impelled dimensions of ethics. As we have already noted, the love-impelled dimension entails seeking the greatest benefit for the most people, albeit within the bounds of God-given reality. So seeking not only to protect life but to protect it for as many people as possible is quite appropriate from this perspective. In fact, furthering freedom and justice as well as life tends to be beneficial for people in the long run, for these are basic components of the environment in which God intends for people to flourish. Accordingly, most of the six criteria we have considered in this chapter are undergirded by the love-impelled dimension of ethics (in its narrower, neighbor-love sense) as well as by the framework provided by the reality-bounded dimension.

The six criteria work together in the process of patient selection as follows:

1. Only patients who satisfy the medical-benefit and willingness criteria are to be considered eligible.
2. Available resources are to be given first to eligible patients who satisfy the imminent-death, vital-responsibilities, or resources-required criterion.[14]
3. If resources are still available, recipients should be impartially selected, generally by lottery, from among the remaining eligible patients.[15]

We should also keep in mind two exceptional circumstances that we considered in Chapter 10. On the limited occasions when a favored-group criterion is legitimate, it should serve as a prerequisite criterion — alongside of medical benefit and willingness — that must be satisfied by any recipient of the resource involved. Legitimate applications of the ability-to-pay criterion, on the other hand, should not be made until after a patient has been chosen according to the selection procedure outlined above.

The overall approach described here will have various implications depending on the setting. In particular, the considerations involved in establishing medical benefit (perhaps including age, environment, psychological ability, geographical location, etc.) will vary from resource to resource. For instance, medical-benefit considerations that are relevant with respect to organ transplants may differ markedly from those relevant in the setting of intensive care. In fact, even within a single medical setting, a determination of which (forms of) selection criteria are relevant will depend on the particular circumstances of each patient, including the larger social contexts in which they live. Nevertheless, despite the variations in medical settings, patients, and social contexts, patient selection remains ethically consistent so long as it continues to be anchored in the God-centered, reality-bounded, and love-impelled dimensions of ethics.

Conclusion:
Ending Lives and
Allocating Resources

Although we have been looking at the topics of ending lives and allocating resources separately to this point, they are in fact significantly related. Both do have their own central issues which warrant focused attention. However, neither can be understood in an overall sense without an appreciation of its interrelationship with the other and with the larger context of health care.

For instance, those who fear that so-called euthanasia will ultimately become a vehicle that society uses to get rid of the burden of unwanted groups of people would do well to realize that patient selection criteria can be used to the same end. There are few more effective ways to dispose of poor, old, and odd people than by using ability-to-pay, age, and social-value criteria to channel resources away from them.

In the context of an aging population such as that of the United States, the connections between ending lives and allocating resources become particularly significant. When today's

235

15-year-olds reach age 65, they will probably make up 20 percent of the U.S. population, as compared with 11 percent today. By 2040, in fact, more than 13 million people in the United States are likely to be over 85 — five times the number of people that age today.[1] Since older people tend to incur a disproportionate share of health care costs, the rising number of elderly persons means that there will be tremendous financial pressure on an already pressured health care system. It will be much more tempting in such a context to use age criteria for patient selection and to encourage elderly people to forgo treatment or even life itself. With both alternatives potentially available, it will be increasingly difficult to address issues of resource allocation without addressing issues of ending lives.

The relationship between the two, though, is even more complex. Resource allocation problems themselves constitute one of the most potent forces behind the movement toward ending lives. The most likely candidates for termination of treatment or of life more directly are those in the last year of life — people who consume a large share of society's health care resources with relatively limited benefit. The prospect of saving resources on a large scale makes it tempting to encourage — perhaps subtly coerce — people to end their lives when long-term survival appears doubtful.

But according to the described perspective, there are better responses to resource limitations than encouraging premature death. First of all, we can encourage efforts to increase the available supply of health care resources. Adopting criteria for patient selection is a moral enterprise only if such criteria provide a way of coping with the underlying problem — scarcity of resources — in an interim way while the underlying problem itself is being addressed in a responsible fashion. If we make no sustained effort to eliminate the need for leaving some patients without treatment, our efforts to develop ethical patient selection criteria will divert our attention from the crucial matter of eliminating the need for such criteria in the first place. How much better it is to remove a problem than merely to allocate its harmful effects ethically.

We can undertake a variety of efforts to reduce scarcity significantly. For example, we should continue and even intensify current efforts to identify and eliminate unnecessary and useless treatments. Technology assessment remains an important tool to help guard against inappropriate treatment. While the savings involved in eliminating waste may be considerable, few expect that realistically achievable savings will be sufficient to provide universal access to all life-sustaining medical technologies.[2] Accordingly, we will have to either augment current funding for health care or determine explicit priorities within the realm of health care. The first of these alternatives has much to be said for it. In the face of such ethical guides as life, freedom, truth, and justice, a good case can be made for increasing the portion of public and private (including church) expenditures presently devoted to health care. There is nothing sacred about the percentage of GNP currently spent on health care in the United States, for example, particularly in light of some of the other uses to which funds are put.

Proper Priorities

Funding for health care may remain limited, however, due to misplaced priorities or because of the amount of resources needed for other worthy pursuits such as housing and education. If such is the case, then it becomes all the more important that we carefully establish priorities for the use of available health care funds. For instance, advanced, expensive technologies can be fascinating, but they seldom offer as much health benefit for the dollar as relatively inexpensive health maintenance or preventive care. If there are no better alternatives, society as a whole may have to forgo certain life-sustaining treatments — in much the same way an individual does — because their moral cost is too great.[3]

In establishing our priorities, we must also take care to ensure that we do not slight certain groups of people. We have already noted the importance of avoiding social-value patient selection criteria in order to protect neglected minority groups in society. Such considerations are also important as we establish funding priorities, however: if our priorities unjustly impact certain groups before selection criteria even come into play, then ethical patient selection criteria cannot prevent the harm from occurring.

An example of this danger may be helpful here. Consider health care near the beginning of life — which is also, sadly, the end of life for many infants. The United States has decided through the years to devote massive amounts of money to marvelous new technologies that are able to save the lives of infants born prematurely. It may not have been anyone's intent in funding such technologies to reduce funding for more standard prenatal care to pregnant women, but that has in fact been the result. One study has reported that 74,000 women annually are delivering children in the United States without even one prenatal visit to a physician. A particularly grievous result of this lack of prenatal care is that many more low-birth-weight infants are being born. These infants can be extremely expensive to treat medically, and they are more likely to die despite treatment.[4]

Low-birth-weight infants have been grouped according to weight (500-749 grams, 750-999 grams, etc.) by the National Perinatal Information Center. The heavier the birth-weight group, the lower the financial cost of enabling the infants to live. The Center concludes that if just 20 percent of these infants were born one weight group heavier, the monetary savings would be $70-90 million. The cost of the prenatal care needed to bring about such a shift is estimated at $9-28 million.[5] And quantifiable monetary losses are not all that is at stake. It has been said that statistics are human beings without the tears.[6] These figures do not give an accounting of what is perhaps the most important factor: the suffering on the part of newborns, their families, and others who care. It should be our priority to sustain life and to stress that the lives of all are equally important irrespective of their ability to afford expensive medical technology. Current allocation priorities regarding prenatal and postnatal care do not appear to serve these ends adequately.

To compound the problem, certain disadvantaged groups in society are unfairly burdened by these allocation priorities. For example, whereas 79 percent of white women receive prenatal care during the first trimester of pregnancy, only 61 percent of black women receive such care. As a result, the percentage of black babies born weighing less than 2500 grams is twice as high as that of white babies, and the ratio goes from 2:1 to 3:1 for newborns weighing less than 1500 grams. One result is a black infant mortality rate of seventeen deaths per thousand births, as compared with the white rate of nine.[7]

Not all groups in society, then, are affected in the same ways by the limited availability of certain resources.[8] The same biases subject certain groups to greater pressures to forgo treatment in order to conserve limited societal resources. Improving allocation priorities is much preferable to jeopardizing the lives of certain groups unfairly by allowing them to continue to bear a disproportionately high share of the burden of such financial pressures.

Sufficient Support

There are other ways in which a wise use of resources can lower the pressures on patients, families, and society to forgo life. One has to do with providing sufficient palliative (or "comfort") care. Premature death may be sought by patients out of a fear of the pain and alienation that the dying process will entail. This fear may be well-founded in the actual experience of friends and family members who have gone before them.

Addressing this issue effectively will require the concerted efforts of patients, families, health care professionals, church congregations, and government. Resources must be made available to provide the kind of caring support that dying patients need. After all, the dying *are* living. There is a critical need for relatively inexpensive forms of palliative care such as effective pain medication. Particularly in the last weeks of life, expensive "lifesaving" technologies tend to offer little benefit to the patient. Resources invested in better palliative care, on the other hand, often benefit the patient substantially.

More is needed than just additional money from governments and churches, however. There is also a great need for the love of God, including that love incarnated in human relationships. Family members, friends, health care professionals, and other believers are in a particularly good position to make a definitive difference at this point. They can make God's presence known and be present themselves in whatever ways patients require. Such love can cast out patients' fears.

These fears are not always self-directed; they often involve a concern that family members not be burdened with the demands that caregiving entails. However, it is far from clear that family members are helped more by a patient's premature exit from life than they are by caring for their loved one to the end. A family's and church's communication of unconditional, unwavering love despite the demands of the dying process is a priceless gift that can go a long way toward rendering premature death unnecessary. Even in such trying circumstances, it remains true that the greater blessing goes to the giver.

Appropriate Control

In a variety of ways, then, better resource allocation can help prevent problems associated with forgoing life. The reverse is also true: a better approach to end-of-life decisions can help avoid difficulties with regard to resource allocation. We have noted that the final days and weeks of dying can be extremely expensive. Our reluctance to release life into God's hands at this point only adds to the suffering and cost, with little gain. Admittedly, there are exceptional situations in which an extra day or two is valuable for personal or family reasons. For the most part, however, these eleventh-hour struggles needlessly consume resources that are badly needed elsewhere.

Allowing patients, families, and other caregivers to forgo treatment under the conditions outlined in Chapters 6 and 7 is a matter of good stewardship of available resources. In most situations, forgoing impotent treatment is not only acceptable but is in fact morally the better course of action.[9] If society as a whole could accept this, it would have the effect not only of freeing up resources for better use but also of promoting a climate in which patients would feel that they had a measure of control over their dying process.

People cannot absolutely control their dying any more than they can their living. However, aspiring to play God, they all too often attempt both. The demand for a quick technological fix for every problem in life, including sickness, is widespread; and if such a fix is not available, the same mentality undergirds the attempt to control death by causing it. Indeed, preserving a proper measure of control over the use of health care resources in the dying process may have a greater impact than any other factor in reducing the temptation of so-called voluntary active euthanasia. It is better to address the problems that make choosing death attractive than to compound those problems with problematic "solutions." As the recent analysis of choosing death by the Park

Ridge Center for the Study of Health, Faith, and Ethics concludes, "it would be shortsighted at best to opt for direct termination of life before we have made a serious attempt to change the factors contributing to a desire for euthanasia."[10]

The issues we have explored in Parts II and III of this book are indeed interrelated in many ways, both with one another and with other issues in the larger context of health care. These are matters that the Bible does not discuss directly for the most part. Yet the biblical writings do offer a perspective on life — a way of thinking and being and doing — that provides a way of negotiating these troubled waters.

Thinking, being, and doing are not neatly separable spheres of living, and we cannot afford to overlook any of them. It is essential, for example, that our attempts to understand what God intends for our lives be accompanied by the cultivation of moral character. Moral character is vital in disposing us not only to seek God's purposes continually but also to act on what we discover.

Moreover, attending to the purposes of God, as best those can be understood, must involve more than mere abstract thinking removed from the particulars of the individual patient and unique circumstances at hand. In fact, attentiveness to the particular situation is crucial and must encompass the entire situation — not just those aspects most immediately observable. The situation includes the reality of God and the way God has created the world to be. If such realities sometimes seem to limit the directions that love can take in the situation, it is only because love must not be limited to a partial understanding of the situation. At the same time, we will not be able to determine the relevance of larger realities in a particular situation unless we pay very close attention to the unique patient and the particular circumstances present.

The approach to ending patients' lives and allocating vital resources that we have examined here will not please all. It sanctions neither the direct taking of life nor always giving treatment to the last possible moment. It calls for neither the allocation of lifesaving resources according to people's social value nor merely the random distribution of them to all in need. It provides some justification for the decisions made by Bill's caregivers (see the Introduction) to treat pain aggressively, to withhold other treatments, and to resist the temptation to intend Bill's death. Yet it challenges both their decision not to give Bill the opportunity to participate in discussions about his dying and their apparently unquestioning compliance with transplant allocation criteria that may well be morally dubious.

The purpose of the described approach, however, is not to buttress presently popular positions but rather to reflect, at least in some small measure, the purposes of God. Discerning those purposes at the bedside of suffering patients or in the public policy arena is not easy and requires all of the wisdom that the community can bring to bear. Few occasions in life, though, warrant more concerted effort than when life itself is on the line.

Notes

Introduction

1. In distinguishing between "personal" and "social" issues, I am not suggesting that primarily personal issues such as decisions to end life do not have social policy dimensions or that primarily social issues such as resource allocation do not raise issues at a personal level. I make an effort to address both aspects of all the issues that are examined in these pages.

2. The terms *ethical* and *moral* are used almost interchangeably in common speech, and in keeping with that I do not make any fastidious distinction between them in this book. Generally speaking, however, the term *ethical* as I use it has more reflective or analytical connotations than *moral*, ethics being the study or science of that which is moral.

3. John F. Kilner, "Selecting Patients When Resources Are Limited: A Study of U.S. Medical Directors of Kidney Dialysis and Transplantation Facilities," *American Journal of Public Health* 78 (February 1988): 144-47.

4. John F. Kilner, *Who Lives? Who Dies? Ethical Criteria in Patient Selection* (New Haven: Yale University, 1990).

5. I use the term *lifesaving* with some frequency in this book for two reasons. Not only is the term more familiar than alternatives such as "life-sustaining," but it also serves to emphasize that the alternative to the treatments being discussed here is death. Technically, "lifesaving" suggests treatment of an acute problem that can be completely alleviated, whereas "life-sustaining" suggests ongoing treatment for a chronic condition. However, since both are commonly used as umbrella terms to indicate all treatments in which life is at stake, I use both in this generic sense.

6. Among the excellent sources addressing this issue, see Margaret A.

Farley, "Feminist Consciousness and the Interpretation of Scripture," in *Feminist Interpretation of Scripture*, ed. Letty Russell (Philadelphia: Westminster Press, 1985), pp. 41-51; Emily Chandler, "Theology and Ethics: A Feminist Perspective," in *Health Care and Its Costs*, ed. Walter Wiest (Lanham, Md.: University Press of America, 1988), pp. 229-43; Robert M. Brown, *Unexpected News: Reading the Bible with Third World Eyes* (Louisville: Westminster/John Knox, 1984); and Bruce C. Birch and Larry L. Rasmussen, *Bible and Ethics in the Christian Life*, rev. ed. (Minneapolis: Augsburg Press, 1989), pp. 117-19. See also books in the Health/Medicine and the Faith Traditions series published by the Park Ridge Center for the Study of Health, Faith, and Ethics in Chicago.

Chapter 1

1. As others have suggested, it might be more accurate to refer to the two major parts of the Christian Scriptures as the New*er* and Old*er* Testaments. Compared with most writings widely available today, neither is very new in terms of date of authorship.

2. For a survey of this diversity, see Victor P. Furnish, *Theology and Ethics in Paul* (Nashville: Abingdon Press, 1968). Since Romans, 1 and 2 Corinthians, Galatians, Philippians, 1 Thessalonians, and Philemon are most widely accepted as having been written by Paul, my analysis in this chapter will focus on these letters.

3. As Raymond F. Collins notes, the expression "let us do evil that good may result" (Rom. 3:8) is not purely ethical in nature (*Christian Morality: Biblical Foundations* [Notre Dame, Ind.: University of Notre Dame Press, 1986]). While "evil" *(ta kaka)* is an ethical term, "good" *(ta agatha)* may not strictly be so. It is often more theological, and especially eschatological, than specifically ethical in Paul's and other New Testament writings. Cf. Walter Grundmann, "ἀγαθός . . . ," in *Theological Dictionary of the New Testament*, vol. 1, ed. Gerhard Kittel, trans. Geoffrey Bromiley (Grand Rapids: William B. Eerdmans, 1964), pp. 15-17. Yet this mix of the ethical and the theological is very characteristic of Paul. It suggests that in the ethical and theological realms alike, that which is good or bad is so because of its essential nature (especially its degree of God-relatedness), not primarily because of its beneficial consequences.

4. While this concluding statement in v. 8 appears to be a judgment on those who would (and do) employ mistaken reasoning, a different reading is suggested by Paul J. Achtemeier (" 'Some Things in Them Hard to Understand': Reflections on an Approach to Paul," *Interpretation* 38 [1984]: 254-67). Based on the logical structure of the passage, Achtemeier contends that Paul is defending God's justice in condemning sinners generally (cf. v. 7). This is a valuable insight, although Paul probably has his immediate opponents in view as examples of those whom God rightly condemns. For detailed support

of this interpretation, see David R. Hall, "Romans 3:1-8 Reconsidered," *New Testament Studies* 29 (1983): 192-95.

5. For some of Paul's views on the implications of Adam's sin for all of humanity, see Rom. 5:17-19. The implications of fallenness for knowing and doing are highlighted in Rom. 1:18; 3:10, 19-20, 23.

6. The term used in Rom. 12:2 is *metamorphousthe*, a present imperative, suggesting continual or repeated action. Cf. Paul W. Gooch, "Authority and Justification in Theological Ethics: A Study in I Corinthians 7," *Journal of Religious Ethics* 11 (Spring 1983): 68.

7. The *oun* near the beginning of Rom. 12:1 links what follows to what precedes as a logical or appropriate outflow.

8. Günther Bornkamm, *Paul*, trans. D. M. G. Stalker (New York: Harper & Row, 1971), p. 203.

9. See Stephen Westerholm, "Letter and Spirit: The Foundation of Pauline Ethics," *New Testament Studies* 30 (April 1984): 229-48. As Thomas Aquinas and many since him have suggested, the letter of the law referred to in 2 Cor. 3:6 and elsewhere may well include any set of sayings or commands that we must obey in order to be saved (*Summa Theologica*, IaIIae, q.106, a.2).

10. Paul is assuming here that the believer will be discerning God's will as it is manifested through a variety of sources — Scripture, human counsel, inner promptings by God, circumstances, and so forth. Whatever the immediate source, however, discernment is key. Because of God, accurate discernment is possible; but because of sin, it cannot be taken for granted. See Robin Scroggs, *Paul for a New Day* (Philadelphia: Fortress Press, 1977), p. 69.

11. Cf. Birger Gerhardsson, *The Ethos of the Bible* (Philadelphia: Fortress Press, 1981), pp. 65-66.

12. In Romans alone, see 2:7, 10, 18; 3:12; 12:9, 21 for the notion of intrinsic good, and 1:28; 2:8, 9; 12:9, 17, 21 for the notion of intrinsic evil. These categories correspond basically to the notions of right and wrong when actions are in view, although Paul does explicitly employ the notion of right in a determinate sense as well (e.g., in Rom. 13:3).

13. Cf. the introduction to and quotation of Ps. 51:4 in Rom. 3:4.

14. It is possible to overemphasize the significance of Paul's eschatology for his ethics. For instance, some have contended that Paul's ethics depends on his opinion that the end of the world is imminent — and they conclude that since Paul was mistaken on this score, his ethics is largely irrelevant today (see, e.g., Jack T. Sanders, *Ethics in the New Testament* [Philadelphia: Fortress Press, 1975], pp. 56-61). However, Paul's ethics emerges as much (if not more) from his understanding of present and past realities as from his view of the future. Moreover, his eschatology contains many elements that stand independent of his opinion that Christ's return is imminent (see Victor P. Furnish, *The Moral*

Teaching of Paul: Selected Issues, 2d ed. [Nashville: Abingdon Press, 1985], pp. 22-24). In fact, even the assertion that some of Paul's writings indicate that he believed he would live to see Christ's return is open to question. In 1 Thess. 4:15, for example, he does use the phrase "we who are still alive, who are left till the coming of the Lord," but elsewhere he affirms that God "will raise us also" from the dead (1 Cor. 6:14) and says, "we make it our goal to please [the Lord], whether we are [alive or dead]" (2 Cor. 5:9). In each of these cases, as elsewhere, Paul uses the words *we* and *us* to refer to Christians generally, without necessarily identifying himself specifically with the group. It may be the case that Paul did expect to live to see the end of the world, but the evidence is by no means clear-cut, and certainly not so substantial that his ethics can be said to depend on it.

15. The fact that much of Paul's moral exhortation is directed to Christians and based on who they are as Christians indicates that he was not concerned with developing a "secular ethics" even in a limited sense. His ethics is for the Christian alone. Any instruction for unbelievers is directed to their need for Jesus Christ. For more on this, see Wolfgang Schrage, *Ethik des Neuen Testaments,* Grundrisse zum Neuen Testament, NTD 4 (Göttingen: Vandenhoeck & Ruprecht, 1982), p. 203. For a discussion of these matters in the context of love commands, see Jean-François Collange, *De Jesus à Paul: L'ethique du Nouveau Testament* (Geneva: Labor et Fides, 1980). In making this observation, I am by no means implying that Paul's ethics is not relevant to the problems of a secularized culture; I am merely suggesting that such an application was not part of Paul's own apostolic, pastoral concern. For indications that Paul did consider it potentially worthwhile to appeal to the ethical sensitivities of unbelievers, see Rom. 12:17; 1 Cor. 10:32-33; 2 Cor. 8:21; 1 Thess. 4:12.

16. Paul's language in 1 Thess. 2 especially reflects this type of family relationship. He describes his relation to the Thessalonians as that of a mother and father to children (vv. 7, 11). He shares his life with them, not just his teaching (v. 8). He addresses them as brothers four times (vv. 1, 9, 14, 17). He even describes himself and his companions as having been orphaned (*aporphanisthentes,* v. 17) when they were separated from the Thessalonians (see Wayne A. Meeks, *The Moral World of the First Christians* [Philadelphia: Westminster Press, 1986], pp. 125-30). Cf. Philem. 8, 16, 21.

17. The fact that Christians are presently children not of the night but of the eschatological day (1 Thess. 5:5ff.; cf. Rom. 13:12ff.) reflects the present in-breaking of future reality. This "already" dimension of Paul's eschatology blurs the neat distinction between future and present realities. I am using the categories of past, present, and future in this discussion for convenience' sake and not to suggest that an absolute distinction is possible. On heavenly citizenship, see Gal. 4:25ff.; Phil. 3:19ff.; cf. Robert Banks, *Paul's Idea of Community* (Grand Rapids: William B. Eerdmans, 1980), pp. 44ff.

18. The classic formulation of this relationship is Rudolf Bultmann's slogan "become what you are!" ("Werde, der du bist" — *Theologie des Neuen Testaments* [Tübingen: J. C. B. Mohr, 1953], p. 329). And yet this formulation invites misinterpretation. Bultmann apparently suggests that essentially one is not something yet but must become it. Paul's argument is different: he exhorts believers to be what they already are. If it had to be reduced to a slogan, "be who you are" would be closer to the mark. It is also true, though, that Paul's readers were not acting fully in accordance with who they were in Christ. So the indicative can exist without the realization of the imperative, even though the indicative cannot exist apart from its imperative force.

19. On the Galatian-Corinthian situation, see Terence J. Keegan, "Paul's Dying/Rising Ethics in I Corinthians," in *Christian Biblical Ethics,* ed. Robert J. Daly (New York: Paulist Press, 1984). For the importance of understanding moral living as a fruit rather than a source of new life, see Herman Ridderbos, *Paul: An Outline of His Theology,* trans. John R. de Witt (Grand Rapids: William B. Eerdmans, 1975), pp. 254-55; cf. Leander E. Keck, *Paul and His Letters* (Philadelphia: Fortress Press, 1979), p. 90.

20. See John E. Stambaugh and David L. Balch, *The New Testament in Its Social Environment* (Philadelphia: Westminster Press, 1986), p. 55; Elisabeth Schüssler Fiorenza, *In Memory of Her* (New York: Crossroad, 1983), p. 234; and Dieter Luhrmann, "Neutestamentliche Haustafeln und antike Okonomie," *New Testament Studies* 27 (October 1980): 83-97.

21. See Keegan, "Paul's Dying/Rising Ethics in I Corinthians," p. 231; cf. Bengt Holmberg, *Paul and Power* (Lund, Sweden: C. W. K. Gleerup, 1978), p. 85. For a discussion of freedom within limits, see Robert Jewett, *Christian Tolerance: Paul's Message to the Modern Church* (Philadelphia: Westminster Press, 1982), pp. 51ff. — though note Jewett's casual association of Paul with the concept of autonomy.

22. Paul is much more concerned that people fulfill their duty to others than that others (or they themselves) claim their rights. That is why he does not simply claim his own rights in 1 Cor. 9 but brings up the issue in a way that will help the Corinthians better understand their duty. Paul himself was not always averse to exercising his rights — especially political rights — when there was no reason not to (see Acts 22:25; 25:11). In certain situations, though, other realities intervened. For example, Paul was appalled that the Corinthians would exercise their rights to sue each other in court rather than relying on the judgment of the Christian community. To do so was to disregard the reality that God's people will judge the world — even angels — and so should be better judges than those who lack a spiritual frame of reference (1 Cor. 6:2-3).

23. According to 1 Corinthians, concern for the good of others may involve refraining from harming them (8:9ff.; 10:28ff.; 11:22) — even if one must suffer wrong in the process (6:7-8) — as well as seeking their good in a

more positive sense (13:4-7 and verses in text). See Peter Richardson, *Paul's Ethic of Freedom* (Philadelphia: Westminster Press, 1979), pp. 118-19.

24. Sandwiched immediately between these two verses is 1 Cor. 13, which reinforces both points.

25. Accordingly, the suggestion of some (e.g., J. L. Houlden, *Ethics and the New Testament* [Baltimore: Penguin, 1973], p. 33) that at the coming of Christ the ceremonial law was jettisoned and the moral law retained is misleading. The notions of law and moral obligation are different for Paul. Whereas moral obligation remains, law as legal requirements — whether moral or ceremonial in nature — does not. Cf. Keck, *Paul and His Letters*, p. 86.

26. There is a danger in reacting so strongly to the notion of legal obligation that the "command" character of God's rule is overly diminished. In Christ we enjoy freedom from the tyranny of the law but not freedom from living in love in accordance with God-given realities. So Paul can say that "keeping God's commands is what counts" (1 Cor. 7:19). We are to be obedient directly to God rather than to the external requirements of law. Such obedience does not contradict our responsibility to live in love toward people (as Sanders suggests in *Ethics in the New Testament*, p. 66). To the contrary, it is the first responsibility of love and one that ultimately directs all of its expressions. See Victor P. Furnish, *The Love Command in the New Testament* (Nashville: Abingdon Press, 1972), pp. 95ff. Cf. T. J. Deidun, *New Covenant Morality in Paul* (Rome: Biblical Institute, 1982), pp. 183ff.

27. For an elaboration of the relationship between love and freedom, see Allen Verhey, *The Great Reversal: Ethics and the New Testament* (Grand Rapids: William B. Eerdmans, 1984), pp. 107-9.

Chapter 2

1. Although the debates over authorship continue, many see the authors of the Gospels of Mark and Luke as the Mark and Luke associated with Paul in Acts. Whereas Paul was "the apostle to the Gentiles" (Rom. 11:13), Matthew wrote primarily to a Jewish audience (as suggested by his Jewish terminology, lack of explanation of Jewish customs, many references to the Old Testament, tracing of Jesus' descent from Abraham, and emphasis on Jesus as the "Son of David").

2. The teachings of Jesus present a difficulty not encountered in the letters of Paul. Whereas Paul composed his material essentially in the form in which it survives today, Jesus' teachings are mediated through the writings of others such as Matthew who received oral and written accounts of what Jesus taught. In one sense this circumstance creates no problem with respect to my purpose here, in that Matthew himself constitutes a biblical writer other than Paul and, accordingly, provides a second biblical perspective.

Nevertheless, if we were interested in getting a sense of Jesus' own outlook that would be widely acknowledged as such, we would do well to focus on passages in Matthew that are considered by biblical scholars to preserve the perspective of Jesus and that are central to his teaching. The four passages selected here fit these criteria. On Jesus as the source of Matt. 5:43-48, see David Wenham, "Paul's Use of the Jesus Tradition: Three Samples," in *The Jesus Tradition outside the Gospels*, ed. David Wenham (Sheffield, Eng.: JSOT Press, 1985), pp. 20-22; Pheme Perkins, *Love Commands in the New Testament* (New York: Paulist Press, 1982), pp. 39-40; John Piper, *Love Your Enemies* (Cambridge: Cambridge University Press, 1979), pp. 53-55, 59-63; and (following Bultmann) Victor P. Furnish, *The Love Command in the New Testament* (Nashville: Abingdon Press, 1972), pp. 24, 61. On Matt. 6:19-34, see Hans D. Betz, "Cosmogony and Ethics in the Sermon on the Mount," in *Cosmogony and Ethical Order*, ed. Robin Lovin and Frank Reynolds (Chicago: University of Chicago Press, 1985), pp. 158-76. On Matt. 12:1-14, see John M. Hicks, "The Sabbath Controversy in Matthew: An Exegesis of Matthew 12:1-14," *Restoration Quarterly* 27 (1984): 85. On Matt. 22:34-40, see Piper (following Bornkamm), *Love Your Enemies*, pp. 92-94; and Furnish, *The Love Command in the New Testament*, pp. 24, 62.

3. For more extended treatments of these themes, see Lisa S. Cahill, "The Ethical Implications of the Sermon on the Mount," *Interpretation* 41 (April 1987): 149; Bonnie B. Thurston, "Matthew 5:43-48," *Interpretation* 41 (April 1987): 171-73; John R. Levison, "Responsible Initiative in Matthew 5:21-48," *Expository Times* 98 (May 1987): 234; Brice L. Martin, "Matthew on Christ and the Law," *Theological Studies* 34 (April 1983): 62-63; Piper, *Love Your Enemies*, pp. 143-45; and Eduard Schweizer, *The Good News according to Matthew* (Atlanta: John Knox Press, 1975), pp. 133-35.

4. On the debate over the meaning of loving the enemy, see Richard Horsley, "Ethics and Exegesis: 'Love Your Enemies' and the Doctrine of Non-Violence," *Journal of the American Academy of Religion* 54 (Spring 1986): 3-31. For additional explorations of the scope of love in this passage, see Cahill, "The Ethical Implications of the Sermon on the Mount," p. 150; Brice L. Martin, "Matthew on Christ and the Law," *Theological Studies* 34 (April 1983): 62-63; Piper, *Love Your Enemies*, p. 144; and Furnish, *The Love Command in the New Testament*, p. 54.

5. On the preoccupation of the hellenistic world with worrying, see Hans D. Betz, "Cosmogony and Ethics in the Sermon on the Mount," in *Cosmogony and Ethical Order*, ed. Robin Lovin and Frank Reynolds (Chicago: University of Chicago Press, 1985), p. 166. On the God-centered dimension of Jesus' teaching here, see Charles E. Carlston, "Matthew 6:24-34," *Interpretation* 41 (April 1987): 181; Betz, *Cosmogony and Ethical Order*, p. 173; and Schweizer, *The Good News according to Matthew*, p. 165.

6. Regarding the significance of the eternal dimension at this point, see

G. E. Okeke, "The After-Life in St. Matthew as an Aspect of Matthean Ethic," *Communio Viatorum* 31 (Summer 1988): 159ff.

7. In light of the similar contrast between "pagan" and godly perspectives in 5:47 and 6:32, Piper also sees a strong tie between the "love" language of 5:43-48 and the call to kingdom righteousness in the latter part of chap. 6 (*Love Your Enemies*, pp. 149-51).

8. In the original Greek, the word for Lord *(kyrios)* appears at the outset of the affirmation in v. 8 — emphasizing the authority of Jesus to interpret God's intentions underlying the scriptural Sabbath law. Similarly, "for" at the start of v. 8 ties that verse to the quotation from Hosea and emphasizes the oneness of God and Christ (the Son of Man). See Hicks, "The Sabbath Controversy in Matthew," p. 88; and Schweizer, *The Good News according to Matthew,* p. 277.

9. There is some debate over whether in v. 6 Jesus is saying that "something" (reflecting a neuter gender in the Greek text) or "someone" greater than the temple is present. In light of the chapter as a whole, the idea seems to be a combination of the two — that the reign of God centered in the person and life of Jesus has arrived (cf. v. 28: "if I drive out demons by the Spirit of God, then the reign of God has come upon you"). See Hicks, "The Sabbath Controversy in Matthew," p. 86; Schweizer, *The Good News according to Matthew,* p. 278. On the challenge to the authority of the temple and the Pharisees implicit in the controversy over Sabbath observance, see Etan Levine, "The Sabbath Controversy according to Matthew," *New Testament Studies* 22 (1976): 482; B. Rod Doyle, "A Concern of the Evangelist: Pharisees in Matthew 12," *Australian Biblical Review* 34 (October 1986): 17-34; and Hicks, "The Sabbath Controversy in Matthew," pp. 83-84.

10. On the nature of the hunger and disability involved in this passage, particularly their significance as examples of major (as opposed to frivolous) "needs," see Luise Schottroff and Wolfgang Stegemann, "The Sabbath Was Made for Man," in *God of the Lowly,* ed. Willy Schottroff and Wolfgang Stegemann (Maryknoll, N.Y.: Orbis Books, 1984), pp. 121-25; and Samuele Bacchiocchi, "Matthew 11:28-30: Jesus' Rest and the Sabbath," *Andrews University Seminary Studies* 22 (Autumn 1984): 307. While Jesus uses people's valuing of animals to show them their own inconsistency, he is not making a systematic statement here about the signficance of animal life.

11. Cf. Bacchiocchi, "Matthew 11:28-30: Jesus' Rest and the Sabbath," pp. 305-6; Martin, "Matthew on Christ and the Law," p. 56.

12. On right thinking as an important aspect of loving God, and the loss entailed by reducing love for God to love for the neighbor, see Klaus Bockmuehl, "The Great Commandment," *Crux* 23 (September 1987): 10-14.

13. As Jesus has already explained in chapter 5, "do not think that I have come to abolish the Law or the Prophets; I have not come to abolish them but to fulfill them" (v. 17). Cf. v. 19b: "whoever practices and teaches

these commands [of the Law] will be called great in the realm of heaven."
On the determinate moral content of the command to love, see Furnish, *The
Love Command in the New Testament*, p. 34. On the significance of the claim
that love is the "greatest commandment," see Eugene Lemcio, "Pirke 'Abot
1:2(3) and the Synoptic Redactions of the Commands to Love God and Neighbor," *Asbury Theological Journal* 43 (Spring 1988): 43-53.

14. On the precedence of love for God over all other commandments,
including the commandment to love one's neighbor, see Martin, "Matthew
on Christ and the Law," p. 63. On the likeness of the two love commands,
see Furnish, *The Love Command in the New Testament*, p. 31. Cf. Johannes
Schneider, "ὅμοιος . . . ," in *Theological Dictionary of the New Testament*, vol. 5,
ed. Gerhard Kittel and Gerhard Friedrich, trans. Geoffrey Bromiley (Grand
Rapids: William B. Eerdmans, 1967), pp. 186-99; Schneider provides a careful
analysis of the word *like (homoia)*.

15. The natural-law tradition is rooted in such Scripture passages as
Rom. 1:19, 32, which indicate that knowledge about God and morality are
available to all. Classic proponents of this tradition include Thomas Aquinas
and his followers (see, e.g., his *Summa Theologica*, IaIIae, q.94; cf. Marvin R.
O'Connell, "The Roman Catholic Tradition since 1545," in *Caring and Curing*,
ed. Ronald Numbers and Darrel Amundsen [New York: Macmillan, 1986],
pp. 138ff.). The prevenient-grace tradition is rooted in such texts as John 1:9
which suggest that God illumines the understanding of every person. Classic
proponents of this tradition include John Wesley and his followers (see, e.g.,
Wesley's sermon "On Working out Our Own Salvation," in *The Works of the
Reverend John Wesley*, vol. 2, ed. John Emery [New York: J. Emery and
B. Waugh, 1831]; cf. E. Brooks Holifield, *Health and Medicine in the Methodist
Tradition* [New York: Crossroad, 1986], pp. 112ff.).

16. For assessments of the utilitarian approach, see the following:
George P. Smith II, "Death Be Not Proud: Medical, Ethical and Legal Dilemmas in Resource Allocation," *Journal of Contemporary Health Law and Policy* 3
(Spring 1987): 50-51; Don S. Browning, "Hospital Chaplaincy as Public Ministry," *Second Opinion* 1 (1986): 73; John F. Kilner, "Who Shall Be Saved? An
African Answer," *Hastings Center Report* 14 (June 1984): 19-21; Mark Siegler,
"Should Age Be a Criterion in Health Care?" *Hastings Center Report* 14 (October 1984): 25; Richard B. Brandt, "The Real and Alleged Problem of Utilitarianism," *Hastings Center Report* 13 (April 1983): 37; Ruth B. Purtilo, "Justice
in the Distribution of Health Care Resources: The Position of Physical Therapists in the United States and Sweden," *Physical Therapy* 62 (January 1982):
48; Kenneth L. Vaux, "Theological Foundations of Medical Ethics," in
Health/Medicine and the Faith Traditions, ed. Martin Marty and Kenneth Vaux
(Philadelphia: Fortress Press, 1982), p. 220; and Thomas C. Oden, *Should Treatment Be Terminated?* (New York: Harper & Row, 1976), p. 89.

17. See, e.g., Joseph Fletcher, *Situation Ethics* (Philadelphia: Westminster

Press, 1966), pp. 81, 95, 152. Robin Scroggs characterizes Paul's ethics as "close to" utilitarian situation ethics, though he does acknowledge several differences (*Paul for a New Day* [Philadelphia: Fortress Press, 1977], pp. 70-71). On the other hand, Pheme Perkins suggests that those whom Paul is correcting are much more utilitarian in their thinking than Paul ("Paul and Ethics," *Interpretation* 38 [July 1984]: 279).

18. E.g., John Stuart Mill, "Utility of Religion," in *The Philosophy of John Stuart Mill*, ed. Marshall Cohen (New York: Random House, 1961), pp. 488-524.

19. For more on the relationship between God and utilitarianism, see Gilbert Meilaender, "Euthanasia and Christian Vision," in *On Moral Medicine: Theological Perspectives in Medical Ethics*, ed. Stephen Lammers and Allen Verhey (Grand Rapids: William B. Eerdmans, 1987), pp. 455-56; James M. Gustafson, "The Transcendence of God and the Value of Human Life," in *On Moral Medicine*, p. 125; and Francis A. Schaeffer and C. Everett Koop, *Whatever Happened to the Human Race?* (Old Tappan, N.J.: Fleming H. Revell, 1979), p. 101.

20. As in the deontological ethics of W. David Ross; see *The Right and the Good* (Oxford: Oxford University Press, 1973), especially pp. 21, 42.

21. Immanuel Kant uses such a basis in *Foundations of the Metaphysics of Morals* (Indianapolis: Bobbs-Merrill, 1969). For a discussion of the "hurdle of reason," see John F. Kilner, "Hurdles for Natural Law Ethics: Lessons from Grotius," *American Journal of Jurisprudence* 28 (1983): 149-67.

22. See Larry R. Churchill and Jose J. Siman, "Principles and the Search for Moral Certainty," *Social Science and Medicine* 23 (1986): 462-65; and John M. Frame, *Medical Ethics: Principles, Persons, and Problems* (Grand Rapids: Baker Book House, 1988), p. 28. Cf. Harmon L. Smith, "Dying with Style," *Anglican Theological Review* 70 (October 1988): 327-45; and Kenneth S. Kantzer, "Biomedical Decision Making: We Dare Not Retreat," *Christianity Today*, 21 March 1986, p. 161.

23. Even the commonality between deontological ethics and the described approach, though, is subject to some important qualifications. Whereas deontologists are prone to speak of the moral "law," proponents of the described approach join Paul in resisting that understanding of obligation for reasons explained in Chapter 1. See Thomas W. Ogletree, *The Use of the Bible in Christian Ethics* (Philadelphia: Fortress Press, 1983), pp. 169, 199-200; cf. Kantzer, "Biomedical Decision Making," p. 161. Moreover, Paul and many of the other biblical writers emphasize the communal nature of ethical decision making, as opposed to the individualistic character of much of deontological ethics. See Perkins, "Paul and Ethics," pp. 270-71, 278; and Victor P. Furnish, *Theology and Ethics in Paul* (Nashville: Abingdon Press, 1968), pp. 233ff. See also Karen Lebacqz, "Bio-ethics: Some Challenges from a Liberation Perspective," in *On Moral Medicine: Theological Perspectives in Medical Ethics*,

ed. Stephen Lammers and Allen Verhey (Grand Rapids: William B. Eerdmans, 1987), pp. 64-69.

24. On narrative, see Arthur Kleinman, *The Illness Narratives: Suffering, Healing and the Human Condition* (New York: Basic Books, 1988); Kathryn M. Hunter, "Making a Case," *Literature and Medicine* 7 (1988): 66-79; and Howard Brody, *Stories of Sickness* (New Haven: Yale University Press, 1987). On phenomenology, see Richard M. Zaner, *Ethics and the Clinical Encounter* (Englewood Cliffs, N.J.: Prentice-Hall, 1988); and S. Kay Toombs, "The Meaning of Illness: A Phenomenological Approach to the Physician-Patient Relationship," *Journal of Medicine and Philosophy* 12 (August 1987): 219-40. On hermeneutics, see Ronald A. Carson, "Interpretive Bioethics: The Way of Discernment," *Theoretical Medicine* 11 (March 1990): 51-59; and Stephen L. Daniel, "The Patient as Text: A Model of Clinical Hermeneutics," *Theoretical Medicine* (June 1986): 195-210.

25. Nevertheless, it must be emphasized that the *agape* love that the Bible speaks of cannot be considered solely in terms of concern for the wellbeing of the neighbor; such concern must not be divorced from the God-centered and reality-bounded dimensions of ethical decision making.

26. The classic exposition of this outlook can be found in Aristotle's *Nichomachean Ethics*, especially book 2.

27. The ethics of virtue characterizes love as a quality of activity in that it is kind, courteous, and selfless; a quality of thinking in that it is humble, sincere, and optimistic; and a quality of suffering in that it is patient and persevering, not bitter or vengeful. See R. E. O. White, *Biblical Ethics* (Atlanta: John Knox Press, 1979), p. 159.

28. In other words, the described approach, in line with Paul's ethics, is more relational at this point. See J. L. Houlden, *Ethics and the New Testament* (Baltimore: Penguin, 1973), p. 26; and Ogletree, *The Use of the Bible in Christian Ethics*, pp. 194-95. As Kenneth E. Schemmer adds, it is easier for us to understand God's intentions for human being (i.e., for how we as people are to be) if we can see them modeled in people whose struggles are similar to our own (*Between Life and Death* [Wheaton, Ill.: Victor Books, 1988]). Moreover, the goal of the described ethics is not to become the ideal person that one is not but rather to be the new creation that one is (cf. Leander E. Keck, *Paul and His Letters* [Philadelphia: Fortress Press, 1979], p. 90). Human beings were created in the image of God, and we retain that image; in consequence, God's moral character remains the standard for our moral character (G. R. Dunstan, *The Artifice of Ethics* [London: SCM Press, 1974], p. 70; and Arthur F. Holmes, *Ethics: Approaching Moral Decisions* [Downers Grove, Ill.: InterVarsity Press, 1984], p. 118).

29. For an elaboration of these virtues in the context of medicine, see James F. Drane, *Becoming a Good Doctor* (Kansas City: Sheed & Ward, 1988); Hessel Bouma III et al., *Christian Faith, Health, and Medical Practice* (Grand

Rapids: William B. Eerdmans, 1989), pp. 142-43; and Edmund Pellegrino, "Character, Virtue, and Self-Interest in the Ethics of the Professions," *Journal of Contemporary Health Policy and Law* 5 (Spring 1989): 53-73.

30. For several New Testment perspectives on good character and its implications for right actions, see D. Glenn Saul, "The Ethics of Decision Making," in *Understanding Christian Ethics*, ed. William Tillman, Jr. (Nashville: Broadman Press, 1988), pp. 90-96. Cf. Arthur F. Holmes, *Shaping Character* (Grand Rapids: William B. Eerdmans, 1991), pp. 58-72.

31. Even John Wesley, with his emphasis on right intention ("perfect love"), acknowledged that good intentions will sometimes fall short of the mark if they are not joined with a careful consideration of what God intends ("truth"). See, for example, Wesley, "An Israelite Indeed," in *The Works of the Reverend John Wesley*, vol. 2, ed. John Emery (New York: J. Emery and B. Waugh, 1831); cf. E. Brooks Holifield, *Health and Medicine in the Methodist Tradition* (New York: Crossroad, 1986), pp. 113-14. Bruce C. Birch and Larry L. Rasmussen have noted the danger of self-deception if virtuous intent is allowed to justify action with no other standards by which to distinguish right actions from wrong (*Bible and Ethics in the Christian Life*, rev. ed. [Minneapolis: Augsburg Press, 1989], pp. 46-47).

32. The Incarnation itself reflects this integration, just as Jesus' summary command to be "perfect" (Matt. 5:48) is literally a call to "maturity" and "wholeness." See Paul D. Simmons, *Birth and Death: Bioethical Decision-Making* (Philadelphia: Westminster Press, 1983), pp. 54-55; cf. Stephen C. Mott, "The Use of the New Testament for Social Ethics," *Journal of Religious Ethics* 15 (Fall 1988): 240; and Rudolf Schnackenburg, "Neutestamentliche Ethik im Kontext heutiger Wirklichkeit," in *Anspruch der Wirklichkeit und christlicher Glaube: Festschrift für A. Auer*, ed. H. Weber and D. Mieth (Düsseldorf: Patmos, 1980), p. 204.

33. On the place of explicitly religious perspectives in public policy discussions of ethical issues in health care, see Brendan P. Minogue, "The Exclusion of Theology from Public Policy: The Case of Euthanasia," *Second Opinion* 14 (July 1990): 90-92; cf. Laurence J. O'Connell, "The Preferential Option for the Poor and Health Care in the United States," in *Medical Ethics*, ed. John Monagle and David Thomasma (Rockville, Md.: Aspen, 1987), pp. 306-13. Birch and Rasmussen develop the notion of vision as one of the hallmarks of ethics in the Bible (*Bible and Ethics in the Christian Life*, pp. 58-62).

Chapter 3

1. Recall the discussion of the idolatrous propensity of the mind (Rom. 1:21-25) in Chapter 1. An analogous problem arises on the human level if we focus on principles to the exclusion of the persons whom those principles are

supposed to serve. See Larry R. Churchill and Jose J. Siman, "Principles and the Search for Moral Certainty," *Social Science and Medicine* 23 (1986): 463.

2. The debate between Donald Bloesch (*Freedom for Obedience* [San Francisco: Harper & Row, 1987], pp. 182-83) and Norman Geisler (*Options in Contemporary Christian Ethics* [Grand Rapids: Baker Book House, 1981], pp. 25-26) is instructive at this point in that they each identify dangerous tendencies in the other's approach. Bloesch is concerned that Geisler's reliance on principles applied by reason has the potential to distance one from God. Geisler, meanwhile, is worried that the subjectivism of a Barthian rejection of ethical principles as authoritative denies one of the most important tools God has given people through the Bible for ethical analysis. For further discussion of this matter, see Stanley Hauerwas, *A Community of Character* (Notre Dame, Ind.: University of Notre Dame Press, 1981), p. 58; and Dennis Hollinger, "Can Bioethics Be Evangelical?" *Journal of Religious Ethics* 17 (Fall 1989): 161-79. Hauerwas highlights the danger of removing ethical principles from their narrative context in the Bible, and Hollinger supports the idea of ethical principles as long as the biblical context is preserved.

3. For examples of scholars who attempt to break down the image of God into its component parts, even while acknowledging the dangers of doing so, see Conrad G. Brunk, "In the Image of God," in *Medical Ethics, Human Choices: A Christian Perspective*, ed. John Rogers (Scottdale, Pa.: Herald Press, 1988), pp. 31-33; and Paul D. Simmons, *Birth and Death: Bioethical Decision-Making* (Philadelphia: Westminster Press, 1983), pp. 60, 127. For developments of the holiness dimension of the image of God, see D. Gareth Jones, *Brave New People*, rev. ed. (Grand Rapids: William B. Eerdmans, 1985), pp. 13-14; John M. Frame, *Medical Ethics: Principles, Persons, and Problems* (Grand Rapids: Baker Book House, 1988), p. 35; G. C. Berkouwer, *Man: The Image of God* (Grand Rapids: William B. Eerdmans, 1962), pp. 349-63; and Norman Anderson, *Issues of Life and Death* (Downers Grove, Ill.: InterVarsity Press, 1976), pp. 21-22.

4. For more on the implications of the Good Samaritan story for medical ethics generally and the image of God in particular, see Arthur J. Dyck, *On Human Care* (Nashville: Abingdon Press, 1977) and "The Image of God: An Ethical Foundation for Medicine," *Linacre Quarterly* 57 (February 1990): 35-45.

5. Acccordingly, the fact that human beings are created in the image of God does not suggest that they are divine — that is to say, on a par with God. See John B. Cobb, Jr., *Matters of Life and Death* (Louisville: Westminster/John Knox, 1991), p. 52.

6. For an elaboration of these New Testament themes, see Karl Barth, *Church Dogmatics*, III/4, trans. A. T. Mackay et al. (Edinburgh: T. & T. Clark, 1961), pp. 324-43.

7. For further discussion of appropriate terminology with regard to the

significance of life, see David C. Thomasma, *Human Life in the Balance* (Louisville: Westminster/John Knox Press, 1990), chap. 1; John Kleinig, *Valuing Life* (Princeton: Princeton University Press, 1991), chap. 1; Richard Stith, "Toward Freedom from Value," in *On Moral Medicine: Theological Perspectives in Medical Ethics,* ed. Stephen Lammers and Allen Verhey (Grand Rapids: William B. Eerdmans, 1987), pp. 129-35; and Stanley Hauerwas, "Rational Suicide and Reasons for Living," in *On Moral Medicine,* p. 463.

8. 1 Cor. 7:21 reads, "Were you a slave when you were called? Don't let it trouble you — although if you can gain your freedom, do so." While there is some debate over the proper translation of this verse — and in the immediate context Paul is indeed arguing that those who are trapped in slavery should not be distraught over it — several considerations support the translation suggested here. First, the "although" (Greek *all'*, a strong adversative that might better be translated "but") that introduces the last part of the verse suggests that what is to follow is in contrast to the preceding generalities. Second, the final "do so" *(chresai)* — literally "make use of it" — is an aorist imperative verb that more naturally indicates a specific action that would change one's present state than a continuation of one's present condition. Finally, translated as above, the verse mirrors the structure of the wider passage on marriage and divorce in which Paul has just been arguing that there should generally be no divorce — but if an unbelieving spouse leaves, it is fine to break free from the relationship (v. 15).

In Philemon 16, Paul expresses his hope (and intention) that Philemon receive Onesimus back "no longer as a slave, but better than a slave, as a dear brother." Paul adds, "he is very dear to me but even dearer to you, both as a man and as a brother in the Lord." Elsewhere in the letter Paul makes it clear that he need not return Onesimus to Philemon, but he is doing so in order that Onesimus's new status will be willingly accepted by Philemon and not simply imposed on him by Onesimus's escape from slavery. Paul explicitly indicates that Onesimus is no longer a slave *(ouketi)* — a judgment that is reaffirmed by Paul's classifying him as a "man" (rather than a slave) and a brother in the Lord.

9. In John 8:34, Jesus introduces his statement to this effect with the words *amen, amen*. These words indicate that an especially solemn and significant truth is about to follow — one that may not readily correlate with the common way of thinking.

10. For further discussion of this contention, see Henry Stob, *The Christian Concept of Freedom* (Grand Rapids: Grand Rapids International Publications, 1957), p. 20.

11. According to Jesus, the evil "strong man" is bound (Mark 3:27). Paul told the Romans, "you have been set free from sin" (Rom. 6:18), echoing Jesus' teaching in John 8:31-36, where the related freedom from self-deception is also in view (cf. 2 Cor. 3:14-16). Jesus speaks of becoming "truly free" (v. 36) as

opposed to obtaining only the superficial freedom from restrictions heralded by the world. Similarly, the stranglehold of the religious law is broken (Rom. 7:3-6; 8:2; Gal. 2:4; 4:21-31; 5:1, 13), signifying that bondage to all humanly imposed religious regulations is ended (cf. Matt. 17:24-26). Eternal death (Rom. 6:21-23) and final judgment (James 2:12-13) also lose their power to terrorize. Calvin (*Institutes of the Christian Religion*, 3.19.9) and Ernst Käsemann (*Jesus Means Freedom*, trans. F. Clarke [Philadelphia: Fortress Press, 1969], pp. 115-16) add the important freedom from the tyranny of circumstances (good or bad) which they find celebrated especially by Paul (Phil. 4:12-13).

12. On this theme, see Jürgen Moltmann, *Theology and Joy*, trans. D. E. Jenkins (London: SCM Press, 1973), p. 67. For more on the somewhat paradoxical character of freedom as binding oneself to God and God's direction, see Jacques Ellul, *The Ethics of Freedom* (Grand Rapids: William B. Eerdmans, 1976), p. 14; and Helmut Thielicke, *The Freedom of the Christian Man* (New York: Harper & Row, 1963), pp. 14-15. As 1 Pet. 2:16 suggests particularly clearly, genuine freedom originates in serving God (cf. Heinrich Schlier, "ἐλεύθερος . . . ," in *Theological Dictionary of the New Testament*, vol. 2, ed. Gerhard Kittel, trans. Geoffrey Bromiley [Grand Rapids: William B. Eerdmans, 1964], p. 500; and Paul Sherer, *The Plight of Freedom* [New York: Harper, 1948], p. 3). God alone is sufficiently powerful to free people from their various bondages (cf. James H. Cone, *A Black Theology of Liberation* [Philadelphia: Lippincott, 1970], p. 209).

13. See Dietrich Bonhoeffer, *Ethics*, ed. Eberhard Bethge, trans. Neville Smith (New York: Macmillan, 1955), pp. 365-72.

14. See John Wesley, "An Israelite Indeed," in *The Works of the Reverend John Wesley*, vol. 2, ed. John Emery (New York: J. Emery and B. Waugh, 1831), p. 277.

15. So Bonhoeffer, *Ethics*, pp. 368-71. Cf. John Murray, *Principles of Conduct* (Philadelphia: Westminster Press, 1957), pp. 145-47, as well as the immediately preceding pages where Murray addresses the biblical events discussed here, among others.

16. Cf. Franklin E. Payne, Jr., *Biblical/Medical Ethics* (Milford, Mich.: Mott Media, 1985), p. 119.

17. Mott, *Biblical Ethics and Social Change* (New York: Oxford University Press, 1982), p. 59 (and see the pages that follow for a perceptive analysis of justice). Cf. Earl E. Shelp, "Justice: A Moral Test for Health Care and Health Policy," in *Justice and Health Care*, ed. Earl Shelp (Boston: D. Reidel, 1981), p. 219.

18. Moreover, those who underestimate the importance of justice thereby indicate that they have failed to understand the essence of people as creations of God whose needs matter greatly to God. See David C. Thomasma, "The Basis of Medicine and Religion: Respect for Persons," in *On Moral Medicine: Theological Perspectives in Medical Ethics*, ed. Stephen Lammers and

Allen Verhey (Grand Rapids: William B. Eerdmans, 1987), p. 291. For the insight that injustice is the context within which justice becomes a significant notion, see Karen Lebacqz, *Foundations of Justice* (Minneapolis: Augsburg Press, 1987), p. 151.

19. On justice as an abstract standard, see Stephen C. Mott, "The Use of the New Testament for Social Ethics," *Journal of Religious Ethics* 15 (Fall 1987): 244-45.

20. The impartiality of God is attested in a number of different contexts, some of which are explicitly justice-related. See Deut. 1:17; Matt. 5:45; Rom. 2:11.

21. Cf. J. Philip Wogaman, "Economics and Medicine: Theological Reflections," *Second Opinion* 8 (July 1988): 72. Furthermore, as Thomas C. Oden has suggested, egalitarian decisions may seem to overlook important considerations in particular instances, but they do so in order to preserve more important values in the long run ("George and Marion: A Theological Brief," in *Christian Theology: A Case Method Approach*, ed. Robert Evans and Thomas Parker [New York: Harper & Row, 1987], p. 59).

22. On the importance of moral imagination, see Arthur F. Holmes, *Shaping Character* (Grand Rapids: William B. Eerdmans, 1991), pp. 42-43.

23. Similarly, although Jesus says we are not to resist an evil person (Matt. 5:39), he did so when he forcibly cleared the Jerusalem temple (Mark 11:15-18). Moreover, he called the Pharisees "fools" (Matt. 23:17) despite his teaching not to call people "fools" (Matt. 5:22 — the same Greek word is used in both verses). For an analysis of how living in a fallen world can necessitate decisions that fall short of what God ultimately wants for the world, see John Piper, *Love Your Enemies* (Cambridge: Cambridge University Press, 1979), pp. 96-99.

24. For different accounts of the guilt involved when making decisions in the face of ethical dilemmas, see Frame, *Medical Ethics*, pp. 9ff.; and Geisler, *Options in Contemporary Christian Ethics*, pp. 99ff.

25. For more on the community orientation of ethics in the Bible, see Bruce C. Birch and Larry L. Rasmussen, *Bible and Ethics in the Christian Life*, rev. ed. (Minneapolis: Augsburg, 1989), chap. 2.

26. For an extended discussion of vision and values in the biblical writings, see Birch and Rasmussen, *Bible and Ethics in the Christian Life*, pp. 47-62.

Chapter 4

1. American Medical Association estimate, reported by Aaron Epstein in "Lawyer Pleads for 'Liberty' of Coma Victim," Lexington *Herald-Leader*, 7 December 1989, pp. 1, 6.

2. Based on an American Medical Association survey of physicians, reported in "'Right-to-Die' Case Reflects Thorny Privacy Issue," *Lexington Herald-Leader,* 25 July 1989, p. 2.

3. Gallup poll conducted for *Hospitals* magazine, reported in "New Poll Shows Americans Prefer Care Withdrawal in Irreversible Coma Cases," *Medical Ethics Advisor* (May 1987).

4. President's Commission for the Study of Ethical Problems in Medicine and Biomedical and Behavioral Research, *Deciding to Forego Life-Sustaining Treatment* (Washington: U.S. Government Printing Office, 1983).

5. E.g., a study by Steven Neu and Carl M. Kjellstrand documents that by 1985, kidney dialysis was already being discontinued in one out of every eleven patients who had begun it ("Stopping Long-Term Dialysis," *New England Journal of Medicine,* 2 January 1986, pp. 14-20). The authors suggest, moreover, that this figure may be understated. For an analysis of why the refusal of available treatment is underreported, see Alonzo L. Plough and Susanne Salem, "Social and Contextual Factors in the Analysis of Mortality in End-Stage Renal Disease Patients: Implications for Health Policy," *American Journal of Public Health* 72 (November 1982): 1293-95.

6. Mervin D. Field, "California Poll: Strong Public Support for the Right to Die," San Francisco *Chronicle,* 21 July 1983, p. 12.

7. For a discussion of a 1986 Gallup poll and 1986 and 1988 Roper polls conducted in California, see Allan Parachini, "The California Humane and Dignified Death Initiative," *Hastings Center Report* 19 (January/February 1989): S11.

8. See Marcia Angell, "Euthanasia," *New England Journal of Medicine,* 17 November 1988, pp. 1348-50; and "The 1988 Roper Poll on Attitudes toward Active Voluntary Euthanasia" (Los Angeles: National Hemlock Society, 1988). In addition, 49 percent of the people sampled in 1989 by the Chicago-based National Opinion Research Center agreed with the statement that people with incurable diseases have the right to end their lives ("View of Suicide as a Right Disturbs Philosophers," *Bulletin of the Park Ridge Center,* September 1990, pp. 6-7). On a related issue, a 1990 New York *Times*/CBS News poll of 573 persons found that 53 percent agreed that physicians should be allowed to help patients take their own lives. A Roper poll that same year put the figure at 64 percent. On these and other polls, see *Active Euthanasia, Religion, and the Public Debate* (Chicago: Park Ridge Center, 1991), pp. 31-32.

9. See, for example, the apparently real case reported in the *Journal of the American Medical Association,* "It's Over, Debbie" (8 January 1988, p. 272), and the subsequent letters to the editor published in the journal (8 April 1988, pp. 2094-98; 12 August 1988, pp. 787-89). For an actual case more recently reported in the *New England Journal of Medicine,* see Timothy E. Quill, "Death and Dignity — A Case of Individualized Decision-Making," *New England Journal of Medicine,* 7 March 1991, pp. 691-94, and subsequent letters to the

editor (29 August 1991, pp. 658-60). Regarding suicide devices, see "Suicide Device for Terminally Ill Raises Legal, Ethical Concerns," Lexington *Herald-Leader,* 29 October 1989, p. E6; and Isabel Wilkerson, "Rage and Support for Doctor's Role in Suicide," New York *Times,* 25 October 1991, p. A1.

10. Sidney H. Wanzer et al., "The Physician's Responsibility toward Hopelessly Ill Patients: A Second Look," *New England Journal of Medicine,* 30 March 1989, pp. 844-49; and Daniel Q. Haney, "Panel Backs Doctors' Aiding in Suicides of Terminally Ill," Lexington *Herald-Leader,* 30 March 1989, pp. 1, 5.

11. Courtney S. Campbell and Bette-Jane Crigger, "Mercy, Murder, and Morality," *Hastings Center Report* 19 (January/February 1989): S1; Parachini, "The California Humane and Dignified Death Initiative," S12.

12. See Stanley J. Reiser, "The Dilemma of Euthanasia in Modern Medical History," in *The Dilemma of Euthanasia,* ed. A. Behnke and S. Bok (New York: Anchor Books, 1975); and Leo Alexander, "Medical Science under Dictatorship," *New England Journal of Medicine,* 14 July 1949, pp. 39-47.

13. See Angell, "Euthanasia," p. 1349; and Gregory E. Pence, "Do Not Go Slowly into That Dark Night: Mercy Killing in Holland," *American Journal of Medicine* 84 (January 1988): 139. Regarding a national opinion poll conducted in September 1989, see Henk Rigter, "Mercy, Murder, and Morality," *Hastings Center Report* 19 (November/December 1989): 52.

14. For estimates and studies, see Paul J. Van der Maas et al., "Euthanasia and Other Medical Decisions concerning the End of Life," *Lancet,* 14 September 1991, pp. 673; Carlos F. Gomez, *Regulating Death: The Case of the Netherlands* (New York: Free Press, 1991); Henk A. M. J. Ten Have, "Euthanasia in the Netherlands: The Legal Context and the Cases," *HEC Forum* 1 (1989): 41; M. A. M. De Wachter, "Active Euthanasia in the Netherlands," *Journal of the American Medical Association,* 15 December 1989, pp. 3316-19; Eben Alexander, "Euthanasia," *Surgical Neurology* 31 (June 1989): 480; Angell, "Euthanasia," p. 1349; and Henk Rigter, "Euthanasia in the Netherlands: Distinguishing Facts from Fiction," *Hastings Center Report* 19 (January/February 1989): 32. These numbers include an estimated 11 percent of patients with AIDS; see Richard Fenigsen, "A Case against Dutch Euthanasia," *Hastings Center Report* 19 (January/February 1989): 522. On the Dutch Medical Association guidelines, see Central Committee of the Royal Dutch Medical Association, "Vision on Euthanasia," *Medisch Contact* 39 (1984): 990-98; Angell, "Euthanasia," p. 1349.

15. "Final Report of the Netherlands State Commission on Euthanasia: An English Summary," *Bioethics* 1 (1987): 163-74; Pence, "Do Not Go Slowly into That Dark Night," p. 140; Angell, "Euthanasia," p. 1349.

16. This total is the sum of figures in four subcategories: direct killing of patients (2,300 cases), physician-assisted suicide (400 cases), provision of morphine in excessive doses with an intent to end life (3,159 cases), and the removal or withholding of life-prolonging treatment with an intent to end

life (4,756 cases). See Richard Fenigsen, "The Report of the Dutch Governmental Committee on Euthanasia," *Issues in Law and Medicine* 7 (Winter 1991): 339-44.

17. The total of 14,691 cases is the sum of figures in three subcategories: direct killing of patients (1,000 cases), provision of morphine in excessive doses with an intent to end life (4,941 cases), and the removal or withholding of life-prolonging treatment with an intent to end life (8,750 cases). In the 1,000 cases of direct killing, 14 percent of the patients had complete mental capability and 11 percent had partial mental capability. In the 4,941 cases in which excessive amounts of morphine were administered, 27 percent of the patients had complete mental capability. See Fenigsen, "The Report of the Dutch Governmental Committee on Euthanasia."

18. See F. C. B. Van Wijmen, *Artsen en zelfgekozen levenseinde* (Maastricht: Vakgroep Gezondheidsrecht Rijksuniversiteit Limburg, 1989), p. 24; H. W. A. Hilhorst, *Euthanasia in het ziekenhuis* (Lochem-Poperinge: De Tijdstroom, 1983), pp. 174-80; Fenigsen, "A Case against Dutch Euthanasia," p. 50; Michael Fumento, "The Dying Dutchman: Coming Soon to a Nursing Home Near You," *American Spectator*, October 1991, pp. 18-22.

19. Royal Dutch Society of Medicine, "Reactie op vragen Staatscommissee Euthanasie," *Medisch Contact* 31 (1984): 999-1002; Fenigsen, "A Case against Dutch Euthanasia," p. 50.

20. C. I. Dessaur and C. J. C. Rutenfrans, "Mag de dokter doden?" (Amsterdam: Querido, 1986); Fenigsen, "A Case against Dutch Euthanasia," p. 51.

21. See Rigter, "Euthanasia in the Netherlands," S32.

22. See H. J. J. Leenen, "The Definition of Euthanasia," *Medicine and Law* 3 (1984): 333-38; John M. Frame, *Medical Ethics: Principles, Persons, and Problems* (Grand Rapids: Baker Book House, 1988), p. 68.

23. See J. Robert Nelson, "Live and Let Live . . . and Die When You Must," *Perkins Journal* 39 (January 1986): 7; and Thomas C. Oden, *Should Treatment Be Terminated?* (New York: Harper & Row, 1976), p. 19.

24. For a more detailed account of a larger number of models, see William F. May, *The Physician's Covenant* (Philadelphia: Westminster Press, 1983).

25. See J. Grimley Evans, "Age and Equality," *Annals of the New York Academy of Sciences* 530 (1988): 119; U.S. Congress Office of Technology Assessment, *Life-Sustaining Technologies and the Elderly*, OTA-BA-306 (Washington: U.S. Government Printing Office, 1987), pp. 261-62; Carol E. Ferrans, "Quality of Life as a Criterion for Allocation of Life-Sustaining Treatment: The Case of Hemodialysis," in *Health Care Ethics*, ed. Gary Anderson and Valerie Glesnes-Anderson (Rockville, Md.: Aspen, 1987), p. 120; William M. Sage et al., "Intensive Care for the Elderly: Outcome of Elective and Nonelective Admissions," *Journal of the American Geriatrics Society* 35 (April 1987): 316; *National*

Kidney Dialysis and Kidney Transplantation Study (Seattle: Battelle Human Affairs Research Centers, 1986), chap. 6, pp. 25-27; T. Jolene Starr et al., "Quality of Life and Rescuscitation Decisions in Elderly Patients," *Journal of General Internal Medicine* 1 (November-December 1986): 373-79; Steven Neu and Carl M. Kjellstrand, "Stopping Long-Term Dialysis," *New England Journal of Medicine,* 2 January 1986, p. 18; Roger W. Evans et al., "The Quality of Life of Patients with End-Stage Renal Disease," *New England Journal of Medicine,* 28 February 1985, pp. 557-58; and Robert A. Pearlman and Albert R. Jonsen, "The Use of Quality-of-Life Considerations in Medical Decision Making," *Journal of the American Geriatrics Society* 33 (May 1985): 349.

26. See John F. Kilner, "Selecting Patients When Resources Are Limited: A Study of U.S. Medical Directors of Kidney Dialysis and Transplantation Facilities," *American Journal of Public Health* 78 (February 1988): 145; Claudia J. Coulton, "Resource Limits and Allocation in Critical Care," in *Human Values in Critical Care Medicine,* ed. Stuart J. Youngner (New York: Praeger, 1986), p. 97; George J. Annas, "The Prostitute, the Playboy, and the Poet: Rationing Schemes for Organ Transplantation," *American Journal of Public Health* 75 (February 1985): 189; Massachusetts Task Force on Organ Transplantation, *Report* (Boston: Boston University Schools of Public Health and Medicine, October 1984), p. 83; Terrie Wetle and Sue E. Levkoff, "Attitudes and Behaviors of Service Providers toward Elder Patients in the VA System," in *Older Veterans: Linking VA and Community Resources,* ed. Terrie Wetle and John Rowe (Cambridge: Harvard University Press, 1984), p. 224; and *National Heart Transplantation Study* (Seattle: Battelle Human Affairs Research Centers, 1984), chap. 8, pp. 30-31.

27. See *Guidelines on the Termination of Life-Sustaining Treatment and the Care of the Dying* (Briarcliff Manor, N.Y.: Hastings Center, 1987), p. 23.

28. Office of Technology Assessment, *Life-Sustaining Technologies and the Elderly,* p. 22.

29. This point will be discussed at greater length in Chapter 5. See also Richard J. Mouw, "Biblical Revelation and Medical Decisions," in *On Moral Medicine: Theological Perspectives in Medical Ethics,* ed. Stephen Lammers and Allen Verhey (Grand Rapids: William B. Eerdmans, 1987), pp. 62-63.

30. Office of Technology Assessment, *Life-Sustaining Technologies and the Elderly,* p. 24.

31. Versions of these two documents can be found in the fall 1985 edition of the *Journal of Christian Nursing.* For other explicitly Christian discussions, see Jean De Blois et al., "Advance Directives for Healthcare Decisions," *Health Progress* (July-August 1991): 27-31; and James F. Bresnahan, "Catholic Spirituality and Medical Interventions in Dying," *America,* 29 June 1991, pp. 670-75.

32. See Charles Green, "Government Might Step into Fray, Push 'Living Wills,'" Lexington *Herald-Leader,* 12 January 1990, p. A2; Jane E. Brody, "Living

Will Lets Individual Dictate Terminally Ill Treatment," Lexington *Herald-Leader*, 7 October 1989, p. C4; and "New Poll Shows Americans Prefer Care Withdrawal in Irreversible Coma Cases," *Medical Ethics Advisor* (May 1987).

33. See Allan S. Brett, "Limitations of Listing Specific Medical Interventions in Advance Directives," *Journal of the American Medical Association*, 14 August 1991, pp. 825-28; Kevin D. O'Rourke and Dennis Brodeur, *Medical Ethics: Common Ground for Understanding*, vol. 2. (St. Louis: Catholic Health Association of the U.S., 1989), pp. 202-3; Frame, *Medical Ethics*, p. 71; Ed Larson and Beth Spring, "Life-Defying Acts: Do Modern Medical Technologies Sustain Life or Merely Prolong Dying?" *Christianity Today*, 6 March 1987, p. 21; Franklin E. Payne, Jr., *Biblical/Medical Ethics* (Milford, Mich.: Mott Media, 1985), pp. 200-201; and Oden, *Should Treatment Be Terminated?* pp. 16-17. For a study documenting the incomplete knowledge of physicians (and, indirectly, patients) concerning living wills, see David J. Doukas et al., "The Living Will: A National Survey," *Family Medicine* 23 (July 1991): 354-56.

34. Linda L. Emanuel and Ezekiel J. Emanuel, "The Medical Directive: A New Comprehensive Advance Care Document," *Journal of the American Medical Association*, 9 June 1989, pp. 3288-93.

35. Cf. George J. Annas, "The Health Care Proxy and the Living Will," *New England Journal of Medicine*, 25 April 1991, p. 1212. On the reasons people resist signing donor cards, see *Organ Transplantation: Issues and Recommendations* (Rockville, Md.: U.S. Department of Health and Human Services, 1986), p. 38.

36. Copies can be obtained from the American Medical Association, 515 North State Street, Chicago, Illinois 60610.

37. Ashwin Sehgal et al., "How Strictly Do Dialysis Patients Want Their Advance Directives Followed?" *Journal of the American Medical Association*, 1 January 1992, pp. 59-63; Carl M. Kjellstrand, "Who Should Decide about Your Death?" *Journal of the American Medical Association*, 1 January 1992, pp. 103-4.

38. For examples of this approach, see David J. Doukas and Laurence B. McCullough, "The Values History: The Evaluation of the Patient's Values and Advance Directives," *Journal of Family Practice* 32 (1991): 145-53; and P. Lambert et al., "The Values History: An Innovation in Surrogate Medical Decision-Making," *Law, Medicine and Health Care* 18 (Fall 1990): 202-12.

39. See, e.g., SRI Gallup poll data reported in "New Poll Shows Americans Prefer Care Withdrawal in Irreversible Coma Cases."

40. For discussions of the Act, see John Miles, "Protecting Patient Self-Determination," *Health Progress*, April 1991, pp. 26-30; Elizabeth L. McCloskey, "The Patient Self-Determination Act," *Kennedy Institute of Ethics Journal* 1 (June 1991): 163-69; John La Puma et al., "Advance Directives on Admission," *Journal of the American Medical Association*, 17 July 1991, pp. 402-5; and Margot L. White and John C. Fletcher, "The Patient Self-Determination Act," *Journal of the American Medical Association*, 17 July 1991, pp. 410-12.

41. Family language is commonly used within the body of Christ (e.g., in Acts 1:16; Rom. 1:13; 1 Cor. 1:10). Cf. Frame, *Medical Ethics*, pp. 38-39. In fact, the church itself is referred to as the family of believers (Gal. 6:10).

42. As Jesus put it, "whoever does the will of my Father in heaven is my brother and sister and mother" (Matt. 12:50). In Jesus' day, as today, people sometimes had to leave their human families in order to live a life of faithfulness to God; however, God provides a much larger family in Christ (Mark 10:29-30).

43. While I am implicitly speaking about adult patients in most of the discussions throughout this book, much of this material applies to infants and other children as well as it does to adults whose decision-making capacity is limited or nonexistent. While children are different from adults in certain ways, these differences can easily be overemphasized in a culture that devalues the elderly and exalts youth, as explained in Chapters 8 and 9.

Chapter 5

1. Regarding the medical resident's actions to end the life of a cancer patient, see "It's Over, Debbie," *Journal of the American Medical Association*, 8 January 1988, p. 272, and associated letters to the editor published in the journal (8 April 1988, pp. 2094-98; 12 August 1988, pp. 787-89); see also Kenneth L. Vaux, "Debbie's Dying: Euthanasia Reconsidered," *Christian Century*, 16 March 1988, pp. 269-71; and "The Theologic Ethics of Euthanasia," *Hastings Center Report* 19 (January/February 1989): 19-22. Regarding the actions of Dr. Kevorkian, see "Suicide Device for Terminally Ill Raises Legal, Ethical Concerns," Lexington *Herald-Leader*, 29 October 1989, p. E6; Isabel Wilkerson, "Rage and Support for Doctor's Role in Suicide," New York *Times*, 25 October 1991, p. A1; and Kevorkian, *Prescription: Medicide* (Buffalo: Prometheus Books, 1991). Regarding the how-to book on suicide, see Derek Humphrey, *Final Exit* (Eugene, Or.: Hemlock Society, 1991); and Katrine Ames et al., "Last Rights," *Newsweek*, 26 August 1991, pp. 40-41. On Dr. Quill's action, see Timothy E. Quill, "Death and Dignity — A Case of Individualized Decision-Making," *New England Journal of Medicine*, 7 March 1991, pp. 691-94, and associated letters to the editor (29 August 1991, pp. 658-60). Regarding Washington state legislative initiative, see Robert I. Misbin, "Physicians' Aid in Dying," *New England Journal of Medicine*, 31 October 1991, pp. 1307-11; and Peter Steinfels, "Beliefs: In Cold Print, the Euthanasia Issue Can Take on Many Shades of Color," New York *Times*, 9 November 1991, p. A8.

2. Kenneth L. Vaux, "Theological Foundations of Medical Ethics," in *Health/Medicine and the Faith Traditions*, ed. Martin Marty and Kenneth Vaux (Philadelphia: Fortress Press, 1982), p. 220.

3. For example, see Paul D. Simmons, *Birth and Death: Bioethical Decision-Making* (Philadelphia: Westminster Press, 1983), pp. 138-39; Dale Moody, *The Word of Truth* (Grand Rapids: William B. Eerdmans, 1981), p. 295; Reinhold Niebuhr, *The Nature and Destiny of Man*, vol. 1 (New York: Scribner's, 1941), pp. 173-76; and Leon R. Kass, "Averting One's Eyes, or Facing the Music? — On Dignity and Death," in *Death Inside Out*, ed. Peter Steinfels and Robert Veatch (New York: Harper & Row, 1974), p. 113.

4. See Lloyd R. Bailey, Sr., *Biblical Perspectives on Death* (Philadelphia: Fortress Press, 1979), p. 38; and E. Brooks Holifield, *Health and Medicine in the Methodist Tradition* (New York: Crossroad, 1986), p. 96. Paul Ramsey affirms this biblical/historical perspective ("The Indignity of 'Death with Dignity,'" in *Death Inside Out*, pp. 81-96), and Robert S. Morison ("The Dignity of the Inevitable and Necessary," in Death inside Out, pp. 97-100) as well as H. Tristram Engelhardt, Jr. ("The Counsels of Finitude," in *Death Inside Out*, pp. 115-25), admits that Ramsey is in line with Christian tradition. Kass prefers to see this view as one of multiple Christian options, citing Thomas Aquinas and Reinhold Niebuhr in support ("Averting One's Eyes, or Facing the Music?" p. 113). While Niebuhr himself rejects the idea, he does acknowledge that the belief that physical death is the result of human disobedience "remains a consistent doctrine of Christian orthodoxy" and even includes Aquinas as part of this tradition (*The Nature and Destiny of Man*, p. 176).

5. That God intended for people to experience unending life does not imply that people were intended to have physical or nonphysical life independent of the daily sustaining provision of God. See Bailey, *Biblical Perspectives on Death*, pp. 36-38; and Norman Anderson, *Issues of Life and Death* (Downers Grove, Ill.: InterVarsity Press, 1976), p. 28.

6. See, e.g., Simmons, *Birth and Death*, pp. 142-44.

7. For more on this, see Larry Richards and Paul Johnson, *Death and the Caring Community* (Portland: Multnomah Press, 1980), p. 31; Ramsey, "The Indignity of 'Death with Dignity,'" pp. 82, 90; and Paul Tournier, *A Doctor's Casebook in the Light of the Bible*, trans. Edwin Hudson (New York: Harper & Row, 1960), pp. 165-67. On similar grounds, Franklin E. Payne, Jr., objects to the contention of Elisabeth Kübler-Ross that death should be completely accepted, as if it were in no sense an enemy (*Biblical/Medical Ethics* [Milford, Mich.: Mott Media, 1985], p. 183).

8. For further development of these contrasts, see Harold O. J. Brown, "Why Will Ye Die, O House of Israel?" in *The Death Decision*, ed. Leonard J. Nelson (Ann Arbor: Servant Publications, 1984), p. 108; Holifield, *Health and Medicine in the Methodist Tradition*, p. 99; and Daniel B. McGee, "Issues of Life and Death," in *Understanding Christian Ethics*, ed. William Tillman, Jr. (Nashville: Broadman Press, 1988), p. 238. Bonnie J. Miller-McLemore makes a distinction between natural and unnatural death (see *Death, Sin and the Moral Life* [Atlanta: Scholars Press, 1988], pp. 176-77) which can be helpful in this

context so long as "natural" is clearly defined as that which people typically experience as opposed to that which God originally intended.

9. For related reflections, see Martin E. Marty, "The Tradition of the Church in Health and Healing," *Second Opinion* 13 (March 1990): 69; Donald F. Duclow, "Into the Whirlwind of Suffering: Resistance and Transformation," *Second Opinion* 9 (November 1988): 10-27; and especially Stanley Hauerwas, *Naming the Silences* (Grand Rapids: William B. Eerdmans, 1990), pp. 73-74. Hauerwas is suspicious of attempts to "explain" suffering on the grounds that such explanations provide little understanding or comfort for those struggling with a particular instance of suffering. In other words, "Why suffering?" is a very different question from "Why me?"

10. Cf. Thomas C. Oden, *Should Treatment Be Terminated?* (New York: Harper & Row, 1976), pp. 71-83.

11. Jesus' paradoxical statement about how to gain life receives an emphasis in the Gospels unlike any other statement. It appears in all four Gospels and in two of them more than once (Matt. 10:38-39; 16:24-25; Mark 8:34-35; Luke 9:23-24; 14:26-27; 17:33; John 12:25). This paradox is at the heart of obtaining much that is valuable in life. We can seldom obtain the most deeply satisfying benefits for ourselves by seeking them directly for their own sake.

12. For a sweeping statement about God's working for human good in every circumstance of life, see Rom. 8:28. See 1 Pet. 1 for the added perspective that when suffering demonstrates that faith in God is genuine, the result is "praise, glory, and honor" to God (v. 7).

13. For illustrations of the divine and communal value of suffering, see Thomas C. Oden, "George and Marion: A Theological Brief," in *Christian Theology: A Case Method Approach,* ed. Robert Evans and Thomas Parker (New York: Harper & Row, 1976), p. 102; and C. Donald Cole, *Christian Perspectives on Controversial Issues* (Chicago: Moody Press, 1982), p. 105. For a related critique of the selfishness of an exclusive focus on one's own happiness when making end-of-life decisions, see Miller-McLemore, *Death, Sin and the Moral Life,* p. 3.

14. For a critique of the attempt to justify suffering as (merely) an occasion to grow, see Stanley Hauerwas, *Suffering Presence* (Notre Dame, Ind.: University of Notre Dame Press, 1986), p. 26.

15. Consider, for example, God's identification with the needy in Matt. 25:31-46, an idea suggested in the Old Testament as well (Prov. 14:31; 19:17; cf. Jer. 22:15-16).

16. Jesus Christ paved the way and set the example (Heb. 12:2; cf. 11:26 regarding Moses); people experience God's gift of maturity and character in the midst of suffering (Rom. 5:3-5; James 1:2-4); and faithful suffering will bring its future reward (Matt. 5:10-12; Rom. 8:18; James 1:12; 1 Pet. 5:10). In a sense people can already participate in the future reward — in its joy —

because God's rule is already a reality even though it will not be fully evident until later. In the biblical writings, suffering and hope are held together — see J. Christiaan Beker, *Suffering and Hope* (Philadelphia: Fortress Press, 1987), p. 85; and Robert D. Orr et al., *Life and Death Decisions* (Colorado Springs: NavPress, 1990), p. 165.

17. Paul's example is instructive here. His life was full of suffering, humanly speaking (Phil. 1:13-17; cf. 2 Cor. 11:24-33), such that he thought it would have been better for him personally to die and be with Christ in a way not possible until after death (Phil. 1:23). Nevertheless, for the sake of others who would benefit from his continued living, he was willing to continue (Phil. 1:24-26).

18. See also Hauerwas, *Suffering Presence*, p. 24; and Oden, *Should Treatment Be Terminated?* p. 74. These observations help to explain the discomfort many experience reading Joseph Bayly's novel *Winterflight* (Word Books, 1981). The book portrays a future United States in which "active euthanasia" at age 75 is mandatory and is carried out in the very pleasant surroundings of "thanotels." The scenario is unsettling not simply because some are killed against their will. Even with regard to the many who willingly submit, there is something chilling about seeing relief of suffering placed in the service of death. This perspective explains, in part, David's hostile reception of the man who claims to have spared King Saul a painful and shameful death by killing him (2 Sam. 1:1-16). The man explains that Saul was badly wounded and suffering, and that Saul had asked the man to kill him in order to spare him from the agonizing death that lay ahead (v. 9; cf. 1 Sam. 31:4). Regardless of these circumstances, David considers killing Saul an outrageous murder and orders the man killed on the spot. Admittedly, Saul was special in David's eyes because he was "the Lord's anointed" (v. 16). However, that fact only intensifies the point: when precious lives are at stake, sparing people from the agony and shame of an extended dying process by killing them does not diminish the evil but multiplies it.

19. For a related discussion of aims vs. motivations, including a discussion of the fundamental moral difference between martyrdom and a patient choosing death, see Gilbert Meilaender, "Euthanasia and Christian Vision," in *On Moral Medicine: Theological Perspectives in Medical Ethics*, ed. Stephen Lammers and Allen Verhey (Grand Rapids: William B. Eerdmans, 1987), pp. 456-59.

20. As we have already noted, no one is truly innocent and undeserving of death. However, some engage in unjust aggression or commit serious crimes that make them morally culpable to a degree that others are not. Whether or not such culpability warrants killing them is an important issue, but it lies beyond the scope of this book.

21. As Richard A. McCormick has observed, where autonomy is emphasized, people become intolerant of dependence and cut themselves off

from the sustaining power of God and others ("Physician-Assisted Suicide: Flight from Compassion," *Christian Century,* 4 December 1991, pp. 1132-33). For more reflections on the "right to die," see J. Kerby Anderson, "Euthanasia: A Biblical Appraisal," *Bibliotheca Sacra* 144 (April-June 1987): 216; Payne, *Biblical/Medical Ethics,* p. 202; and Cole, *Christian Perspectives on Controversial Issues,* p. 106. James J. McCartney has noted the reluctance of most Christians to speak of a right to die because they view death as a negativity rather than as something that one has a right to ("The Right to Die: Perspectives from the Catholic and Jewish Traditions," in *To Die or Not to Die,* ed. Arthur Berger and Joyce Berger [New York: Praeger, 1990], p. 14).

22. Cf. Ramsey, "The Indignity of 'Death with Dignity' "; Oden, *Should Treatment Be Terminated?* pp. 71, 88; and Richard A. McCormick, "George and Marion: A Theological Brief," in Robert Evans and Thomas Parker, *Christian Theology: A Case Method Approach* (New York: Harper & Row, 1976), pp. 90-91. Part of the tragedy of severe illness and the way people are sometimes treated in such situations stems from the fact that they are not always made aware of all of the treatment alternatives that are available to them. However, whatever else a good response to suffering may include, it cannot include intending death, according to the described perspective.

23. For an analysis of the oath from a Christian perspective that finds this commitment to be common ground between them, see Allen Verhey, "The Doctor's Oath — and a Christian Swearing It," in *On Moral Medicine: Theological Perspectives in Medical Ethics,* ed. Stephen Lammers and Allen Verhey (Grand Rapids: William B. Eerdmans, 1987), pp. 72-82.

24. Leon R. Kass makes some interesting points along these lines in "Neither for Love nor Money: Why Doctors Should Not Kill," a paper presented at the annual meeting of the American Association of Medical Colleges, Chicago, Illinois, 13 November 1988. For more on this issue, see Willard Gaylin et al., " 'Doctors Must Not Kill,' " *Journal of the American Medical Association,* 8 April 1988, pp. 2139-40; Albert R. Jonsen et al., *Clinical Ethics* (New York: Macmillan, 1988), pp. 126-27; Richard M. Gula, *What Are They Saying about Euthanasia?* (New York: Paulist Press, 1986), p. 71; Robert Twycross, "Decisions about Death and Dying," in *Decision Making in Medicine: The Practice of Its Ethics,* ed. Gordon Scorer and Antony Wing (London: Edward Arnold, 1979), p. 108; Norman Anderson, *Issues of Life and Death* (Downers Grove, Ill.: InterVarsity, 1976), p. 96; and G. R. Dunstan, *The Artifice of Ethics* (London: SCM Press, 1974), p. 92.

25. See Hauerwas, *Suffering Presence,* p. 36.

26. See George L. Chalmers, "Life Issues: Euthanasia," in *Medicine in Crisis: A Christian Response,* ed. Ian Brown and Nigel Cameron (Edinburgh: Rutherford House, 1988), pp. 114-15; Twycross, "Decisions about Death and Dying," p. 107; Francis A. Schaeffer and C. Everett Koop, *Whatever Happened to the Human Race?* (Old Tappan, NJ: Fleming H. Revell, 1979), p. 99; and

Benedict M. Ashley and Kevin D. O'Rourke, *Health Care Ethics: A Theological Analysis,* 3d ed. (St. Louis: Catholic Hospital Association, 1989), §13.6.

27. See Richard John Neuhaus, "The Way They Were, the Way We Are: Bioethics and the Holocaust," *First Things* (March 1990): 31-37; David C. Thomasma and Glenn C. Graber, *Euthanasia: Toward an Ethical Social Policy* (New York: Continuum, 1990), pp. 175-78; John J. Davis, "Brophy vs. New England Sinai Hospital," *Journal of Biblical Ethics in Medicine* 1 (July 1987): 53-56; Harold O. J. Brown, "Euthanasia: Lessons from Nazism," *Human Life Review* 13 (Spring 1987): 88-99; Payne, *Biblical/Medical Ethics,* p. 201; William Brennan, *Medical Holocausts I: Exterminative Medicine in Nazi Germany and Contemporary America* (Boston: Nordland, 1980), pp. 80ff.; Schaeffer and Koop, *Whatever Happened to the Human Race?* pp. 102ff.; Oden, *Should Treatment Be Terminated?* p. 62; Paul Ramsey, *The Patient as Person* (New Haven: Yale University Press, 1970), p. 164; and Leo Alexander, "Medical Science under Dictatorship," *New England Journal of Medicine,* 14 July 1949, pp. 39-47.

28. For more evidence specifically in the context of ending patients' lives, see sources in note 27 as well as DebbieLynne Simmons, "Created for Life," *The Plough,* March-April 1985, p. 13.

29. See J. Robert Nelson, "The Question of Euthanasia," *Engage/Social Action* 4 (April 1976): 30.

30. Cf. Richard Stith, "Toward Freedom from Value," in *On Moral Medicine: Theological Perspectives in Medical Ethics,* ed. Stephen Lammers and Allen Verhey (Grand Rapids: William B. Eerdmans, 1987), pp. 127-43. There are pragmatic difficulties associated with attempts to place a value on life as well, such as the difficulty of comparing very precisely the negative value of killing with that of continued suffering. See Arthur J. Dyck, *On Human Care* (Nashville: Abingdon Press, 1977), p. 88.

31. Cf. Guy I. Benrubi, "Euthanasia — The Need for Procedural Safeguards," *New England Journal of Medicine,* 16 January 1992, pp. 197-98; and Vaux, "The Theologic Ethics of Euthanasia." The harmful influence of society, however, justifies efforts to prevent that harm or to provide constructive recompense — not the compounding of that harm by fostering death.

Chapter 6

1. On Cruzan, see Larry Gostin and Robert F. Weir, "Life and Death Choices after *Cruzan:* Case Law and Standards of Professional Conduct," *Milbank Quarterly* 69 (1991): 143-73; and "A Time to Die: The Cases of Nancy Cruzan and Janet Adkins," *Bulletin of the Park Ridge Center* 5 (September 1990): 16-31. See also the entire Spring-Summer 1991 issue of *Law, Medicine and Health Care.* On Wanglie, see Ronald E. Cranford et al., "Helga Wanglie's Ventilator," *Hastings Center Report* 21 (July-August 1991): 23-29; and Lisa

Belkin, "Patient's Death Sought against Family's Wishes," Lexington *Herald-Leader,* 11 January 1991, pp. A3, 7.

2. The potential moral similarity between so-called active and passive euthanasia is most often pressed by those intending to justify some instances of active euthanasia. However, the implications of the similarity run the other way as well. Some decisions to act are indeed morally similar to some decisions not to act. When death is intended, though, both types of decision run contrary to a God-centered, reality-bounded, love-impelled approach.

3. For some classical treatments of the moral problems associated with suicide, see Augustine, *The City of God,* bk. 1; Aquinas, *Summa Theologica,* IIaIIae, q.64; and Dietrich Bonhoeffer, *Ethics,* ed. Eberhard Bethge, trans. Neville Smith (New York: Macmillan, 1955), chap. 4. And for elaborations of these arguments, see Gilbert Meilaender, "Euthanasia and Christian Vision," in *On Moral Medicine: Theological Perspectives in Medical Ethics,* ed. Stephen Lammers and Allen Verhey (Grand Rapids: William B. Eerdmans, 1987), p. 455; Germain Grisez and Joseph M. Boyle, Jr., "The Morality of Killing: A Traditional View," in *Bioethics: Reading and Cases,* ed. Baruch Brody and H. Tristram Engelhardt, Jr. (Englewood Cliffs, N.J.: Prentice-Hall, 1987), p. 157; Joseph L. Lombardi, "Suicide and the Service of God," *Ethics* 95 (October 1984): 65-67; Benedict M. Ashley and Kevin D. O'Rourke, *Health Care Ethics: A Theological Analysis,* 3d ed. (St. Louis: Catholic Hospital Association, 1989), pp. 374-80; Sidney Callahan, "The Limits on Self-Destruction," *Health Progress* 73 (April 1992): 72-73; Thomas C. Oden, "George and Marion: A Theological Brief," in *Christian Theology: A Case Method Approach,* ed. Robert Evans and Thomas Parker (New York: Harper & Row, 1976), p. 100; and Thomas C. Oden, *Should Treatment Be Terminated?* (New York: Harper & Row, 1976), p. 32.

4. For additional justifications of suicide, particularly those addressing dignified dying and the questionable origins of Christian prohibitions against suicide, see Paul D. Simmons, *Birth and Death: Bioethical Decision-Making* (Philadelphia: Westminster Press, 1983), p. 154; and Kenneth Boyd, "Terminal Care, Euthanasia and Suicide," *Modern Churchmen* 30 (1988): 13. Cf. Margaret P. Battin, *Ethical Issues in Suicide* (Englewood Cliffs, N.J.: Prentice-Hall, 1982). For expanded refutations of these arguments, see Bonhoeffer, *Ethics,* p. 170; Richard M. Gula, *What Are They Saying about Euthanasia?* (New York: Paulist Press, 1986), p. 100; Stanley Hauerwas, "Rational Suicide and Reasons for Living," in *On Moral Medicine: Theological Perspectives in Medical Ethics,* ed. Stephen Lammers and Allen Verhey (Grand Rapids: William B. Eerdmans, 1987), p. 462; Ashley and O'Rourke, *Health Care Ethics,* pp. 374ff.; and Robert N. Wennberg, *Terminal Choices* (Grand Rapids: William B. Eerdmans, 1989), pp. 81-82.

5. E.g., the deaths of Saul and his armor-bearer (1 Sam. 31), Ahithophel (2 Sam. 17), Zimri (1 Kings 16), Samson (Judg. 16), and Judas (Matt. 27); cf.

Abimelech (Judg. 9). For an analysis of these suicides, see James T. Clemons, *What Does the Bible Say about Suicide?* (Minneapolis: Fortress Press, 1990); Niceto Blazquez, "The Church's Traditional Moral Teaching on Suicide," in *Suicide and the Right to Die,* ed. Jacques Pohier and Dietmer Mieth (Edinburgh: T. & T. Clark, 1985), pp. 63-74. On the death of Jesus, see Harry Kuitert, "Have Christians the Right to Kill Themselves? From Self-Murder to Self-Killing," in *Suicide and the Right to Die,* pp. 100-106.

6. For assessments of the pragmatic drawbacks of quality-of-life thinking, see John R. Connery, "Quality of Life," *Linacre Quarterly* 53 (February 1986): 32; Simmons, *Birth and Death,* p. 123; and Richard A. McCormick, "George and Marion: A Theological Brief," in *Christian Theology: A Case Method Approach,* ed. Robert Evans and Thomas Parker (New York: Harper & Row, 1976), p. 91.

7. A broad range of people have suggested that a permanent loss of consciousness — especially self-consciousness — signals death. See, for example, Helmut Thielicke, "The Doctor as Judge of Who Shall Live and Who Shall Die," in *Who Shall Live?* ed. Kenneth Vaux (Philadelphia: Fortress Press, 1970), p. 162; Norman Anderson, *Issues of Life and Death* (Downers Grove, Ill.: InterVarsity Press, 1976), p. 102; Stanley Hauerwas, "Religious Concepts of Brain Death and Associated Problems," in *Brain Death,* ed. Julius Korein (New York: New York Academy of Sciences, 1978), pp. 329-38; Karen G. Gervais, *Redefining Death* (New Haven: Yale University Press, 1986); Robert M. Veatch, *Death, Dying, and the Biological Revolution,* rev. ed. (New Haven: Yale University Press, 1988); *Death: Beyond Whole-Brain Criteria,* ed. Richard M. Zaner, Hingham, Mass.: Kluwer, 1989); Tony Campolo, *Twenty Hot Potatoes Christians Are Afraid to Touch* (Dallas: Word Books, 1988), pp. 143-47; and Daniel Wikler, "Not Dead, Not Dying? Ethical Categories and Persistent Vegetative State," *Hastings Center Report* 18 (February/March 1988): 41-47. While this criterion for death is conceptually attractive, its usefulness hinges on the possibility of knowing for sure whether or not a patient's loss of consciousness is truly irreversible. On the inconclusiveness of the biblical materials with respect to this issue, see Simmons, *Birth and Death,* p. 132; and John M. Frame, *Medical Ethics: Principles, Persons, and Problems* (Grand Rapids: Baker Book House, 1988), p. 58.

8. John J. Cobb has argued that many people understand a person classified as a "vegetable" to be less than fully human and, "in the interests of society," are more likely to protect the dignity of someone else they consider fully human (*Matters of Life and Death* [Louisville: Westminster/John Knox, 1991], p. 66).

9. For examples of such cases in Minnesota and New Mexico, see Ronald E. Cranford, "The Persistent Vegetative State: The Medical Reality (Getting the Facts Straight)," *Hastings Center Report* 18 (February/March 1988): 29-30. For other accounts and cases, see Keith Andrews, "Persistent Vegetative State," *British Medical Journal* 303 (July 1991): 121; David S. Short,

"The Persistent Vegetative State," *Ethics and Medicine* 7 (Autumn 1991): 39; "Dental Drug 'Awakens' Man in Vegetative State," Lexington *Herald-Leader,* 29 March 1990, p. A3; Bonnie Steinbock, "Recovery from Persistent Vegetative State? The Case of Carrie Coons," *Hastings Center Report* 19 (July/August 1989): 14-15; Harry A. Cole, "Deciding on a Time to Die: A Fitting Response," *Second Opinion* 7 (March 1988): 11-25; Frame, *Medical Ethics,* p. 76; and James B. Nelson and Jo Anne Rohricht, *Human Medicine,* rev. ed. (Minneapolis: Augsburg Press, 1984), p. 148. An alternative reading of these cases is that they are supernatural interventions of God. More research is necessary so that the natural possibilities of such cases occurring can be better understood.

10. On the idolatrous rebellion at issue here, see Daniel B. McGee, "Issues of Life and Death" in *Understanding Christian Ethics* (Nashville: Broadman Press, 1988), p. 232; Willard S. Krabill, "Death and Dying: Prevailing Medical Perspectives," in *Medical Ethics, Human Choices: A Christian Perspective,* ed. John Rogers (Scottdale, Pa.: Herald Press, 1988), p. 61; Gula, *What Are They Saying about Euthanasia?* p. 137; and Thielicke, "The Doctor as Judge of Who Shall Live and Who Shall Die," p. 166.

11. For more on the implications of a Christian understanding of life and death for withholding and withdrawing treatment, see Jesse H. Ziegler, "Prolonging Life, Prolonging Death," in *Medical Ethics, Human Choices,* ed. John Rogers (Scottdale, Pa.: Herald Press, 1988), p. 90; Frame, *Medical Ethics,* p. 63; Howard J. Loewen, "The Clinic, the Church, and the Kingdom," in *Medical Ethics, Human Choices,* p. 46; J. Kerby Anderson, "Euthanasia: A Biblical Appraisal," *Bibliotheca Sacra* 144 (April-June 1987): 216-17; Richard A. McCormick, "Theology and Bioethics: Christian Foundations," in *Theology and Bioethics,* ed. Earl Shelp (Boston: D. Reidel, 1985), pp. 97-98; and Gilbert Meilaender, "The Distinction between Killing and Allowing to Die," *Theological Studies* 37 (September 1976): 469-70.

12. On the caring involved here, see Paul Ramsey, *The Patient as Person* (New Haven: Yale University Press, 1970), pp. 113-64; Ashley and O'Rourke, *Health Care Ethics,* pp. 374-80. On the difference that the presence or absence of caring can produce in the course of action taken, see J. Stuart Showalter and Brian L. Andrew, *To Treat or Not to Treat: A Working Document for Making Critical Life Decisions* (St. Louis: Catholic Health Association of the United States, 1984), p. 3; and Allen I. Hyman, "Commentary on Belliotti's 'Allocation of Resources,' " *Values and Ethics in Health Care* 5 (1980): 264. Compare, for instance, with an eye toward the issue of withdrawing treatment, the stances of two literary characters, the Earl of Kent in Shakespeare's *King Lear* and Agatha in T. S. Eliot's *The Family Reunion.* As Lear nears death, Kent says, "vex not his ghost. O, let him pass! He hates him that would upon the rack of this tough world stretch him out longer." Eliot's Agatha, on the other hand, wants to do something "not for the good that it will do, but that nothing may be left undone on the margin of the impossible."

Chapter 7

1. The term received special attention around the time that the first living-will legislation was passed (the California Natural Death Act, 1976). See, for example, S. A. Levenson et al., "Ethical Considerations in Critical and Terminal Illness in the Elderly," *Journal of the American Geriatrics Society* 29 (1981): 564; Tom L. Beauchamp, "Can We Stop or Withhold Dialysis?" in *Controversies in Nephrology — 1979*, ed. George Schreiner (Washington: Georgetown University Press, 1979), p. 168; Paul Ramsey, *Ethics at the Edges of Life* (New Haven: Yale University Press, 1978), p. 327; Robert M. Veatch, "Death and Dying: The Legislative Options," *Hastings Center Report* 7 (October 1977): 6-8; Thomas A. Shannon, "What Guidance from the Guidelines?" *Hastings Center Report* 7 (June 1977): 28; Mitchell Rabkin et al., "Orders Not to Resuscitate," *New England Journal of Medicine*, 21 August 1976, pp. 364-66; and Robert M. Byrn, "Compulsory Lifesaving Treatment for the Competent Adult," *Fordham Law Review* 44 (October 1975): 13-16. More recent support for the term is documented in notes 4 and 5 of Chapter 11. For details about similar legislation that was passed during the next decade in thirty-six states, see George P. Smith II, "Death Be Not Proud: Medical, Ethical and Legal Dilemmas in Resource Allocation," *Journal of Contemporary Health Law and Policy* 3 (Spring 1987): 47-63. For further discussion of the term in a Christian context, see John M. Frame, *Medical Ethics: Principles, Persons, and Problems* (Grand Rapids: Baker Book House, 1988), p. 63; and Thomas C. Oden, *Should Treatment Be Terminated?* (New York: Harper & Row 1976), p. 44.

2. Cf. Richard Stith, in *On Moral Medicine: Theological Perspectives in Medical Ethics*, ed. Stephen Lammers and Allen Verhey (Grand Rapids: William B. Eerdmans, 1987), p. 127; Lennart Molin, "Christian Ethics and Human Life," *Covenant Quarterly* 45 (August 1987): 118, 121; Lewis B. Smedes, "Respect for Human Life: 'Thou Shalt Not Kill,'" in *On Moral Medicine*, p. 147; and Karl Barth, *Church Dogmatics*, III/4, trans. A. T. Mackay et al. (Edinburgh: T. & T. Clark, 1961), pp. 116, 119.

3. This is not to suggest that the freedom of the patient is unbounded. For one thing, any individual's freedom is limited by the fact that the freedoms of others must also be protected. Accordingly, there is moral warrant for restraining people by legal means or otherwise from actions that would bring significant harm to others.

4. For more on providing patients with the resources of faith in the midst of illness, see Frame, *Medical Ethics*, pp. 23-24; David Schroeder, "Life and Death: Biblical-Theological Perspectives," in *Medical Ethics, Human Choices: A Christian Perspective*, ed. John Rogers (Scottdale, Pa.: Herald Press, 1988), p. 71; Franklin E. Payne, Jr., *Biblical/Medical Ethics* (Milford, Mich.: Mott Media, 1985), pp. 184, 226-27; and Paul D. Simmons, *Birth and Death: Bioethical Decision-Making* (Philadelphia: Westminster Press, 1983), p. 130.

5. Concerns regarding the ethical implications of withdrawing treatment are legitimate; however, it is not valid to equate withdrawal of treatment with "active euthanasia" in all cases. For examples of statements in which the two *are* equated, see Payne, *Biblical/Medical Ethics*, p. 198; William C. Mays, "Christian Ethics and Biomedical Issues: A Chaplain's Perspective," in *A Matter of Life and Death*, ed. Harry Hollis (Nashville: Broadman Press, 1977), p. 63; and C. Everett Koop, *Right to Live, Right to Die* (Wheaton, Ill.: Tyndale Press, 1976), p. 135.

6. For further development and illustration of these ideas, see John F. Kilner, "Ethical Issues in the Initiation and Termination of Treatment," *American Journal of Kidney Diseases* 15 (March 1990): 222ff.; and John Fletcher, "Ethical Issues," in *Current Therapy in Critical Care Medicine*, ed. Joseph Parrillo (Philadelphia: B. C. Decker, 1987), p. 343.

7. On these contributions of the hospice movement, see Nina M. Fish, "Hospice: Terminal Illness, Teamwork and the Quality of Life," in *Social Work in Health Settings*, ed. Toba Kerson (New York: Haworth Press, 1989), pp. 449-69; *Hospice Care: Principles and Practice*, ed. Charles A. Corr and Donna M. Corr (New York: Springer, 1983); Anne Munley, *The Hospice Alternative* (New York: Basic Books, 1983); Robert W. Buckingham, *The Complete Hospice Guide* (New York: Harper & Row, 1983); and Norman Anderson, *Issues of Life and Death* (Downers Grove, Ill.: InterVarsity Press, 1976), p. 99. On the inadequate training of the vast majority of physicians in pain management, see Kathleen M. Foley, "The Relationship of Pain and Symptom Management to Patient Requests for Physician-Assisted Suicide," *Journal of Pain and Symptom Management* 6 (July 1991): 289-97; and Richard A. McCormick, "Physician-Assisted Suicide: Flight from Compassion," *Christian Century*, 4 December 1991, p. 1133.

8. Some discussions of the ethics of pain medication introduce the so-called "principle of double effect." See, for example, the October 1991 issue of the *Journal of Medicine and Philosophy*. Robert N. Wennberg has identified numerous individuals who have written about the principle, some in favor and some opposed (*Terminal Choices* [Grand Rapids: William B. Eerdmans, 1989], pp. 102-6). For more on the topic, see A. Van den Beld, "Killing and the Principle of Double Effect," *Scottish Journal of Theology* 41 (1988): 93-116; Stith, "Toward Freedom from Value," p. 137; Edward J. Bayer, "Perspectives from Catholic Theology," in *By No Extraordinary Means: The Choice to Forgo Life-Sustaining Food and Water*, ed. Joanne Lynn (Bloomington, Ind.: Indiana University Press, 1986), pp. 94-95; and Robert Twycross, "Decisions about Death and Dying," in *Decision Making in Medicine: The Practice of Its Ethics*, ed. Gordon Scorer and Antony Wing (London: Edward Arnold, 1979), p. 107. Proponents of this principle argue that as long as one intends something moral by an action (its primary effect), one is not morally culpable for an unintended secondary effect — particularly if that secondary effect is not

directly caused by the action. The principle can be helpful as long as something as morally significant as life is not at stake (as it is not, for example, when death is imminent even with treatment). However, it is not always so easy to escape responsibility for certain aspects of one's choices. Motivations, intentions, and actions are all ethically important. Even if we have the best of motivations and intentions, our actions can be wrong if they conflict with the reality-bounded dimension of ethics (which includes the life guide). The issue is then the presence of the conflict, not its primary or secondary nature. For example, there is nothing wrong with jumping into the air for fun, but there is something wrong with jumping off a bridge to one's death. If one were to jump off a bridge solely with the intention of experiencing the thrill of jumping into the air — not killing oneself — then the action might not seem as bad morally. It would still be wrong according to the described perspective, however, since a result of the action is that life is destroyed, even though it could be argued that gravity is the direct cause of death rather than the jump per se.

9. See Twycross, "Decisions about Death and Dying," p. 107; Anderson, *Issues of Life and Death*, p. 95; Paul Ramsey, *The Patient as Person* (New Haven: Yale University Press, 1970), p. 129; and the sources cited by these authors. A recent study of pain medication in conjunction with withholding or withdrawing life support buttresses the idea that the administration of pain medication does not generally accelerate dying. The study found that "death was not hastened by drug administration. . . . The median time until death following the initiation of the withholding or withdrawal of life support was 3.5 hours in the patients who received drugs and 1.3 hours in those patients who did not." See William C. Wilson et al., "Ordering and Administration of Sedatives and Analgesics during the Withholding and Withdrawal of Life Support from Critically Ill Patients," *Journal of the American Medical Association,* 19 February 1992, p. 949.

10. On the history of the extraordinary/ordinary distinction, see James J. McCartney, "The Development of the Doctrine of Ordinary and Extraordinary Means of Preserving Life in Catholic Moral Theology before the Karen Quinlan Case," *Linacre Quarterly* 47 (August 1980): 215-24; and Richard M. Gula, *What Are They Saying about Euthanasia?* (New York: Paulist Press, 1986), pp. 45-60. For an analysis of the distinction, see Ramsey, *The Patient as Person*, pp. 118-24; David Braine, *Medical Ethics and Human Life* (Aberdeen: Palladio, 1983), p. 44; Fletcher, "Ethical Issues," p. 342; Stith, "Toward Freedom from Value," p. 139; and William B. Smith, "Judeo-Christian Teaching on Euthanasia: Definitions, Distinctions and Decisions," *Linacre Quarterly* 54 (February 1987): 28-32.

11. Many people plausibly contend that artificial nutrition and hydration (tube-feeding and intravenous fluids) are medical treatments with the same moral status as any other potentially life-sustaining treatment. These

treatments provide basic food and water in much the same manner that a respirator provides air. Withholding them no more changes the basic medical cause of death than does withholding a respirator. If the underlying medical condition renders part of the digestive or respiratory system inoperative, then a decision has to be made in either case about whether artificial means should be used to try to compensate. Claims that withholding nutrition and hydration results in a very painful death for the patient, some argue, are unfounded as long as good nursing care (especially moisture for lips, mouth, and eyes) is provided (see Ronald E. Cranford, "The Persistent Vegetative State: The Medical Reality (Getting the Facts Straight)," *Hastings Center Report* 18 [February/March 1988]: 31; and Willard S. Krabill, "Death and Dying: Prevailing Medical Perspectives," in *Medical Ethics, Human Choices: A Christian Perspective,* ed. John Rogers [Scottdale, Pa.: Herald Press, 1988], p. 57).

Others consider providing food and water to have such symbolic value that it cannot merely be considered medical treatment (see, e.g., Gilbert Meilaender, "On Removing Food and Water: Against the Stream," *Hastings Center Report* 14 [December 1984]: 11-12; and Daniel Callahan, "On Feeding the Dying," *Hastings Center Report* 13 [October 1983]: 22). They maintain that it represents the minimum nurturing support that every member of the human community is due until the moment of death. In the end, however, this view of artificial nutrition and hydration is not very convincing. Most individuals and commissions discussing the issue are more persuaded that artificial nutrition and hydration — automatically provided through tubes with little if any personal interaction between patient and caregiver — do not effectively preserve for most people the symbolic value of giving a cup of water and piece of bread to one in need. They see enough diversity of perspective to argue for freedom of judgment on the part of those making a particular treatment decision (see, e.g., Wennberg, *Terminal Choices,* pp. 134-36; *Guidelines on the Termination of Life-Sustaining Treatment and the Care of the Dying* [Briarcliff Manor, N.Y.: Hastings Center, 1987], pp. 59-60; President's Commission for the Study of Ethical Problems in Medicine and Biomedical and Behavioral Research, *Deciding to Forego Life-Sustaining Treatment* [Washington: U.S. Government Printing Office, 1983], p. 190; and Joanne Lynn and James F. Childress, "Must Patients Always Be Given Food and Water?" *Hastings Center Report* 13 [October 1983]: 17-21). R. J. Connelly has even proposed conditions under which forgoing artificial nutrition and hydration may be viewed as a legitimate form of Christian fasting ("Natural Death and Christian Fasting," *Journal of Religion and Health* 25 [Fall 1986]: 227-36). I would argue, however, that the same ethical frame of reference applies to food and water as to other life-sustaining care: as long as the patient needs them (i.e., death is imminent only if they are not provided) and administering them does not go against the patient's wishes, they should be provided.

12. In Chapter 3 we noted passages in the Bible that speak of this

general responsibility to meet people's vital needs. The special responsibility of those in the household of faith for one another is suggested in Paul's appeal to the Galatians, among other places: "let us do good to all people, especially to those who belong to the family of believers" (Gal. 6:10). A special responsibility for one's own biological family members is affirmed explicitly in 1 Tim. 5:8. Other aspects of this special responsibility for one's parents can be readily traced back through Jesus into the Old Testament (see Matt. 15:3-6; Deut. 5:16; Exod. 20:12). For further analysis of the responsibility to meet the vital needs of others in the context of medical treatment decisions, see Frame, *Medical Ethics*, pp. 24-25, 47-48.

13. This standard — being expected to give only according to one's means (2 Cor. 8:11) — is also invoked elsewhere (e.g., in Acts 11:29 and 1 Cor. 16:2). For more detailed examinations of the Jerusalem collection(s), see Wilhelm C. Linss, "The First World Hunger Appeal," *Currents in Theology and Mission* 12 (August 1985): 211-19; and Dieter Georgi, *Die Geschichte der Kollekte des Paulus für Jerusalem* (Hamburg-Bergstedt: Reich, 1965).

14. For further exploration of these factors in the context of life-or-death decisions focusing on God, see Smedes, "Respect for Human Life," p. 17; Dietrich Bonhoeffer, *Ethics*, ed. Eberhard Bethge, trans. Neville Smith (New York: Macmillan, 1955), pp. 169-70; Germain Grisez and Joseph M. Boyle, Jr., "The Morality of Killing: A Traditional View," in *Bioethics: Reading and Cases*, ed. Baruch Brody and H. Tristram Engelhardt, Jr. (Englewood Cliffs, N.J.: Prentice-Hall, 1987), p. 160; and Douglas MacG. Jackson and David S. Short, "The Distinctive Christian Ethic in Medical Practice," in *Medical Ethics: A Christian View*, 2d ed., ed. Vincent Edmunds and C. Gorden Scorer (London: Tyndale Press, 1966), p. 25. For a focus on community in this context, see Stephen G. Post, "Family Caretaking: Moral Commitments and the Burden of Care," *Second Opinion* 8 (July 1988): 116-25; Stanley Hauerwas, "Rational Suicide and Reasons for Living," in *On Moral Medicine: Theological Perspectives in Medical Ethics*, ed. Stephen Lammers and Allen Verhey (Grand Rapids: William B. Eerdmans, 1987), p. 463; and Lowell O. Erdahl, *Pro-Life/Pro-Peace* (Minneapolis: Augsburg Press, 1986), pp. 111-12.

Chapter 8

1. For a more extended treatment of the problem of the allocation of vital resources, see John F. Kilner, *Who Lives? Who Dies? — Ethical Criteria in Patient Selection* (New Haven: Yale University Press, 1990).

2. Paul E. Kalb and David H. Miller, "Utilization Strategies for Intensive Care Units," *Journal of the American Medical Association*, 28 April 1989, pp. 2389-95; Robert H. Blank, *Rationing Medicine* (New York: Columbia University Press, 1988); Stan Godshall, "Allocating Limited Medical Resources," in *Medi-*

cal Ethics, Human Choices: A Christian Perspective, ed. John Rogers (Scottdale, Pa.: Herald Press, 1988), pp. 121-31; Robert Reinhold, "Crisis in Emergency Rooms: More Symptoms Than Cures," New York *Times*, 28 July 1988, pp. A1, 20; Thomas E. Starzl et al., "Equitable Allocation of Extrarenal Organs: With Special Reference to the Liver," *Transplantation Proceedings* 20 (February 1988): 131-38; Fredrick R. Abrams, "Access to Health Care," in *Health Care Ethics*, ed. Gary Anderson and Valerie Glesnes-Anderson (Rockville, Md.: Aspen, 1987), pp. 49-68; Arthur L. Caplan, "Obtaining and Allocating Organs for Transplantation," in *Human Organ Transplantation*, ed. Dale H. Cowan et al. (Ann Arbor: Health Administration Press, 1987), pp. 5-17; Larry R. Churchill, *Rationing Health Care in America: Perceptions and Principles of Justice* (South Bend, Ind.: University of Notre Dame Press, 1987); Howard H. Hiatt, *America's Health in the Balance: Choice or Chance?* (New York: Harper & Row, 1987); Stanley R. Ingman et al., "ESRD and the Elderly: Cross-National Perspective on Distributive Justice," in *Ethical Dimensions of Geriatric Care*, ed. Stuart Spicker et al. (Boston: D. Reidel, 1987), pp. 223-62; Ruth Macklin, *Mortal Choices* (New York: Pantheon Books, 1987); Felix T. Rapaport, "Living Donor Kidney Transplantation," *Transplantation Proceedings* 19 (February 1987): 169-73; William R. Hendee, "Rationing Health Care," in *Life and Death Issues*, ed. James Hamner III and Barbara Jacobs (Memphis: University of Tennessee Press, 1986), pp. 1-10; Thomas C. King, "Ethical Dilemmas of Restricted Resources," in *Human and Ethical Issues in the Surgical Care of Patients with Life-Threatening Disease*, ed. Frederic Herter et al. (Springfield, Ill.: Charles C. Thomas, 1986), pp. 169-75; Michael J. Strauss et al., "Rationing of Intensive Care Unit Services: An Everyday Occurrence," *Journal of the American Medical Association*, 7 March 1986, pp. 1143-46; Christine K. Cassel, "Doctors and Allocation Decisions: A New Role in the New Medicare," *Journal of Health Politics, Policy, and Law* 10 (Fall 1985): 549-64; Maxwell J. Mehlman, "Rationing Expensive Lifesaving Medical Treatments," *Wisconsin Law Review*, no. 2 (1985): 239-303; Frances H. Miller, "Reflections on Organ Transplantation in the United Kingdom," *Law Medicine and Health Care* 13 (February 1985): 31-32; Arthur Parsons, "Allocating Health Care Resources: A Moral Dilemma," *Canadian Medical Association Journal*, 15 February 1985, pp. 466-69; Drummond Rennie et al., "Limited Resources and the Treatment of End-stage Renal Failure in Britain and the United States," *Quarterly Journal of Medicine*, n.s., 56 (July 1985): 321-36; Working Group on Mechanical Circulatory Support, National Heart, Lung and Blood Institute, *Artificial Heart and Assist Devices: Directions, Needs, Costs, Societal and Ethical Issues* (Bethesda, Md.: National Institutes of Health, 1985); Bruce E. Zawacki, "ICU Physician's Ethical Role in Distributing Scarce Resources," *Critical Care Medicine* 13 (January 1985): 57-60.

3. UNICEF, *The State of the World's Children 1988* (New York: Oxford University Press, 1988); *Poverty in Latin America* (Washington: World Bank, 1986); Nancy B. Cummings, "Uremia Therapy: The Resource Allocation

Dilemma from a Global Perspective," *Kidney International* 28, Suppl. 17 (1985): S133-35; John F. Kilner, "Who Shall Be Saved? An African Answer," *Hastings Center Report* 14 (June 1984): 18-22.

4. U.S. Department of Commerce, *1992 U.S. Industrial Outlook* (Washington: U.S. Government Printing Office, 1992); Lavinia Edmunds, "The Long Wait for a New Life," *Johns Hopkins Magazine* 41 (February 1989): IX-XVI; United Network for Organ Sharing (UNOS), "Memorandum on UNOS Policy regarding Utilization of the Point System for Cadaveric Kidney Allocation," 11 November 1988; Jeremiah A. Barondess et al., "Clinical Decision-Making in Catastrophic Situations: The Relevance of Age," *Journal of American Geriatrics Society* 36 (October 1988): 919-37; Blank, *Rationing Medicine;* Dale Jamieson, "The Artificial Heart: Reevaluating the Investment," in *Organ Substitution Technology,* ed. Deborah Mathieu (Boulder: Westview Press, 1988), pp. 277-93; Richard A. McCormick, "'A Clean Heart Create for Me, O God': Impact Questions on the Artificial Heart," in *Medical Ethics,* ed. John Monagle and David Thomasma (Rockville, Md.: Aspen, 1988), pp. 122-26; Steven H. Miles et al., "The Total Artificial Heart: An Ethics Perspective on Current Clinical Research and Deployment," *Chest* 94 (August 1988): 409-13; Daniel Callahan, *Setting Limits: Medical Goals in an Aging Society* (New York: Simon & Schuster, 1987); Churchill, *Rationing Health Care in America;* Theodore Cooper, "Survey of Development, Current Status, and Future Prospects for Organ Transplantation," in *Human Organ Transplantation,* ed. Dale Cowan et al. (Ann Arbor: Health Administration Press, 1987), pp. 18-26; Jack G. Copeland et al., "Selection of Patients for Cardiac Transplantation," *Circulation* 75 (1987): 1-9; Roger W. Evans and Junichi Yagi, "Social and Medical Considerations Affecting Selection of Transplant Recipients: The Case of Heart Transplantation," in *Human Organ Transplantation,* pp. 27-41; John Hardwig, "Robin Hoods and Good Samaritans: The Role of Patients in Health Care Distribution," *Theoretical Medicine* 8 (February 1987): 47-59; Howard H. Hiatt, *America's Health in the Balance: Choice or Chance?* (New York: Harper & Row, 1987); Macklin, *Mortal Choices;* John C. Moskop, "The Moral Limits to Federal Funding for Kidney Disease," *Hastings Center Report* 17 (April 1987): 11-15; Rapaport, "Living Donor Kidney Transplantation"; John A. Robertson, "Supply and Distribution of Hearts for Transplantation: Legal, Ethical, and Policy Issues," *Circulation* 75 (January 1987): 77-87; David J. Rothman, "Ethical and Social Issues in the Development of New Drugs and Vaccines," *Bulletin of the New York Academy of Medicine* 63 (July-August 1987): 557-68; Timothy M. Smeeding, "Artificial Organs, Transplants and Long-Term Care for the Elderly: What's Covered? Who Pays?" in *Should Medical Care Be Rationed by Age?* ed. Timothy M. Smeeding (Totowa, N.J.: Rowman & Littlefield, 1987), pp. 140-55.

5. See Kilner, "Who Shall Be Saved?"

6. As a rule, it is probably best to avoid expressions such as "the elderly" and "the poor." When we use such terms, we reduce the individuals

we are describing to a single characteristic, typically to their detriment. Even just modifying the phrase to "elderly people" would be an improvement, a small step toward underscoring the fact that we are talking about real people with real differences. But the problem with age criteria is precisely that they demean elderly people by reducing them to a single characteristic, their age. In this context, references to "the elderly" accurately symbolize this problem, and I have intentionally chosen to use the term here for that reason.

7. See William R. Hendee, "Rationing Health Care," in *Life and Death Issues*, ed. James Hamner III and Barbara Jacobs (Memphis: University of Tennessee Press, 1986), p. 8; Joseph Meissner, "Legal Services and Medical Treatment for Poor People: A Need for Advocacy," *Issues in Law and Medicine* 2 (July 1986): 6; Basile J. Uddo, "The Withdrawal or Refusal of Food and Hydration as Age Discrimination: Some Possibilities," *Issues in Law and Medicine* 2 (July 1986): 40.

8. One national survey reported that 35 percent of the respondents supported age criteria and 58 percent opposed them ("Who Lives, Who Dies, Who Decides? — National Poll Results" [San Francisco: Pacific Presbyterian Medical Center, 1987]); another national survey reported that 57 percent of the respondents supported them (Roger W. Evans and Diane L. Manninen, "Public Opinion concerning Organ Donation, Procurement, and Distribution," results of a 1987 survey conducted for UNOS by Battelle Human Affairs Research Centers, Seattle, partially published in *Transplantation Proceedings* 20 [October 1988]: 781-85). One state survey reported 19 percent in support and 57 percent opposed ("Preliminary Analysis — Small Group Meetings" [Tustin, Cal.: California Health Decisions, 1986]); another reported 40 percent in support and 43 percent opposed (Washington Health Choices, *Executive Report* [Seattle: Puget Sound Health Systems Agency, 1986]).

9. On heart transplantation, see *National Heart Transplantation Study* (Seattle: Battelle Human Affairs Research Centers, 1984), chap. 8, pp. 18, 30, 50, 58, 66; chap. 9, pp. 2, 4; chap. 10, p. 25; and Evans and Yagi, "Social and Medical Considerations Affecting Selection of Transplant Recipients," pp. 27, 29. The difficulty of obtaining a heart transplant for those over fifty is one of the reasons pioneer artificial heart recipients Barney Clark and William Schroeder wanted the new device. The upper age limit then being placed upon artificial heart recipients was sixty-five. See Smeeding, "Artificial Organs, Transplants and Long-Term Care for the Elderly," p. 144; William C. DeVries et al., "Clinical Use of the Total Artificial Heart," *New England Journal of Medicine*, 2 February 1984, p. 278; and Otto Friedrich, "One Miracle, Many Doubts," *Time*, 10 December 1984, p. 73.

On intensive care, see Barondess et al., "Clinical Decision-Making in Catastrophic Situations," pp. 920-21; Donna K. McClish et al., "The Impact of Age on Utilization of Intensive Care Resources," *Journal of the American Geriatrics Society* 35 (November 1987): 983; and Mary E. Charlson et al., "Resuscitation: How Do We Decide?" *Journal of the American Medical Association*, 14 March 1986, p. 1319; cf. Anne A. Scitovsky, "Medical Care Expenditures in the Last Twelve Months of Life," final report to the John A. Hartford Foundation, March 1986.

On kidney dialysis and transplantation, see Carl M. Kjellstrand, "Age, Sex, and Race Inequality in Renal Transplantation," *Archives of Internal Medicine* 148 (June 1988): 1305-9; Carl M. Kjellstrand and George M. Logan, *Racial, Sexual and Age Inequalities in Chronic Dialysis,"* *Nephron* 45 (1987): 257-63; Jeanie S. Kayser-Jones, "Distributive Justice and the Treatment of Acute Illness in Nursing Homes," *Social Science and Medicine* 23 (1986): 1282; Lindsey Gruson, "Some Doctors Move to Bar Transplants to Foreign Patients," New York *Times*, 18 August 1985, p. 5; and Roger W. Evans, "Health Care Technology and the Inevitability of Resource Allocation and Rationing Decisions," *Journal of the American Medical Association*, 22/29 April 1983, p. 2209. Regarding organ transplantation generally, see David A. Ogden, "Organ Procurement and Transplantation," in *Health Care Clinics*, ed. Gary Anderson and Valerie Glesnes-Anderson (Rockville, Md.: Aspen, 1987), p. 104; and Miller, "Reflections on Organ Transplantation in the United Kingdom," p. 31.

10. Regarding treatment of breast cancer, see Sheldon Greenfield et al., "Patterns of Care Related to Age of Breast Cancer Patients," *Journal of the American Medical Association*, 22/29 May 1987, pp. 2766-70; cf. Jonathan Samet et al., "Choice of Cancer Therapy Varies with Age of Patient," *Journal of the American Medical Association*, 27 June 1986, pp. 3385-90; and Terrie Wetle, "Age as a Risk Factor for Inadequate Treatment," *Journal of the American Medical Association*, 2 July 1987, p. 516. Regarding treatment of acute illnesses, see Kayser-Jones, "Distributive Justice and the Treatment of Acute Illness in Nursing Homes."

11. See Kjellstrand, "Age, Sex, and Race Inequality in Renal Transplantation," p. 1308; William M. Sage et al., "Intensive Care for the Elderly: Outcome of Elective and Nonelective Admissions," *Journal of the American Geriatrics Society* 35 (April 1987): 316; Roger W. Evans et al., "National Policies for the Treatment of End-Stage Renal Disease" (Seattle: Battelle Human Affairs Research Centers, 1984); "European Hospitals Less Technology-Intensive, Less Expensive than U.S.," *Medical World News*, 12 March 1984, p. 24; S. Challah et al., "Negative Selection of Patients for Dialysis and Transplantation in the United Kingdom," *British Medical Journal*, 14 April 1984, p. 1122; Jeffrey M. Prottas et al., "Cross-National Differences in Dialysis Rates," *Health Care Financing Review* 4 (March 1983): 98.

12. J. Grimley Evans, "Age and Equality," *Annals of the New York Academy of Sciences* 530 (1988): 119; Caplan, "Obtaining and Allocating Organs for Transplantation," p. 13; John G. Francis and Leslie P. Francis, "Rationing of Health Care in Britain: An Ethical Critique of Public Policy-Making," in *Should Medical Care Be Rationed by Age?* ed. Timothy M. Smeeding (Totowa,

N.J.: Rowman & Littlefield, 1987), p. 129; Hiatt, *America's Health in the Balance*, p. 105; Ingman et al., "ESRD and the Elderly," p. 227; Joseph A. Califano, Jr., *America's Health Care Revolution: Who Lives? Who Dies? Who Pays?* (New York: Random House, 1986), p. 180; James F. Childress, "Artificial and Transplanted Organs," in *Biolaw*, vol. 1, ed. J. F. Childress et al. (Frederick, Md.: University Publications of America, 1986), p. 318; Leslie P. Francis, "Poverty, Age Discrimination, and Health Care," in *Poverty, Justice, and the Law*, ed. George R. Lucas (Lanham, Md.: University Press of America, 1986), p. 120; Paul A. Haber, "Rationing Is a Reality," *Journal of the American Geriatrics Society* 34 (October 1986): 762; John B. Sanders, "ICU Admission and Discharge Screening Criteria," *Nursing Administration Quarterly* 10 (Spring 1986): 26-27; George J. Annas, "The Prostitute, the Playboy, and the Poet: Rationing Schemes for Organ Transplantation," *American Journal of Public Health* 75 (February 1985): 188; Francis P. Chinard, "Ethics and Technology," *Journal of the Medical Society of New Jersey* 82 (February 1985): 121; Thomas Halper, "Life and Death in a Welfare State: End-Stage Renal Disease in the United Kingdom," *Milbank Memorial Fund Quarterly* 63 (Winter 1985): 55; Robert Schwartz and Andrew Grubb, "Why Britain Can't Afford Informed Consent," *Hastings Center Report* 15 (August 1985): 24; Robert M. Veatch, "Distributive Justice and the Allocation of Technological Resources to the Elderly," contract report prepared for the Office of Technology Assessment, U.S. Congress, Washington, D.C., December 1985.

13. *National Kidney Dialysis and Kidney Transplantation Study* (Seattle: Battelle Human Affairs Research Centers, 1986), chap. 2, p. 17; Haber, "Rationing Is a Reality," p. 762; *National Heart Transplantation Study*, chap. 44, pp. 25-26, 32; Henry J. Aaron and William B. Schwartz, *The Painful Prescription: Rationing Hospital Care* (Washington: Brookings Institution, 1984), p. 110; William B. Schwartz and Henry J. Aaron, "Rationing Hospital Care: Lessons from Britain," *New England Journal of Medicine*, 5 January 1984, p. 53.

14. John F. Kilner, "Selecting Patients When Resources Are Limited: A Study of U.S. Medical Directors of Kidney Dialysis and Transplantation Facilities," *American Journal of Public Health* 78 (February 1988): 144-47.

15. See Norman Daniels, "Is Age-Rationing Just?" paper delivered at the Pacific Section of the American Philosophical Association, San Francisco, March 1986, p. 1; Francis, "Poverty, Age Discrimination, and Health Care," p. 118; Ronald Kotulak, "Never-Say-Die Policy Prompts Rationing Call," Chicago Tribune, 15 July 1986, p. 12; Phillip G. Clark, "The Social Allocation of Health Care Resources: Ethical Dilemmas in Age-Group Competition," *Gerontologist* 25 (April 1985): 119-20; "Rationing of Health Care," *Perspective* 20 (Summer 1985): 9; Arthur L. Caplan, "The Selection of Patients for Dialytic Therapy — Should Treatment Be Left to Chance?" *Dialysis and Transplantation* 13 (March 1984): 161; Norman G. Levinsky, "The Doctor's Master," *New England Journal of Medicine*, 13 December 1984, p. 1574.

16. Severe illness may also diminish the capacity of people of any age to *communicate* their wisdom.

17. See J. Gordon Harris, *God and the Elderly* (Philadelphia: Fortress Press, 1987), p. 108.

18. See Childress, "Artificial and Transplanted Organs," p. 318; Task Force on Organ Transplantation, *Organ Transplantation: Issues and Recommendations* (Rockville, Md.: U.S. Dept. of Health and Human Services, 1986), p. 90. On the importance of symbols (such as the provision of lifesaving health care) in shaping the way the elderly are treated throughout society, see David J. Maitland, *Aging: A Time for New Learning* (Atlanta: John Knox Press, 1987).

19. For more on the implications of such passages, see David M. Feldman, *Health and Medicine in the Jewish Tradition* (New York: Crossroad, 1986), pp. 97-99.

20. Nancy Foner, *Ages in Conflict: A Cross-Cultural Perspective on Inequality between Old and Young* (New York: Columbia University Press, 1984).

21. For a general critique of these medical criteria outside the context of the elderly, see chaps. 12-14 of Kilner, *Who Lives? Who Dies?*

22. U.S. Congress Office of Technology Assessment, *Life-Sustaining Technologies and the Elderly,* OTA-BA-306 (Washington: U.S. Government Printing Office, 1987), pp. 19-20; Macklin, *Mortal Choices,* p. 157; Working Group on Mechanical Circulatory Support, National Heart, Lung and Blood Institute, *Artificial Heart and Assist Devices,* p. 26.

23. Guido Calabresi and Philip Bobbitt, *Tragic Choices* (New York: W. W. Norton, 1978).

24. Evans, "Age and Equality," p. 119; U.S. Congress Office of Technology Assessment, *Life-Sustaining Technologies and the Elderly,* pp. 261-62; Sage et al., "Intensive Care for the Elderly," p. 316; "Is Intensive Care Worth It? An Assessment of Input and Outcome for the Critically Ill," *Critical Care Medicine* 14 (September 1986): 782; Carol E. Ferrans, "Quality of Life as a Criterion for Allocation of Life-Sustaining Treatment: The Case of Hemodialysis," in *Health Care Ethics,* ed. Gary Anderson and Valerie Glesnes-Anderson (Rockville, Md.: Aspen, 1987), p. 120; *National Kidney Dialysis and Kidney Transplantation Study,* chap. 6, pp. 25-27; Steven Neu and Carl M. Kjellstrand, "Stopping Long-Term Dialysis," *New England Journal of Medicine,* 2 January 1986, p. 18; David C. Thomasma, "Quality of Life Judgments, Treatment Decisions and Medical Ethics," *Clinics in Geriatric Medicine* 2 (February 1986): 22. A study conducted by M. Powell Lawton et al. of the last year of life of elderly persons shows that their quality of life is substantially higher than would commonly be inferred from their physical health status ("The Quality of the Last Year of Life of Older Persons," *Milbank Quarterly* 68 [1990]: 1-28).

25. Bernard Lo, "Quality of Life Judgments in the Care of the Elderly," in *Medical Ethics,* ed. John Monagle and David Thomasma (Rockville, Md.: Aspen, 1988), p. 141; Michael O'Donnell, "One Man's Burden," *British Medical*

Journal, 5 July 1986, p. 59; Uddo, "The Withdrawal or Refusal of Food and Hydration as Age Discrimination," p. 43.

26. T. Jolene Starr et al., "Quality of Life and Rescuscitation Decisions in Elderly Patients," *Journal of General Internal Medicine* 1 (November/December 1986): 373-79; Kayser-Jones, "Distributive Justice and the Treatment of Acute Illness in Nursing Homes," pp. 1280-85; Robert A. Pearlman and Albert R. Jonsen, "The Use of Quality-of-Life Considerations in Medical Decision Making," *Journal of the American Geriatrics Society* 33 (May 1985): 349.

27. Myra E. Levine, "Ration or Rescue: The Elderly Patient in Critical Care," *Critical Care Nursing Quarterly* 12 (June 1989): 87-88; Ferrans, "Quality of Life as a Criterion for Allocation of Life-Sustaining Treatment," pp. 113-14; John Harris, "QALYfying the Value of Life," *Journal of Medical Ethics* 13 (September 1987): 120-21.

28. Carol Levine, "Stopping Dialysis for 'Low Quality' of Life: A Case from Britain," *Hastings Center Report* 15 (February 1985): 2; Colin Hughes, "Call for Inquiry on Kidney Patient," London *Times*, 8 January 1985, p. 3; Diana Brahams, "When Is Discontinuation of Dialysis Justified?" *Lancet*, 19 January 1985, pp. 176-77.

29. Raanan Gillon, "Justice and Allocation of Medical Resources," *British Medical Journal*, 27 July 1985, p. 267; cf. Michael D. Kirby, "Bioethical Decisions and Opportunity Costs," *Journal of Contemporary Health Law and Policy* 2 (Spring 1986): 20.

30. Lo, "Quality of Life Judgments in the Care of the Elderly," p. 141; Harris, "QALYfying the Value of Life," p. 119; Ferrans, "Quality of Life as a Criterion for Allocation of Life-Sustaining Treatment," pp. 112-13; Meissner, "Legal Services and Medical Treatment for Poor People," pp. 7ff.; Uddo, "The Withdrawal or Refusal of Food and Hydration as Age Discrimination," p. 43; Robert A. Destro, "Quality-of-Life Ethics and Constitutional Jurisprudence: The Demise of Natural Rights and Equal Protection for the Disabled and Incompetent," *Journal of Contemporary Health Law and Policy* 2 (Spring 1986): 71-130; Thomasma, "Quality of Life Judgments, Treatment Decisions and Medical Ethics," p. 22.

31. Regarding freedom, see Stephen G. Post, "Justice for Elderly People in Jewish and Christian Thought," in *Too Old for Health Care?* ed. Robert Benstock and Stephen Post (Baltimore: The Johns Hopkins University Press, 1991), p. 128. On justice, see Alwyn Smith, "Qualms and QALYs," *Lancet*, 16 May 1987, 1135; Ferrans, "Quality of Life as a Criterion for Allocation of Life-Sustaining Treatment," p. 113; Harris, "QALYfying the Value of Life," p. 121; Kenneth Boyd and Brian Potter, "Priorities in the Allocation of Scarce Resources," *Journal of Medical Ethics* 12 (December 1986): 198; Sanders, "ICU Admission and Discharge Screening Criteria," p. 28.

32. Dan W. Brock, "Ethical Issues in Recipient Selection for Organ Transplantation," in *Organ Substitution Technology*, ed. Deborah Mathieu

(Boulder: Westview Press, 1988), p. 94; George Weckman and Richard W. Willy, "Descriptive Medical Ethics and Allocation," *Listening* 22 (Winter 1987): 16; Macklin, *Mortal Choices*, p. 155; King, "Ethical Dilemmas of Restricted Resources," p. 174; Claudia J. Coulton, "Resource Limits and Allocation in Critical Care," in *Human Values in Critical Care Medicine*, ed. Stuart J. Youngner (New York: Praeger, 1986), p. 101; Arthur L. Caplan, "A New Dilemma: Quality, Ethics and Expensive Medical Technologies," *New York Medical Quarterly* 6 (1986): 26; *National Kidney Dialysis and Kidney Transplantation Study*, chap. 1, p. 37.

33. E.g., Gerald R. Winslow, *Triage and Justice* (Berkeley and Los Angeles: University of California Press, 1982), p. 166; Margot J. Fromer, *Ethical Issues in Health Care* (St. Louis: C. V. Mosby, 1981), p. 60; Paul Ramsey, *The Patient as Person* (New Haven: Yale University Press, 1970), p. 249; Nicholas Rescher, "The Allocation of Exotic Medical Lifesaving Therapy," *Ethics* 79 (1969): 181.

34. For further analysis of the notion of need in a medical context, see Glenn C. Graber et al., *Ethical Analysis of Clinical Medicine* (Baltimore: Urban & Schwarzenberg, 1985), p. 209; Gillon, "Justice and Allocation of Medical Resources," p. 267; Mark E. Thompson, "Selection of Candidates for Cardiac Transplantation," *Heart Transplantation* 3 (November 1983): 65.

35. *National Heart Transplantation Study*, chap. 9, pp. 14, 15; Mark Linzer, "Doing What 'Needs' to Be Done," *New England Journal of Medicine*, 16 February 1984, 470.

36. Evans, "Age and Equality," p. 120; *Guidelines on the Termination of Life-Sustaining Treatment and the Care of the Dying* (Briarcliff Manor, N.Y.: Hastings Center, 1987), p. 136; Wetle, "Age as a Risk Factor for Inadequate Treatment," p. 516; Arthur L. Caplan, "Equity in the Selection of Recipients for Cardiac Transplants," *Circulation* 75 (January 1987): 16; Patricia M. McKevitt et al., "The Elderly on Dialysis: Physical and Psychosocial Functioning," *Dialysis and Transplantation* 15 (March 1986): 135.

37. See D. E. R. Sutherland et al., "The High-Risk Recipient in Transplantation," *Transplantation Proceedings* 14 (March 1982): 24-25.

38. U.S. Congress Office of Technology Assessment, *Life-Sustaining Technologies and the Elderly*, p. 19; "Age as a Risk Factor for Inadequate Treatment," p. 516; Hiatt, *America's Health in the Balance*, pp. 50-51; Margaret A. Somerville, "Should the Grandparents Die? Allocation of Medical Resources with an Aging Population," *Law, Medicine and Health Care* 14 (September 1986): 160; Hans-Olov Adami et al., "The Relation between Survival and Age at Diagnosis in Breast Cancer," *New England Journal of Medicine*, 28 August 1986, pp. 559-63.

39. Thomas E. Starzl et al., "Liver Transplantation in Older Patients," *New England Journal of Medicine*, 19 February 1987, 484; Evans and Yagi, "Social and Medical Considerations Affecting Selection of Transplant Recipients," 29;

Ogden, "Organ Procurement and Transplantation," p. 105; Callahan, *Setting Limits*, p. 126. There is evidence that the drug cyclosporine has made it possible for patients 60 years old and older on average to do as well as those 18 to 59 years of age; see John D. Pirsch et al., "Orthotopic Liver Transplantation in Patients 60 Years of Age and Older," *Transplantation* 51 (1991): 431-33.

40. L. Westlie et al., "Mortality, Morbidity and Life Satisfaction in the Very Old Dialysis Patient," *Transactions of the American Society for Artificial Internal Organs* 30 (1984): 21-30; David H. Taube et al., "Successful Treatment of Middle Aged and Elderly Patients with End Stage Renal Disease," *British Medical Journal*, 25 June 1983, 2018-20; John M. Weller et al., "Analysis of Survival of End-Stage Renal Disease Patients," *Kidney International* 21 (January 1982): 78-83; Tom A. Hutchinson et al., "Predicting Survival in Adults with End-Stage Renal Disease: An Age Equivalence Index," *Annals of Internal Medicine* 96 (April 1982): 417-23.

41. Wetle, "Age as a Risk Factor for Inadequate Treatment," p. 516; G. D'Amico, "Treating End-Stage Renal Failure in Italy," in *Renal Failure — Who Cares?* ed. F. M. Parsons and C. S. Ogg (Lancaster, Eng.: MTP, 1983), p. 96; Calabresi and Bobbitt, *Tragic Choices*, p. 230.

Chapter 9

1. U.S. Congress Office of Technology Assessment, *Life-Sustaining Technologies and the Elderly*, OTA-BA-306 (Washington: U.S. Government Printing Office, 1987), p. 157; Terrie Wetle, "Age as a Risk Factor for Inadequate Treatment," *Journal of the American Medical Association*, 2 July 1987, p. 516; David C. Thomasma, "Quality of Life Judgments, Treatment Decisions and Medical Ethics," *Clinics in Geriatric Medicine* 2 (February 1986): 23; Frances H. Miller, "Reflections on Organ Transplantation in the United Kingdom," *Law Medicine and Health Care* 13 (February 1985): 31; John D. Arras, "Utility, Natural Rights, and the Right to Health Care," in *Biomedical Ethics Reviews*, ed. James Humber and Robert Almeder (Clifton, N.J.: Humana Press, 1984), pp. 34-35; Christopher Robbins, "The Ethical Challenge of Health Care Rationing," in *The End of an Illusion: The Future of Health Policy in Western Industrialized Nations*, ed. Jean de Kervasdoue et al. (Berkeley and Los Angeles: University of California Press, 1984), p. 126.

2. C. R. Stiller, "Ethics of Transplantation," *Transplantation Proceedings* 17, Suppl. 3 (December 1985): 135; Robert Young, "Some Criteria for Making Decisions concerning the Distribution of Scarce Medical Resources," *Theory and Decision* 6 (November 1975): 448; Nicholas Rescher, "The Allocation of Exotic Medical Lifesaving Therapy," *Ethics* 79 (1969): 182.

3. David H. Taube et al., "Successful Treatment of Middle Aged and Elderly Patients with End Stage Renal Disease," *British Medical Journal*, 25

June 1983, p. 2020; Albert R. Jonsen et al., *Clinical Ethics* (New York: Macmillan, 1982), p. 31.

4. Michael Waldholz, "Cost of Using Kidney Device Sparks Debate," *Wall Street Journal*, 5 February 1981, p. 32.

5. Allen I. Hyman, "Ethical Considerations in Intensive Care," in *Human and Ethical Issues in The Surgical Care of Patients with Life-Threatening Disease*, ed. Frederic Herter et al. (Springfield, Ill.: Charles C. Thomas, 1986), p. 41; Glenn W. Geelhoed, "Access to Care in a Changing Practice Environment," *Bulletin of the American College of Surgeons* 70 (June 1985): 11; Glenn Richards, "Technology Costs and Rationing Issues," *Hospitals*, 1 June 1984, p. 81.

6. Daniel Callahan, *Setting Limits: Medical Goals in an Aging Society* (New York: Simon & Schuster, 1987), pp. 65ff.; E. Lovell Becker, "Finite Resources and Medical Triage," *American Journal of Medicine* 66 (April 1979): 550.

7. Norman Daniels, *Just Health Care* (London: Cambridge University Press, 1985), pp. 96-97; Jeff Lyon, "Organ Transplants: Conundra without End," *Second Opinion* 2 (March 1986): 59.

8. Phil Gunby, "Media-Abetted Liver Transplants Raise Questions of 'Equity and Decency,' " *Journal of the American Medical Association*, 15 April 1983, 1982; Robert M. Veatch, "Ethical Foundations for Valuing Lives: Implications for Life-Extending Technologies," in *A Technology Assessment of Life-Extending Technologies*, Supplementary Report, vol. 6 (Glastonbury, Conn.: The Futures Group, 1977), p. 232; Hastings Center Research Group, "Values and Life-Extending Technologies," in *Life Span*, ed. Robert M. Veatch (San Francisco: Harper & Row, 1979), pp. 54-56, 82.

9. Paul T. Menzel, *Medical Costs, Moral Choices* (New Haven: Yale University Press, 1983), p. 191.

10. Menzel, *Medical Costs, Moral Choices*, p. 191; Jonathan Glover, *Causing Death and Saving Lives* (New York: Penguin, 1977), p. 220.

11. Callahan, *Setting Limits*, pp. 137ff.; Daniel Callahan, "Aging and the Ends of Medicine," *Annals of the New York Academy of Sciences* 530 (1988): 128-29. Cf. Jeremiah A. Barondess et al., "Clinical Decision-Making in Catastrophic Situations: The Relevance of Age," *Journal of American Geriatrics Society* 36 (October 1988): 935; Stanley R. Ingman et al., "ESRD and the Elderly: Cross-National Perspective on Distributive Justice," in *Ethical Dimensions of Geriatric Care*, ed. Stuart Spicker et al. (Boston: D. Reidel, 1987), p. 246. In support of the idea that there is a fixed human life span that humanity has nearly reached, see James F. Fries, "Aging, Natural Death, and the Compression of Morbidity," *New England Journal of Medicine*, 17 July 1980, pp. 130-35.

12. See Norman Daniels, "Am I My Parents' Keeper?" in *Securing Access to Health Care*, vol. 2 (Washington: U.S. Government Printing Office, 1983), pp. 265-91; *Just Health Care*, pp. 96-97; "Is Age-Rationing Just?" paper delivered at the Pacific Section of the American Philosophical Association, San Francisco, March 1986, pp. 16-20; and chap. 5 of *Am I My Parents' Keeper?*

An Essay on Justice between the Young and Old (New York: Oxford University Press, 1988). See also Robert M. Veatch, "From Fae to Schroeder: The Ethics of Allocating High Technology," *Spectrum* 16 (April 1985): 17-18; and "Distributive Justice and the Allocation of Technological Resources to the Elderly," contract report prepared for the U.S. Congress Office of Technology Assessment, Washington, D.C., December 1985, p. 77.

13. Daniels, *Am I My Parents' Keeper?* pp. 8-9; "Is Age-Rationing Just?" pp. 19-20; and *Just Health Care,* pp. 96-97; *National Heart Transplantation Study* (Seattle: Battelle Human Affairs Research Centers, 1984), chap. 38, p. 26; cf. Callahan, *Setting Limits,* pp. 148ff.

14. Margaret P. Battin, "Age Rationing and the Just Distribution of Health Care: Is There a Duty to Die?" *Ethics* 97 (January 1987): 324ff.

15. Veatch, "Distributive Justice and the Allocation of Technological Resources to the Elderly," p. 43; and *The Foundations of Justice* (New York: Oxford University Press, 1986), p. 146.

16. Even Daniel Callahan, who supports the use of this criterion, admits that "the average life expectancy continues to increase, with no end in sight" ("Aging and the Ends of Medicine," *Annals of the New York Academy of Sciences* 530 [1988]: 128).

17. Callahan, *Setting Limits,* pp. 184-85.

18. See, e.g., Callahan, *Setting Limits,* pp. 66, 172. Accordingly, Callahan does not consider the elderly to be as worthy of attention as younger people; "the primary orientation" of the elderly, he says, "should be to the young" ("Aging and the Ends of Medicine," p. 128).

19. Callahan, *Setting Limits,* pp. 184-85.

20. On selective settings, see Daniels, *Am I My Parents' Keeper?* p. 96; and *Just Health Care,* p. 111; and Battin, "Age Rationing and the Just Distribution of Health Care," p. 340. On political acceptability, see Daniels, *Am I My Parents' Keeper?* p. 97; cf. Wikler, "Comments on Battin's 'Age Rationing,' " in *Should Medical Care Be Rationed by Age?* ed. Timothy M. Smeeding (Totowa, N.J.: Rowman & Littlefield, 1987), p. 98.

21. Daniels, *Am I My Parents' Keeper?* p. 96; *Just Health Care,* p. 113; and "Am I My Parents' Keeper?" pp. 289-91; and Battin, "Age Rationing and the Just Distribution of Health Care," p. 340.

22. Stephen G. Post, "Justice for Elderly People in Jewish and Christian Thought," in *Too Old for Health Care?* ed. Robert Benstock and Stephen Post (Baltimore: The Johns Hopkins University Press, 1991), p. 127; Larry R. Churchill, "Should We Ration Health Care by Age?" *Journal of the American Geriatrics Society* 36 (July 1988): 646-47.

23. Battin, "Age Rationing and the Just Distribution of Health Care," p. 340.

24. Norman Daniels admits that this might be the case (*Just Health Care,* p. 99). Cf. U.S. Congress Office of Technology Assessment, *Life-Sustaining*

Technologies and the Elderly, p. 159; Veatch, "Distributive Justice and the Allocation of Technological Resources to the Elderly," pp. 21, 48.

25. Daniels, *Am I My Parents' Keeper?* p. 129.

26. Battin, "Age Rationing and the Just Distribution of Health Care," p. 337.

27. Sheldon Greenfield et al., "Patterns of Care Related to Age of Breast Cancer Patients," *Journal of the American Medical Association*, 22/29 May 1987, pp. 2766-70; Anne A. Scitovsky and Alexander M. Capron, "Medical Care at the End of Life: The Interaction of Economics and Ethics," *Annual Review of Public Health* 7 (1986): 72-73; Jeanie S. Kayser-Jones, "Distributive Justice and the Treatment of Acute Illness in Nursing Homes," *Social Science and Medicine* 23 (1986): 1279-86. Cf. Wetle, "Age as a Risk Factor for Inadequate Treatment," p. 516; and Jonathan Samet et al., "Choice of Cancer Therapy Varies with Age of Patient," *Journal of the American Medical Association*, 27 June 1986, pp. 3385-90.

28. J. Wesley Robb, "The Allocation of Limited Medical Resources: An Ethical Perspective," *Pharos* 44 (Spring 1981): 29; Gina B. Kolata, "Dialysis after Nearly a Decade," *Science*, 2 May 1980, p. 473.

29. Jerry Avorn, "Benefit and Cost Analysis in Geriatric Care: Turning Age Discrimination into Health Policy," *New England Journal of Medicine*, 17 May 1984, pp. 1294-1301. Cf. Daniels, "Is Age-Rationing Just?" pp. 19-20; and see the comments of Roger Evans in a panel discussion (Canale et al.) recorded in *Life and Death Issues*, ed. James Hamner III and Barbara Jacobs (Memphis: University of Tennessee Press, 1986), pp. 49-50.

30. Barondess et al., "Clinical Decision-Making in Catastrophic Situations," pp. 920, 923; Howard C. Eglit, *Age Discrimination* (Colorado Springs: Shepard's/McGraw-Hill, 1987), p. 1-1; Wetle, "Age as a Risk Factor for Inadequate Treatment," p. 516; David J. Maitland, *Aging: A Time for New Learning* (Atlanta: John Knox Press, 1987), pp. 2ff.; J. Gordon Harris, *God and the Elderly* (Philadelphia: Fortress Press, 1987), p. 110. For an analysis of the history of U.S. culture's preoccupation with economic productivity, see Thomas R. Cole, "The 'Enlightened' View of Aging: Victorian Morality in a New Key," *Hastings Center Report* 13 (June 1983): 34-40.

31. Kivuto Ndeti, *Elements of Akamba Life* (Nairobi: East Africa Publishing House, 1972), pp. 68-69, 104; John S. Mbiti, *Concepts of God in Africa* (London: SPCK, 1970), p. 207.

32. Joseph Muthiani, *Akamba from Within: Egalitarianism in Social Relations* (New York: Exposition Press, 1973), 74; Kivuto Ndeti, "The Role of Akamba Kithitu in Questions of Human Justice," *Proceedings of the Fifth Annual Conference* (Nairobi: University of East Africa, Social Science Council, 1969), p. 1186; W. T. W. Morgan, "Kikuyu and Kamba: The Tribal Background," in *Nairobi: City and Region*, ed. W. T. W. Morgan (Nairobi: Oxford University Press, 1967), p. 65.

33. John F. Kilner, "Who Shall Be Saved? An African Answer," *Hastings*

Center Report 14 (June 1984): 18-22. The expressions here are taken from the interviews with Kiua Mulela (Muvuti Location) and Esther Nthenya (Mbiuni Location).

34. Howard Brody, *Ethical Decisions in Medicine*, 2d ed. (Boston: Little, Brown, 1981), p. 225; Ramon Velez et al., "Treatment of End-Stage Renal Disease," *New England Journal of Medicine*, 5 February 1981, p. 356. For a cross-cultural study documenting the great variety in the ways that elderly people are treated, see Nancy Foner, *Ages in Conflict: A Cross-Cultural Perspective on Inequality between Old and Young* (New York: Columbia University Press, 1984).

35. For more on this perspective, see Nancy S. Jecker and Robert A. Pearlman, "Ethical Constraints on Rationing Medical Care by Age," *Journal of the American Geriatric Society* 37 (November 1989): 1067-75.

36. On the virtues of the elderly, see William F. May, *The Patient's Ordeal* (Bloomington, Ind.: Indiana University Press, 1991), pp. 120-41. Stephen Sapp elaborates their special potential for wisdom in *Full of Years: Aging and the Elderly in the Bible and Today* (Nashville: Abingdon Press, 1987), pp. 72-75. Regarding studies of their mental abilities, see Gary Gillund, "Memory Processes in the Aged," in *Should Medical Care Be Rationed by Age?* ed. Timothy Smeeding (Totowa, N.J.: Reuman & Littlefield, 1987), pp. 48-60; and John L. Horn, "Comments on Gillund's 'Memory Processes in the Aged,'" in *Should Medical Care Be Rationed by Age*, pp. 61-68. In much the same way that every right entails an associated responsibility, the benefit that the elderly receive from the social encouragement and appreciation of their contributions entails a moral obligation for them to contribute in whatever ways they can. See Post, "Justice for Elderly People in Jewish and Christian Thought," pp. 131-32; and Sapp, *Full of Years*, pp. 133, 159.

37. Paul Ramsey, *Ethics at the Edges of Life* (New Haven: Yale University Press, 1978), pp. xii-xiii; and Paul Ramsey, *The Patient as Person* (New Haven: Yale University Press, 1970), pp. 258-59; cf. Sapp, *Full of Years*, pp. 145-47.

38. See, e.g., Battin, "Age Rationing and the Just Distribution of Health Care," p. 335.

39. Battin, "Age Rationing and the Just Distribution of Health Care," p. 336.

40. J. Grimley Evans, "Age and Equality," *Annals of the New York Academy of Sciences* 530 (1988): 120; Wetle, "Age as a Risk Factor for Inadequate Treatment," p. 516; *Guidelines on the Termination of Life-Sustaining Treatment and the Care of the Dying* (Briarcliff Manor, N.Y.: Hastings Center, 1987), p. 136; Arthur L. Caplan, "Equity in the Selection of Recipients for Cardiac Transplants," *Circulation* 75 (January 1987): 16; Thomasma, "Quality of Life Judgments, Treatment Decisions and Medical Ethics," p. 22; Patricia M. McKevitt et al., "The Elderly on Dialysis: Physical and Psychosocial Functioning," *Dialysis and Transplantation* 15 (March 1986): 135.

41. For more extended development of these themes, see Margaret A. Somerville, "Justice across the Generations," *Social Science and Medicine* 29 (1989): 393; and Jecker and Pearlman, "Ethical Constraints on Rationing Medical Care by Age," p. 1073; cf. Churchill, "Should We Ration Health Care by Age?" p. 647.

Chapter 10

1. An international study involving respondents from thirty countries indicates that utilitarian considerations play "a very significant role in the selection process" (Roger W. Evans et al., "National Policies for the Treatment of End-Stage Renal Disease" [Seattle: Battelle Human Affairs Research Centers, 1984], p. 6). More specific studies have established that such considerations play a sizable role in such places as China (Gail E. Henderson et al., "High Technology Medicine in China," *New England Journal of Medicine,* 14 April 1988, pp. 1000-1004), Kenya (John F. Kilner, "Who Shall Be Saved? An African Answer," *Hastings Center Report* 14 [June 1984]: 18-22), Romania ("Human Rights and Scientific and Technological Developments," United Nations 30th Session, Item 70 of the Provisional Agenda, 28 July 1975), Scandinavia (E. Bergsten et al., "A Study of Patients on Haemodialysis," *Scandinavian Journal of Social Medicine* 11, suppl. [1977]: 7), Great Britain (Stanley R. Ingman et al., "ESRD and the Elderly: Cross-National Perspective on Distributive Justice," in *Ethical Dimensions of Geriatric Care,* ed. Stuart Spicker et al. [Boston: D. Reidel, 1987], p. 239; L. Carter-Jones, "Politics, Mortality and Economics — Are There Choices?" in *Renal Failure — Who Cares?* ed. F. M. Parsons and C. S. Ogg [Lancaster, Eng.: MTP, 1983], pp. 99-106; Victor Parsons and P. M. Lock, "Triage and the Patient with Renal Failure," *Journal of Medical Ethics* 6 [December 1980]: 174), and Australia (J. M. Najman et al., "Patient Characteristics Negatively Stereotyped by Doctors," *Social Science and Medicine* 16 [1982]: 1781-82). For comparable studies regarding the situation in the United States, see John F. Kilner, *Who Lives? Who Dies? Ethical Criteria in Patient Selection* (New Haven: Yale University Press, 1990), chap. 3; John F. Kilner, "Selecting Patients When Resources Are Limited: A Study of U.S. Medical Directors of Kidney Dialysis and Transplantation Facilities," *American Journal of Public Health* 78 (February 1988): 145-46; Carl M. Kjellstrand, "Age, Sex, and Race Inequality in Renal Transplantation," *Archives of Internal Medicine* 148 (June 1988): 1305-9; *National Heart Transplantation Study* (Seattle: Battelle Human Affairs Research Centers, 1984), chap. 8, pp. 30-31; chap. 44, p. 15; chap. 45, pp. 29-30; Terrie Wetle and Sue E. Levkoff, "Attitudes and Behaviors of Service Providers toward Elder Patients in the VA System," in *Older Veterans: Linking VA and Community Resources,* ed. Terrie Wetle and John

Rowe (Cambridge: Harvard University Press, 1984), p. 224; Alfred H. Katz, "Patients in Chronic Hemodialysis in the United States: A Preliminary Survey," *Social Science and Medicine* 3 (1970): 676-77; A. H. Katz and D. M. Procter, "Social-Psychological Characteristics of Patients Receiving Hemodialysis Treatment for Chronic Renal Failure" (Washington: U.S. Government Printing Office, 1969), pp. 654, 658. Cf. Larry R. Churchill, "Bone Marrow Transplantation, Physician Bias, and Down Syndrome: Ethical Reflections," *Journal of Pediatrics* 114 (January 1989): 87-88.

2. Ingman et al., "ESRD and the Elderly," p. 231; J. Wauters et al., "Selection Criteria and Physician Bias in the Treatment of End-Stage Renal Failure: Results of a National Survey," report presented at the 4th Congress of the International Society for Artificial Organs, Kyoto, Japan, 1983; Parsons and Lock, "Triage and the Patient with Renal Failure."

3. See, e.g., Marc D. Basson, "Choosing among Candidates for Scarce Medical Resources," *Journal of Medicine and Philosophy* 4 (September 1979): 330; Robert Young, "Some Criteria for Making Decisions concerning the Distribution of Scarce Medical Resources," *Theory and Decision* 6 (November 1975): 451; Nicholas Rescher, "The Allocation of Exotic Medical Lifesaving Therapy," *Ethics* 79 (1969): 179. While the social-value criterion in view here focuses on the value of future contributions, many analogous difficulties apply regarding the consideration of past contributions.

4. Carol E. Ferrans, "Quality of Life as a Criterion for Allocation of Life-Sustaining Treatment: The Case of Hemodialysis," in *Health Care Ethics*, ed. Gary Anderson and Valerie Glesnes-Anderson (Rockville, Md.: Aspen, 1987), p. 113; Emily Friedman, "Rationing and the Identified Life," *Hospitals* 58 (May 1984): 68; Renee C. Fox and Judith P. Swazey, *The Courage to Fail*, 2d ed. (Chicago: University of Chicago Press, 1978), p. 232.

5. James F. Childress, *Priorities in Biomedical Ethics* (Philadelphia: Westminster Press, 1981), p. 94; Maurice Reidy, "Distribution and Choice," *Foundations for a Medical Ethic* (New York: Paulist Press, 1979), p. 77; Helmut Thielicke, "The Doctor as Judge of Who Shall Live and Who Shall Die," in *Who Shall Live?* ed. Kenneth Vaux (Philadelphia: Fortress Press, 1970), pp. 149, 193; "Scarce Medical Resources," *Columbia Law Review* 9 (April 1969): 657; David Sanders and Jesse Dukeminier, Jr., "Medical Advance and Legal Lag: Hemodialysis and Kidney Transplantation," *UCLA Law Review* 15 (February 1968): 375.

6. Fox and Swazey, *The Courage to Fail*, p. 254; Tom Sawyer, interview with authors of "Scarce Medical Resources," dated 29 August 1968, Columbia Law Library archives; Shana Alexander, "They Decide Who Lives, Who Dies," *Life*, 9 November 1962, pp. 117, 124-25.

7. Colin Hughes, "Call for Inquiry on Kidney Patient," London *Times*, 8 January 1985, p. 3; Alexander, "They Decide Who Lives, Who Dies," p. 124.

8. Philip J. Held et al., "Access to Kidney Transplantation: Has the U.S.

Eliminated Income and Racial Differences?" *Archives of Internal Medicine* 148 (December 1988): 2594-2600; Jeff Lyon, "Organ Transplants: Conundra without End," *Second Opinion* 2 (March 1986): 59; Fox and Swazey, *The Courage to Fail,* p. 249; Comptroller General of the United States, "Report to the Congress: Treatment of Chronic Kidney Failure: Dialysis, Transplant, Costs, and the Need for More Vigorous Efforts" (Washington: U.S. Dept. of Health, Education, and Welfare, 1975), pp. 16-17.

9. "Scarce Medical Resources," p. 643.

10. Kilner, "Selecting Patients When Resources Are Limited," pp. 145-46; cf. Kilner, *Who Lives? Who Dies?* pp. 217-20.

11. With regard to limited general support, see Kilner, *Who Lives? Who Dies?* chap. 4; and Kilner, "Selecting Patients When Resources Are Limited," pp. 145-46. With regard to differentiation among candidates for organ transplantation on the basis of locality, see Roger W. Evans and Diane L. Manninen, "Public Opinion concerning Organ Donation, Procurement, and Distribution," survey conducted for UNOS by Battelle Human Affairs Research Centers, Seattle, Washington, 1987, p. 4; John A. Robertson, "Supply and Distribution of Hearts for Transplantation: Legal, Ethical, and Policy Issues," *Circulation* 75 (January 1987): 82; Task Force on Organ Transplantation, *Organ Transplantation: Issues and Recommendations* (Rockville, Md.: U.S. Dept. of Health and Human Services, 1986), p. 86; *The Access of Foreign Nationals to U.S. Cadaver Organs* (Boston: U.S. Dept. of Health and Human Services, 1986), pp. 4, 16; and Stanley R. Mandel, "Setting the Record Straight on Organ Sales," *Hastings Center Report* 16 (August 1986): 48-49. With regard to giving preferential treatment to veterans, see Norman G. Levinsky, "Health Care for Veterans: The Limits of Obligation," *Hastings Center Report* 16 (August 1986): 11; Christina H. Sommers, "Once a Soldier, Always a Dependent," *Hastings Center Report* 16 (August 1986): 16; and *The Price of Life: Ethics and Economics* (Minneapolis: Minnesota Coalition on Health Care Costs, 1984), p. 50.

12. See Olga Jonasson, "In Organ Transplants, Americans First?" *Hastings Center Report* 16 (October 1986): 24. George Shreiner reported an increase in organ donation among the 65,000 ethnic Greeks in Washington, D.C., when Georgetown University opened its kidney transplantation program to Greek nationals in 1983 ("Procurement and Allocation of Human Organs for Transplantation," November 2 and 9 hearings of the U.S. House of Representatives Committee on Science and Technology, Subcommittee on Investigations and Oversight [Washington: U.S. Government Printing Office, 1983], p. 199).

13. For further arguments in favor of a quota system and details regarding how it should function, see Kilner, *Who Lives? Who Dies?* pp. 52-54. Cf. *The Access of Foreign Nationals to U.S. Cadaver Organs,* pp. 5-16; Task Force on Organ Transplantation, *Organ Transplantation: Issues and Recommendations,* pp. 94-95, 137-38; James W. Nickel, "Should Undocumented Aliens Be Entitled to Health Care?" *Hastings Center Report* 16 (December 1986): 22-23;

Jonasson, "In Organ Transplants, Americans First?" p. 24; Jeffrey M. Prottas, "In Organ Transplants, Americans First?" *Hastings Center Report* 16 (October 1986): 24; John I. Kleinig, "In Organ Transplants, Americans First?" *Hastings Center Report* 16 (October 1986): 25.

14. Kilner, *Who Lives? Who Dies?* chap. 8; and "Selecting Patients When Resources Are Limited," pp. 145-46; Jeanie S. Kayser-Jones, "Distributive Justice and the Treatment of Acute Illness in Nursing Homes," *Social Science and Medicine* 23 (1986): 1280-81; William J. Winslade and Judith W. Ross, *Choosing Life or Death* (New York: Free Press, 1986), p. 190; *National Heart Transplantation Study*, chap. 10, p. 25; Roger W. Evans et al., "National Policies for the Treatment of End-Stage Renal Disease," pp. 6, 12; Henry J. Aaron and William B. Schwartz, *The Painful Prescription: Rationing Hospital Care* (Washington: Brookings Institution, 1984), p. 34; Joann Rodgers, "Life on the Cutting Edge," *Psychology Today* 18 (October 1984): 61; Wetle and Levkoff, "Attitudes and Behaviors of Service Providers toward Elder Patients in the VA System," p. 224.

15. Rodgers, "Life on the Cutting Edge," p. 64; Stanley Rabinowitz and Hermanus I. J. van der Spuy, "Selection Criteria for Dialysis and Renal Transplant," *American Journal of Psychiatry* 135 (July 1978): 861. The histories of patient selection for scarce insulin and dialysis in the United States provide vivid examples of the inaccuracy of psychological-ability criteria. See Karen Merriken and Thomas D. Overcast, "Patient Selection for Heart Transplantation: When Is a Discriminating Choice Discrimination?" *Journal of Health Politics, Policy and Law* 10 (Spring 1985): 19-20; Roberta G. Simmons and Richard L. Simmons, "Sociological and Psychological Aspects of Transplantation," in *Transplantation*, ed. J. S. Najarian and R. L. Simmons (Philadelphia: Lea & Febiger, 1972), p. 369.

16. George Weckman and Richard W. Willy, "Descriptive Medical Ethics and Allocation," *Listening* 22 (Winter 1987): 16; Working Group on Mechanical Circulatory Support, National Heart, Lung and Blood Institute, *Artificial Heart and Assist Devices: Directions, Needs, Costs, Societal and Ethical Issues* (Bethesda, Md.: National Institutes of Health, 1985), p. 26.

17. Charles Krauthammer, "Lifeboat Ethics: The Case of Baby Jesse," Washington *Post*, 13 June 1986, p. A19; Samuel Z. Goldhaber et al., "Cardiac Surgery for Adults with Mental Retardation: Dilemmas in Management," *American Journal of Medicine* (October 1985): 405; Christopher Robbins, "The Ethical Challenge of Health Care Rationing," in *The End of an Illusion: The Future of Health Policy in Western Industrialized Nations*, ed. Jean de Kervasdoue et al. (Berkeley and Los Angeles: University of California Press, 1984), p. 124.

18. Sawyer, interview with authors of "Scarce Medical Resources," p. 17.

19. Regarding the degree to which psychological problems can be treated, see Jack G. Copeland et al., "Selection of Patients for Cardiac Trans-

plantation," *Circulation* 75 (1987): 6; and Rodgers, "Life on the Cutting Edge," p. 62. On dialysis, see Parsons and Lock, "Triage and the Patient with Renal Failure," p. 44. On stress, see J. Auer, "Social and Psychological Issues of End-Stage Renal Failure," in *Renal Failure — Who Cares?* ed. F. M. Parsons and C. S. Ogg (Lancaster, Eng.: MTP, 1983), p. 207.

20. For arguments presented in the United States, see Kilner, *Who Lives? Who Dies?* chap. 9; and "Selecting Patients When Resources Are Limited," pp. 145-46; Paul A. Haber, "Rationing Is a Reality," *Journal of the American Geriatrics Society* 34 (October 1986): 763; Sharon M. Paulus, "Suit Filed in Oklahoma Alleging Twenty-Four Infants Died after Being Denied Beneficial Medical Treatment," *Issues in Law and Medicine* 1 (January 1986): 323; and *National Heart Transplantation Study,* chap. 4, pp. 29-30; chap. 8, pp. 6, 58-59, 66; and chap. 10, pp. 22, 24. For arguments presented in other countries, see Kilner, *Who Lives? Who Dies?* chap. 9; Frances H. Miller, "Reflections on Organ Transplantation in the United Kingdom," *Law Medicine and Health Care* 13 (February 1985): 31; Evans et al., "National Policies for the Treatment of End-Stage Renal Disease," pp. 6, 12; and Elizabeth Ward, "Death or Dialysis — A Personal View," *British Medical Journal,* 22/29 December 1984, p. 1712.

21. See Rodgers, "Life on the Cutting Edge," pp. 62-63. More generally, see Working Group on Mechanical Circulatory Support, National Heart, Lung and Blood Institute, *Artificial Heart and Assist Devices,* p. 26.

22. Nora K. Bell, "Triage in Medical Practices: An Unacceptable Model?" *Social Science and Medicine* 15F (December 1981): 155; and "Why Medical Criteria Won't Work in the Allocation of Scarce Medical Resources," *Georgia Journal of Science* 37 (January 1979): 18.

23. Paulus, "Suit Filed in Oklahoma Alleging Twenty-Four Infants Died after Being Denied Beneficial Medical Treatment," p. 323; Working Group on Mechanical Circulatory Support, National Heart, Lung and Blood Institute, *Artificial Heart and Assist Devices,* p. 26.

24. *National Heart Transplantation Study,* chap. 9, p. 37.

25. Roger W. Evans, "Money Matters: Should Ability to Pay Ever Be a Consideration in Gaining Access to Transplantation?" *Transplantation Proceedings* 21 (June 1989): 3419-23; Jeremiah A. Barondess et al., "Clinical Decision-Making in Catastrophic Situations: The Relevance of Age," *Journal of American Geriatrics Society* 36 (October 1988): 934; Howard H. Hiatt, *America's Health in the Balance: Choice or Chance?* (New York: Harper & Row, 1987), p. 4; Larry R. Churchill, *Rationing Health Care in America: Perceptions and Principles of Justice* (South Bend, Ind.: University of Notre Dame Press, 1987), pp. 10-11; E. Richard Brown, "DRGs and the Rationing of Hospital Care," in *Health Care Ethics,* ed. Gary Anderson and Valerie Glesnes-Anderson (Rockville, Md.: Aspen, 1987), pp. 70-71.

26. Regarding dialysis and organ transplantation, see Kilner, *Who Lives? Who Dies?* chap. 16; and "Selecting Patients When Resources Are

Limited," pp. 145-46; Held et al., "Access to Kidney Transplantation"; Timothy M. Smeeding, "Artificial Organs, Transplants and Long-Term Care for the Elderly: What's Covered? Who Pays?" in *Should Medical Care Be Rationed by Age?* ed. Timothy M. Smeeding (Totowa, N.J.: Rowman & Littlefield, 1987), p. 155; Roger W. Evans and Junichi Yagi, "Social and Medical Considerations Affecting Selection of Transplant Recipients: The Case of Heart Transplantation," in *Human Organ Transplantation,* ed. Dale H. Cowan et al. (Ann Arbor: Health Administration Press, 1987), p. 28; Robertson, "Supply and Distribution of Hearts for Transplantation," p. 28; Task Force on Organ Transplantation, *Organ Transplantation: Issues and Recommendations,* pp. 18, 86, 96, 100; and U.S. Department of Health and Human Services Task Force on Organ Transplantation, "Report to the Secretary and the Congress on Immunosuppressive Therapies" (Rockville, Md.: U.S. Government Printing Office, 1985), p. 18. Regarding intensive and emergency care, see Arthur L. Kellermann and Bela B. Hackman, "Emergency Department Patient 'Dumping': An Analysis of Interhospital Transfers to the Regional Medical Center at Memphis, Tennessee," *American Journal of Public Health* 78 (October 1988): 1289-90; David A. Ansell and Robert L. Schiff, "Patient Dumping: Status, Implications, and Policy Recommendations," *Journal of the American Medical Association,* 20 March 1987, p. 1501; Robert L. Schiff et al., "Transfer to a Public Hospital: A Prospective Study of 467 Patients," *New England Journal of Medicine,* 27 February 1986, pp. 554-56; William G. Reed et al., "The Effect of a Public Hospital's Transfer Policy on Patient Care," *New England Journal of Medicine,* 27 November 1986, p. 1431; "For-Profit Hospital Care: Who Profits? Who Cares?" (Washington: National Council of Senior Citizens, 1986), pp. 3-10; Geraldine Dallek and Judith Waxman, " 'Patient Dumping': A Crisis in Emergency Medical Care for the Indigent," *Clearinghouse Review* 19 (April 1986): 1413; and Claudia J. Coulton, "Resource Limits and Allocation in Critical Care," in *Human Values in Critical Care Medicine,* ed. Stuart J. Youngner (New York: Praeger, 1986), p. 97.

27. Henderson et al., "High Technology Medicine in China"; Joyce Bermel, "Organs for Sale: From Marketplace to Jungle," *Hastings Center Report* 16 (February 1986): 3; Transplantation Society (Council), "Commercialisation in Transplantation: The Problems and Some Guidelines for Practice," *Lancet,* 28 September 1985, p. 716; Drummond Rennie et al., "Limited Resources and the Treatment of End-stage Renal Failure in Britain and the United States," *Quarterly Journal of Medicine* 56, n.s. (July 1985): 321-36; Andrew Schneider and Mary P. Flaherty, "The Challenge of a Miracle: Selling the Gift," Pittsburg *Press,* 3-10 November 1985; Evans et al., "National Policies for the Treatment of End-Stage Renal Disease," pp. 6, 12; Victor Fuchs, "The 'Rationing' of Medical Care," *New England Journal of Medicine,* 13 December 1984, p. 1572.

28. Task Force on Organ Transplantation, *Organ Transplantation: Issues and Recommendations,* p. 105; "Preliminary Analysis — Small Group Meet-

ings" (Tustin, Calif.: California Health Decisions, 1986), p. 3; Washington Health Choices, *Executive Report* (Seattle: Puget Sound Health Systems Agency, 1986), p. 5; *National Heart Transplantation Study*, chap. 35, pp. 2-3; chap. 36, p. 22; Evans et al., "National Policies for the Treatment of End-Stage Renal Disease," p. 13; President's Commission for the Study of Ethical Problems in Medicine and Biomedical and Behavioral Research, *Securing Access to Health Care* (Washington: U.S. Government Printing Office, 1983), p. 26.

29. For a more detailed examination of the ethics of buying and selling organs for transplantation, see Kilner, *Who Lives? Who Dies?* pp. 183-84.

30. For analyses of the way this public-appeal form of the ability-to-pay criterion functions, see Robert H. Blank, *Rationing Medicine* (New York: Columbia University Press, 1988), pp. 48, 97; Albert Gore, Jr., "National Transplantation Network: UNOS or NBC," Loma Linda University Ethics Center *Update* 3 (January 1987): 3; Allen R. Dyer, "Patients, Not Costs, Come First," *Hastings Center Report* 16 (February 1986): 5-6; Winslade and Ross, *Choosing Life or Death*, pp. 195-96; and Elizabeth Wehr, "National Health Policy Sought for Organ Transplant Surgery," *Congressional Quarterly*, 25 February 1984, p. 453. For situations in which this form of the criterion has proven decisive, see Marcia Chambers, "Tough Transplant Questions Raised by 'Baby Jesse' Case," New York *Times*, 15 June 1986, p. 16; Kevin D. O'Rourke and Dennis Brodeur, *Medical Ethics: Common Ground for Understanding*, vol. 2 (St. Louis: Catholic Health Association of the U.S., 1989), p. 57; Eugene L. Meyer, "Tax Money for Transplant Operations: Who Pays?" Washington *Post*, 12 September 1984, pp. C1, 8; and John K. Iglehart, "Transplantation: The Problem of Limited Resources," *New England Journal of Medicine*, 14 July 1983, p. 127.

31. For a discussion of funding denied on the basis of skin color, see D'Orsay D. Bryant III, "Spare Part Surgery: The Ethics of Organ Transplantation," *Journal of the National Medical Association* 77 (February 1985): 116. (In fact, statistics show that an overwhelming percentage of organ transplants have gone to white patients — see Gina B. Kolata, "Liver Transplants Endorsed," *Science*, 8 July 1983, p. 139.) For a discussion of funding denied because of a lack of interest on the part of the physician, see H. J. J. Leenen, "The Selection of Patients in the Event of a Scarcity of Medical Facilities — An Unavoidable Dilemma," *International Journal of Medicine and Law* 12 (Fall 1979): 165. For other examples of unsuccessful attempts to raise the funds necessary for treatment, see "Dying for Want of a Transplant: One Man's Plight, Society's Burden," *Medical World News*, 14 November 1983, p. 50.

32. See Loretta M. Kopelman, "Justice and the Hippocratic Tradition of Acting for the Good of the Sick," in *Ethics and Critical Care Medicine*, ed. John C. Moskop and Loretta Kopelman (Boston: D. Reidel, 1985), p. 94; cf. Norman Daniels, "The Ideal Advocate and Limited Resources," *Theoretical Medicine* 8 (February 1987): 77-78. One exceptional example of generosity in the United States is an Ohio consortium of transplant surgeons and institutions who •

agreed to devote 25 percent of transplant-related fees and gifts to transplants for poor persons — see David L. Jackson and George J. Annas, "The Introduction of Major Organ Transplantation on the State Level: Ethical and Practical Considerations in the Development of Public Policy," in *Human Values in Critical Care Medicine,* ed. Stuart Youngner (New York: Praeger, 1986), p. 118.

33. "Dying Friend Extends Life through Heart Transplant," Lexington *Herald-Leader,* 17 November 1988, p. A10; Gore, "National Transplantation Network," p. 3.

Chapter 11

1. John F. Kilner, *Who Lives? Who Dies? — Ethical Criteria in Patient Selection* (New Haven: Yale University, 1990), chap. 15; John F. Kilner, "Ethical Issues in the Initiation and Termination of Treatment," *American Journal of Kidney Diseases* 15 (March 1990): 220; John F. Kilner, "Selecting Patients When Resources Are Limited: A Study of U.S. Medical Directors of Kidney Dialysis and Transplantation Facilities," *American Journal of Public Health* 78 (February 1988): 145-46; Claudia J. Coulton, "Resource Limits and Allocation in Critical Care," in *Human Values in Critical Care Medicine,* ed. Stuart J. Youngner (New York: Praeger, 1986), p. 97; Terrie Wetle and Sue E. Levkoff, "Attitudes and Behaviors of Service Providers toward Elder Patients in the VA System," in *Older Veterans: Linking VA and Community Resources,* ed. Terrie Wetle and John Rowe (Cambridge: Harvard University Press, 1984), p. 224; *National Heart Transplantation Study* (Seattle: Battelle Human Affairs Research Centers, 1984), chap. 8, pp. 30-31.

2. Kilner, *Who Lives? Who Dies?* chap. 10; "Ethical Issues in the Initiation and Termination of Treatment," pp. 220-21; and "Selecting Patients When Resources Are Limited," pp. 145-46; Dan W. Brock, "Ethical Issues in Recipient Selection for Organ Transplantation," in *Organ Substitution Technology,* ed. Deborah Mathieu (Boulder: Westview Press, 1988), p. 88; Working Group on Mechanical Circulatory Support, National Heart, Lung and Blood Institute, *Artificial Heart and Assist Devices: Directions, Needs, Costs, Societal and Ethical Issues* (Bethesda, Md.: National Institutes of Health, 1985), p. 26; Bruce E. Zawacki, "ICU Physician's Ethical Role in Distributing Scarce Resources," *Critical Care Medicine* 13 (January 1985): 59; *National Heart Transplantation Study,* chap. 8.

3. See further discussion in Chapter 7, as well as David L. Jackson and George J. Annas, "The Introduction of Major Organ Transplantation on the State Level: Ethical and Practical Considerations in the Development of Public Policy," in *Human Values in Critical Care Medicine,* ed. Stuart Youngner (New York: Praeger, 1986), p. 119; Albert R. Jonsen et al., *Clinical Ethics* (New York: Macmillan, 1982), pp. 31-32.

4. Kilner, *Who Lives? Who Dies?* chap. 11; John A. Robertson, "Supply and Distribution of Hearts for Transplantation: Legal, Ethical, and Policy Issues," *Circulation* 75 (January 1987): 82; Coulton, "Resource Limits and Allocation in Critical Care," p. 97; Jane Warmbrodt, "Who Gets the Organs?" *Midwest Medical Ethics* 1 (Summer 1985): 3; Frances H. Miller, "Reflections on Organ Transplantation in the United Kingdom," *Law Medicine and Health Care* 13 (February 1985): 32; U.S. House of Representatives Committee on Science and Technology, Subcommittee on Investigations and Oversight, "Procurement and Allocation of Human Organs for Transplantation," November 2 and 9 hearings (Washington: U.S. Government Printing Office, 1983), pp. 19, 80, 106-9; Stuart W. Hinds, "Triage in Medicine," in *Triage in Medicine and Society,* ed. George R. Lucas (Houston: Texas Medical Center Institute of Religion and Human Development, 1975), p. 16; Henry K. Beecher, *Research and the Individual* (Boston: Little, Brown, 1971), p. 279.

5. Roger W. Evans and Diane L. Manninen, "Public Opinion concerning Organ Donation, Procurement, and Distribution," results of a survey conducted for UNOS by Battelle Human Affairs Research Centers, Seattle, Washington, 1987, p. 4.

6. Some have suggested that when vital resources are scarce, the first people to be excluded from treatment should be those who are responsible for their illness. There is considerable difference of opinion about who would fall into this category, but some would nominate alcoholics, heavy smokers, overeaters, AIDS patients, and the like who have engaged in behaviors that they knew posed risks to their health. However, it would probably be too difficult to apply this sort of criterion fairly in the practice of health care with our current level of knowledge. Were such a criterion to be employed, though, the described perspective's commitment to fairness would suggest that people should not be denied treatment unless a number of conditions were met. First, their disorder would have to have been demonstrably caused by their own actions and not by other factors. Second, they would have to have been capable of freely engaging in these actions. Third, they would have to have been aware of the strong possibility that the disorder in question would result. Fourth, the search for all connections between personal behavior and medical disorders should at least be under way, and the criterion would have to be used consistently on the basis of our best knowledge about such connections. We should not require alcoholics to pledge abstinence, for example, if we have no intention of requiring comparable abstinence on the part of those with other destructive behaviors (smoking, overeating, etc.). It would be so difficult to meet these conditions that a fair and workable selection criterion is unlikely in the foreseeable future. For more on this criterion see Kilner, *Who Lives? Who Dies?* chap. 15; and David Orentlicher, "Denying Treatment to the Noncompliant Patient," *Journal of the American Medical Association,* 27 March 1991, pp. 1501-2.

7. Kilner, *Who Lives? Who Dies?* chap. 17; and "Selecting Patients When Resources Are Limited," pp. 145-46; "Memorandum on UNOS Policy regarding Utilization of the Point System for Cadaveric Kidney Allocation," 11 November 1988, p. 24; Gordon F. Snyder, *Tough Choices* (Elgin, Ill.: Brethren Press, 1988), p. 84; Maxwell J. Mehlman, "Rationing Expensive Lifesaving Medical Treatments," *Wisconsin Law Review*, no. 2 (1985): 270; Miller, "Reflections on Organ Transplantation in the United Kingdom," p. 32; Fred Rosner, "Allocation of Scarce Medical Resources," *New York State Journal of Medicine* 83 (March 1983): 357; Gerald R. Winslow, *Triage and Justice* (Berkeley and Los Angeles: University of California Press, 1982), pp. 100, 102, 147; Hinds, "Triage in Medicine," pp. 16-17.

8. Paul A. Haber, "Rationing Is a Reality," *Journal of the American Geriatrics Society* 34 (October 1986): 763; Mehlman, "Rationing Expensive Lifesaving Medical Treatments," p. 271; Christopher Robbins, "The Ethical Challenge of Health Care Rationing," in *The End of an Illusion: The Future of Health Policy in Western Industrialized Nations*, ed. Jean de Kervasdoue et al. (Berkeley and Los Angeles: University of California Press, 1984), p. 126.

9. With respect to special cases such as natural disasters and organ transplantation in which exceptions may be warranted, see Kilner, *Who Lives? Who Dies?* pp. 198-206.

10. For an example of a culture that has traditionally tended to endorse this outlook, see John F. Kilner, "Who Shall Be Saved? An African Answer," *Hastings Center Report* 14 (June 1984), p. 19.

11. Arguments about whether we should distinguish between a patient who has never received an organ transplant and a patient who has received an organ but now needs another are not addressed by the resources-required criterion. The reason for applying the criterion — saving more lives — is not applicable in such a case: no matter who receives the available organ, lives beyond that of the recipient are not likely to be saved. See Kilner, *Who Lives? Who Dies?* pp. 60-61.

12. Kilner, *Who Lives? Who Dies?* chap. 5; and "Selecting Patients When Resources Are Limited," pp. 145-46; Roger W. Evans et al., "National Policies for the Treatment of End-Stage Renal Disease" (Seattle: Battelle Human Affairs Research Centers, 1984), pp. 6, 12; Winslow, *Triage and Justice*, p. 74; Arthur C. Kennedy, "The Problem of ESRD in Developing Countries," in *Proceedings of the 8th International Congress of Nephrology* (Athens: N.p., 1981), pp. 585-86.

13. For wartime examples, see H. G. Pledger, "Triage of Casualties after Nuclear Attack," *Lancet*, 20 September 1986, p. 678; Robbins, "The Ethical Challenge of Health Care Rationing," pp. 125-26; and Henry K. Beecher, *Research and the Individual* (Boston: Little, Brown, 1971), pp. 280-81. For other situations, see Kilner, *Who Lives? Who Dies?* chap. 6; Kilner, "Selecting Patients When Resources Are Limited," pp. 145-46; and Winslow, *Triage and Justice*, pp. 27-28.

14. If not all eligible candidates who satisfy at least one of these criteria can be treated with available resources, the selection that saves the greatest number of lives is to be preferred. When it is not possible to determine on the basis of available information which of several patients should receive treatment, recipients should be selected by means of a lottery.

15. With respect to special cases such as natural disasters and organ transplantation in which exceptions may be warranted, see Kilner, *Who Lives? Who Dies?* pp. 198-206.

Conclusion

1. See Howard H. Hiatt, *America's Health in the Balance: Choice or Chance?* (New York: Harper & Row, 1987), pp. 5-6.

2. For example, a key cost-cutting strategy of the 1980s — eliminating inappropriate in-patient hospital days — has just about reached the limit of its effectiveness. See William B. Schwartz and Daniel N. Mendelson, "Hospital Cost Containment in the 1980's — Hard Lessons Learned and Prospects for the 1990's," *New England Journal of Medicine,* 11 April 1991, pp. 1037-42.

3. For more extended discussion of this idea, see Kevin W. Wildes, "Health Care Rationing and Insured Access: Does the Catholic Tradition Have Anything to Say?" *Linacre Quarterly* 58 (August 1991): 50-58; and John F. Kilner, *Who Lives? Who Dies? Ethical Criteria in Patient Selection* (New Haven: Yale University Press, 1990), pp. 186-87.

4. See Paul R. McGinn, "Infant Mortality Battle: Heroic Saves, Tragic Losses," *American Medical News,* 7 January 1991, pp. 23-24.

5. The National Perinatal Information Center study, from which the birth-weight and monetary figures here are drawn, is summarized by Rebecca Voelker in "Weighing Costs, Benefits in Neonatal Care," *American Medical News,* 7 January 1991, p. 22. It should be noted that if poor pregnant women are to obtain access to prenatal care, funds are needed for more than the direct cost of the care itself. Some women may not be able to afford transportation to the clinic, others may need someone to care for their other children during the office visits, and so on. Also, achieving the kind of cost savings suggested here would require strengthened cooperation among multiple levels of government. The costs of bringing urban women in for prenatal care, for instance, would likely have to be borne by a city government's health care department, whereas the savings realized in reduced neonatal intensive care would likely be enjoyed primarily by state and national governments.

6. A slightly different form of the expression is found in Gerald H. Friedland, "Clinical Care in the AIDS Epidemic," *Daedalus* 118 (Spring 1989): 62.

7. These figures are drawn from the Children's Defense Fund report

"Maternal and Infant Health: Special Interim Report on Prenatal Care, Low-Birthweight Birth, and Public Health Service Year 2000 Objectives" (Washington: Children's Defense Fund, 1990). The ratios cited represent the following figures. Whereas 12 percent of black newborns weigh less than 2500 grams, only 6 percent of white newborns fall into this category. Three percent of black newborns weigh less than 1500 grams; the comparable figure for white newborns is 1 percent.

8. For similar health care financing problems in the United States affecting Native Americans, see *Bridging the Gap: Report of the Task Force on Parity of Indian Health Services* (Washington: Department of Health and Human Services, 1986); regarding health care for mentally retarded persons, see Arnold Birenbaum et al., *Health Care Financing for Severe Developmental Disabilities* (Washington: American Association on Mental Retardation, 1990).

9. Some have described it as a moral duty; see, e.g., Tony Campolo, *Twenty Hot Potatoes Christians Are Afraid to Touch* (Dallas: Word Books, 1988), p. 143; and Paul T. Menzel, *Strong Medicine* (New York: Oxford University Press, 1990), p. 195.

10. *Active Euthanasia, Religion, and the Public Debate* (Chicago: Park Ridge Center for the Study of Health, Faith, and Ethics, 1991), p. 111. Cf. Daniel Callahan, *What Kind of Life?* (New York: Simon & Schuster, 1990), pp. 241-46.

References Cited

Aaron, Henry J., and William B. Schwartz. *The Painful Prescription: Rationing Hospital Care*. Washington: Brookings Institution, 1984.

Abrams, Fredrick R. "Access to Health Care." In *Health Care Ethics*, edited by Gary Anderson and Valerie Glesnes-Anderson, 49-68. Rockville, Md.: Aspen, 1987.

"Account of Assisted Suicide in Journal Advances Debate." *Medical Ethics Advisor* 7 (April 1991): 44-47.

Achtemeier, Paul J. " 'Some Things in Them Hard to Understand': Reflections on an Approach to Paul." *Interpretation* 38 (1984): 254-67.

Adami, Hans-Olov, et al. "The Relation between Survival and Age at Diagnosis in Breast Cancer." *New England Journal of Medicine*, 28 August 1986, 559-63.

Alexander, Eben. "Euthanasia." *Surgical Neurology* 31 (June 1989): 480-81.

Alexander, Leo. "Medical Science under Dictatorship." *New England Journal of Medicine*, 14 July 1949, 39-47.

Alexander, Shana. "They Decide Who Lives, Who Dies." *Life*, 9 November 1962, 102-25.

Ames, Katrine, et al. "Last Rights." *Newsweek*, 26 August 1991, 40-41.

Anderson, J. Kerby. "Euthanasia: A Biblical Appraisal." *Bibliotheca Sacra* 144 (April-June 1987): 208-17.

Anderson, Norman. *Issues of Life and Death*. Downers Grove, Ill.: InterVarsity Press, 1976.

304

Andrews, Keith. "Persistent Vegetative State." *British Medical Journal*
    303 (July 1991): 121.
Angell, Marcia. "Euthanasia." *New England Journal of Medicine*, 17
    November 1988, 1348-50.
Annas, George J. "The Health Care Proxy and the Living Will." *New
    England Journal of Medicine*, 25 April 1991, 1210-13.
————. "The Prostitute, the Playboy, and the Poet: Rationing
    Schemes for Organ Transplantation." *American Journal of Public
    Health* 75 (February 1985): 187-89.
Ansell, David A., and Robert L. Schiff. "Patient Dumping: Status,
    Implications, and Policy Recommendations." *Journal of the
    American Medical Association*, 20 March 1987, 1500-1502.
Aquinas, Thomas. *Summa Theologica*. New York: McGraw-Hill, 1964.
Aristotle. *Nichomachean Ethics*. Indianapolis: Bobbs-Merrill, 1962.
Arras, John D. "Utility, Natural Rights, and the Right to Health
    Care." In *Biomedical Ethics Reviews*, edited by James Humber
    and Robert Almeder, 23-45. Clifton, N.J.: Humana, 1984.
Ashley, Benedict M., and Kevin D. O'Rourke. *Health Care Ethics: A
    Theological Analysis*. 3d ed. St. Louis: Catholic Hospital Asso-
    ciation, 1989.
Augustine of Hippo. *The City of God*. Translated by Marcus Dods.
    New York: Random House, 1950.
Auer, J. "Social and Psychological Issues of End-Stage Renal Failure."
    In *Renal Failure — Who Cares?* edited by F. M. Parsons and C. S.
    Ogg, 205-14. Lancaster, England: MTP, 1983.
Avorn, Jerry. "Benefit and Cost Analysis in Geriatric Care: Turning
    Age Discrimination into Health Policy." *New England Journal
    of Medicine*, 17 May 1984, 1294-1301.
Bacchiocchi, Samuele. "Matthew 11:28-30: Jesus' Rest and the Sab-
    bath." *Andrews University Seminary Studies* 22 (Autumn 1984):
    289-316.
Bailey, Lloyd R., Sr. *Biblical Perspectives on Death*. Philadelphia:
    Fortress Press, 1979.
Banks, Robert. *Paul's Idea of Community*. Grand Rapids: William B.
    Eerdmans, 1980.
Barondess, Jeremiah A., et al. "Clinical Decision-Making in Cata-
    strophic Situations: The Relevance of Age." *Journal of the Amer-
    ican Geriatrics Society* 36 (October 1988): 919-37.
Barth, Karl. *Church Dogmatics*. Vol. 3, part 4, translated by A. T.
    Mackay et al., 324-43. Edinburgh: T. & T. Clark, 1961. Re-
    printed in *On Moral Medicine*, edited by Stephen Lammers and
    Allen Verhey, 109-21. Grand Rapids: William B. Eerdmans,
    1987.

Basson, Marc D. "Choosing among Candidates for Scarce Medical Resources." *The Journal of Medicine and Philosophy* 4 (September 1979): 313-33.

Battin, Margaret P. "Age Rationing and the Just Distribution of Health Care: Is There a Duty to Die?" *Ethics* 97 (January 1987): 317-40.

————. *Ethical Issues in Suicide.* Englewood Cliffs, N.J.: Prentice-Hall, 1982.

Bayer, Edward J. "Perspectives from Catholic Theology." In *By No Extraordinary Means: The Choice to Forgo Life-Sustaining Food and Water,* edited by Joanne Lynn, 89-98. Bloomington, Ind.: Indiana University Press, 1986.

Bayly, Joseph. *Winterflight.* Waco, Tex.: Word Books, 1981.

Beauchamp, Tom L. "Can We Stop or Withhold Dialysis?" In *Controversies in Nephrology — 1979,* edited by George Schreiner, 163-70. Washington: Georgetown University, Nephrology Division, 1979.

Becker, E. Lovell. "Finite Resources and Medical Triage." *American Journal of Medicine* 66 (April 1979): 549-50.

Beecher, Henry K. *Research and the Individual.* Boston: Little, Brown, 1971.

Beker, J. Christiaan. *Suffering and Hope.* Philadelphia: Fortress Press, 1987.

Belkin, Lisa. "Patient's Death Sought against Family's Wishes." *Lexington Herald-Leader,* 11 January 1991, A3, A7.

Bell, Nora K. "Triage in Medical Practices: An Unacceptable Model?" *Social Science and Medicine* 15F (December 1981): 151-56.

————. "Why Medical Criteria Won't Work in the Allocation of Scarce Medical Resources." *Georgia Journal of Science* 37 (January 1979): 13-20.

Benrubi, Guy I. "Euthanasia — The Need for Procedural Safeguards." *New England Journal of Medicine,* 16 January 1992, 197-99.

Berkouwer, G. C. *Man: The Image of God.* Grand Rapids: William B. Eerdmans, 1962.

Bergsten, E., et al. "A Study of Patients on Haemodialysis." *Scandinavian Journal of Social Medicine* 11, Suppl. (1977): 7-31.

Bermel, Joyce. "Organs for Sale: From Marketplace to Jungle." *Hastings Center Report* 16 (February 1986): 3-4.

Betz, Hans D. "Cosmogony and Ethics in the Sermon on the Mount." In *Cosmogony and Ethical Order,* edited by Robin Lovin and Frank Reynolds, 158-76. Chicago: University of Chicago Press, 1985.

Birch, Bruce C., and Larry L. Rasmussen. *Bible and Ethics in the Christian Life*. Rev. ed. Minneapolis: Augsburg Press, 1989.

Birenbaum, Arnold, et al. *Health Care Financing for Severe Developmental Disabilities*. Washington: American Association on Mental Retardation, 1990.

Blank, Robert H. *Rationing Medicine*. New York: Columbia University Press, 1988.

Blazquez, Niceto. "The Church's Traditional Moral Teaching on Suicide." In *Suicide and the Right to Die*, edited by Jacques Pohier and Dietmer Mieth, 63-74. Edinburgh: T. & T. Clark, 1985.

Bloesch, Donald. *Freedom for Obedience*. San Francisco: Harper & Row, 1987.

Bockmuehl, Klaus. "The Great Commandment." *Crux* 23 (September 1987): 10-20.

Bonhoeffer, Dietrich. *Ethics*. Edited by Eberhard Bethge, translated by Neville Smith. New York: Macmillan, 1955.

Bornkamm, Günther. *Paul*. Translated by D. M. G. Stalker. New York: Harper & Row, 1971.

Bouma, Hessel, III, et al. *Christian Faith, Health, and Medical Practice*. Grand Rapids: William B. Eerdmans, 1989.

Boyd, Kenneth. "Terminal Care, Euthanasia and Suicide." *Modern Churchmen* 30 (1988): 9-16.

Boyd, Kenneth, and Brian Potter. "Priorities in the Allocation of Scarce Resources." *Journal of Medical Ethics* 12 (December 1986): 197-200.

Brahams, Diana. "When Is Discontinuation of Dialysis Justified?" *Lancet*, 19 January 1985, 176-77.

Braine, David. *Medical Ethics and Human Life*. Aberdeen: Palladio, 1983.

Brandt, Richard B. "The Real and Alleged Problem of Utilitarianism." *Hastings Center Report* 13 (April 1983): 37-43.

Brennan, William. *Medical Holocausts I: Exterminative Medicine in Nazi Germany and Contemporary America*. Boston: Nordland, 1980.

Bresnahan, James F. "Catholic Spirituality and Medical Interventions in Dying." *America*, 29 June 1991, 670-75.

Brett, Allan S. "Limitations of Listing Specific Medical Interventions in Advance Directives." *Journal of the American Medical Association*, 14 August 1991, 825-28.

Brock, Dan W. "Ethical Issues in Recipient Selection for Organ Transplantation." In *Organ Substitution Technology*, edited by Deborah Mathieu, 86-99. Boulder: Westview, 1988.

Brody, Howard. *Ethical Decisions in Medicine*. 2d ed. Boston: Little, Brown, 1981.

————. *Stories of Sickness.* New Haven: Yale University Press, 1987.

Brody, Jane E. "Living Will Lets Individual Dictate Terminally Ill Treatment." *Lexington Herald-Leader,* 7 October 1989, C1, C4.

Brown, E. Richard. "DRGs and the Rationing of Hospital Care." In *Health Care Ethics,* edited by Gary Anderson and Valerie Glesnes-Anderson, 69-90. Rockville, Md.: Aspen, 1987.

Brown, Harold O. J. " 'Why Will Ye Die, O House of Israel?' " In *The Death Decision,* edited by Leonard J. Nelson, 95-114. Ann Arbor: Servant Publications, 1984.

————. "Euthanasia: Lessons from Nazism." *Human Life Review* 13 (Spring 1987): 88-99.

Brown, Robert M. *Unexpected News: Reading the Bible with Third World Eyes.* Louisville: Westminster/John Knox Press, 1984.

Browning, Don S. "Hospital Chaplaincy as Public Ministry." *Second Opinion* 1 (1986): 66-75.

Brunk, Conrad G. "In the Image of God." In *Medical Ethics, Human Choices: A Christian Perspective,* edited by John Rogers, 29-39. Scottdale, Pa.: Herald Press, 1988.

Bryant, D'Orsay D., III. "Spare Part Surgery: The Ethics of Organ Transplantation." *Journal of the National Medical Association* 77 (February 1985): 113-17.

Buckingham, Robert W. *The Complete Hospice Guide.* New York: Harper & Row, 1983.

Bultmann, Rudolf. *Theologie des Neuen Testaments.* Tübingen: J. C. B. Mohr, 1953.

Byrn, Robert M. "Compulsory Lifesaving Treatment for the Competent Adult." *Fordham Law Review* 44 (October 1975): 1-36.

Cahill, Lisa S. "The Ethical Implications of the Sermon on the Mount." *Interpretation* 41 (April 1987): 144-56.

Calabresi, Guido, and Philip Bobbitt. *Tragic Choices.* New York: W. W. Norton, 1978.

Califano, Joseph A., Jr. *America's Health Care Revolution: Who Lives? Who Dies? Who Pays?* New York: Random House, 1986.

California Health Decisions. "Preliminary Analysis — Small Group Meetings." Tustin, Calif.: California Health Decisions, 1986.

"California Natural Death Act." California Health and Safety Code, div. 7, pt. 1, chap. 3, 9, secs. 7185-7195 (signed into law 1 October 1976). In *Ethics in Medicine,* edited by Stanley Reiser et al., 665-67. Cambridge: M.I.T. Press, 1977.

Callahan, Daniel. "Aging and the Ends of Medicine." *Annals of the New York Academy of Sciences* 530 (1988): 125-32.

————. "On Feeding the Dying." *Hastings Center Report* 13 (October 1983): 22.

————. *Setting Limits: Medical Goals in an Aging Society.* New York: Simon & Schuster, 1987.

————. *What Kind of Life.* New York: Simon & Schuster, 1990.

Callahan, Sidney. "The Limits on Self-Destruction." *Health Progress* 73 (April 1992): 72-73.

Callaway, John, et al. "Diagnosis Critical: Health Care in the 80's" (video). Broadcast on WTTW (Chicago), 29 October 1986.

Calvin, John. *Institutes of the Christian Religion.* Vols. 20-21 of the Library of Christian Classics. Edited by John T. McNeill, translated by Ford Lewis Battles. Philadelphia: Westminster Press, 1960.

Campbell, Courtney S., and Bette-Jane Crigger. "Mercy, Murder, and Morality." *Hastings Center Report* 19 (January/February 1989): S1.

Campolo, Tony. "When Is It OK to Tell the Doctor to Pull the Plug?" In his *Twenty Hot Potatoes Christians Are Afraid to Touch*, 143-47. Dallas: Word Books, 1988.

Canale, Dee J., et al. "Panel Discussion." In *Life and Death Issues*, edited by James Hamner III and Barbara Jacobs, 41-54. Memphis: University of Tennessee Press, 1986.

Caplan, Arthur L. "Equity in the Selection of Recipients for Cardiac Transplants." *Circulation* 75 (January 1987): 10-19.

————. "A New Dilemma: Quality, Ethics and Expensive Medical Technologies." *New York Medical Quarterly* 6 (1986): 23-27.

————. "Obtaining and Allocating Organs for Transplantation." In *Human Organ Transplantation*, edited by Dale H. Cowan et al., 5-17. Ann Arbor: Health Administration, 1987. .

————. "The Selection of Patients for Dialytic Therapy — Should Treatment Be Left to Chance?" *Dialysis and Transplantation* 13 (March 1984): 155-61.

Carlston, Charles E. "Matthew 6:24-34." *Interpretation* 41 (April 1987): 179-83.

Carson, Ronald A. "Interpretive Bioethics: The Way of Discernment." *Theoretical Medicine* 11 (March 1990): 51-59.

Carter-Jones, L. "Politics, Mortality and Economics — Are There Choices?" In *Renal Failure — Who Cares?* edited by F. M. Parsons and C. S. Ogg, 99-106. Lancaster, England: MTP, 1983.

Cassel, Christine K. "Doctors and Allocation Decisions: A New Role in the New Medicare." *Journal of Health Politics, Policy, and Law* 10 (Fall 1985): 549-64.

Central Committee of the Royal Dutch Medical Association. "Vision on Euthanasia." *Medisch Contact* 39 (1984): 990-98.

Challah, S., et al. "Negative Selection of Patients for Dialysis and

Transplantation in the United Kingdom." *British Medical Journal,* 14 April 1984, 1119-22.

Chalmers, George L. "Life Issues: Euthanasia." In *Medicine in Crisis: A Christian Response,* edited by Ian Brown and Nigel Cameron, 102-19. Edinburgh: Rutherford House, 1988.

Chambers, Marcia. "Tough Transplant Questions Raised by 'Baby Jesse' Case." *New York Times,* 15 June 1986, 1+.

Chandler, Emily. "Theology and Ethics: A Feminist and Liberation Theology Perspective." In *Health Care and Its Costs: A Challenge for the Church,* edited by Walter Wiest, 229-43. Lanham, Md.: University of America Press, 1988.

Charlson, Mary E., et al. "Resuscitation: How Do We Decide?" *Journal of the American Medical Association,* 14 March 1986, 1316-22.

Children's Defense Fund. "Maternal and Infant Health: Special Interim Report on Prenatal Care, Low-Birthweight Birth, and Public Health Service Year 2000 Objectives." Washington: Children's Defense Fund, 1990.

Childress, James F. "Allocating Health Care Resources." In *Priorities in Medical Ethics,* 74-97, 129-35. Philadelphia: Westminster Press, 1981.

————. "Artificial and Transplanted Organs." In *Biolaw,* vol. I, edited by J. F. Childress et al., 303-31. Frederick, Md.: University Publications of America, 1986.

Chinard, Francis P. "Ethics and Technology." *Journal of the Medical Society of New Jersey* 82 (February 1985): 119-23.

Churchill, Larry R. "Bone Marrow Transplantation, Physician Bias, and Down Syndrome: Ethical Reflections." *Journal of Pediatrics* 114 (January 1989): 87-88.

————. *Rationing Health Care in America: Perceptions and Principles of Justice.* South Bend, Ind.: University of Notre Dame Press, 1987.

————. "Should We Ration Health Care by Age?" *Journal of the American Geriatrics Society* 36 (July 1988): 644-47.

Churchill, Larry R., and Jose J. Siman. "Principles and the Search for Moral Certainty." *Social Science and Medicine* 23 (1986): 461-68.

Clark, Phillip G. "The Social Allocation of Health Care Resources: Ethical Dilemmas in Age-Group Competition." *Gerontologist* 25 (April 1985): 119-25.

Clemons, James T. *What Does the Bible Say about Suicide?* Minneapolis: Fortress Press, 1990.

Cobb, John B., Jr. *Matters of Life and Death.* Louisville: Westminster/John Knox Press, 1991.

Cole, C. Donald. *Christian Perspectives on Controversial Issues.* Chicago: Moody Press, 1982.

Cole, Harry A. "Deciding on a Time to Die: A Fitting Response." *Second Opinion* 7 (March 1988): 11-25.

Cole, Thomas R. "The 'Enlightened' View of Aging: Victorian Morality in a New Key." *Hastings Center Report* 13 (June 1983): 34-40.

Collange, Jean-François. *De Jesus à Paul: L'ethique du Nouveau Testament.* Geneva: Labor et Fides, 1980.

Collins, Raymond F. *Christian Morality: Biblical Foundations.* Notre Dame, Ind.: University of Notre Dame Press, 1986.

Comptroller General of the United States. "Report to the Congress: Treatment of Chronic Kidney Failure: Dialysis, Transplant, Costs, and the Need for More Vigorous Efforts." Washington: U.S. Department of Health, Education, and Welfare, 1975.

Cone, James H. *A Black Theology of Liberation.* Philadelphia: Lippincott, 1970.

Connelly, R. J. "Natural Death and Christian Fasting." *Journal of Religion and Health* 25 (Fall 1986): 227-36.

Connery, John R. "Quality of Life." *Linacre Quarterly* 53 (February 1986): 26-33.

Cooper, Theodore. "Survey of Development, Current Status, and Future Prospects for Organ Transplantation." In *Human Organ Transplantation,* edited by Dale Cowan et al., 18-26. Ann Arbor: Health Administration Press, 1987.

Copeland, Jack G., et al. "Selection of Patients for Cardiac Transplantation." *Circulation* 75 (1987): 1-9.

Corr, Charles A., and Donna M. Corr, eds. *Hospice Care: Principles and Practice.* New York: Springer, 1983.

Coulton, Claudia J. "Resource Limits and Allocation in Critical Care." In *Human Values in Critical Care Medicine,* edited by Stuart J. Youngner, 87-108. New York: Praeger, 1986.

Cranford, Ronald E. "The Persistent Vegetative State: The Medical Reality (Getting the Facts Straight)." *Hastings Center Report* 18 (February/March 1988): 27-32.

Cranford, Ronald E., et al. "Helga Wanglie's Ventilator." *Hastings Center Report* 21 (July-August 1991): 23-29.

Cummings, Nancy B. "Uremia Therapy: The Resource Allocation Dilemma from a Global Perspective." *Kidney International* 28, Suppl. 17 (1985): S133-35.

Dallek, Geraldine, and Judith Waxman. " 'Patient Dumping': A Crisis in Emergency Medical Care for the Indigent." *Clearinghouse Review* 19 (April 1986): 1413-17.

D'Amico, G. "Treating End-Stage Renal Failure in Italy." In *Renal Failure — Who Cares?* edited by F. M. Parsons and C. S. Ogg, 89-98. Lancaster, England: MTP, 1983.

Daniel, Stephen L. "The Patient as Text: A Model of Clinical Hermeneutics." *Theoretical Medicine*, June 1986, 195-210.

Daniels, Norman. "Am I My Parents' Keeper?" In the President's Commission for the Study of Ethical Problems in Medicine and Biomedical and Behavioral Research, *Securing Access to Health Care*, vol. 2, 265-91. Washington: U.S. Government Printing Office, 1983.

————. *Am I My Parents' Keeper? An Essay on Justice between the Young and Old.* New York: Oxford University Press, 1988.

————. "Is Age-Rationing Just?" Paper delivered at the Pacific Section of the American Philosophical Association, San Francisco, March 1986.

————. "The Ideal Advocate and Limited Resources." *Theoretical Medicine* 8 (February 1987): 69-80.

————. *Just Health Care.* London: Cambridge University Press, 1985.

Davis, John J. "Brophy vs. New England Sinai Hospital." *Journal of Biblical Ethics in Medicine* 1 (July 1987): 53-56.

De Blois, Jean, et al. "Advance Directives for Healthcare Decisions: A Christian Perspective." *Health Progress* 72 (July-August 1991): 27-31.

Deidun, T. J. *New Covenant Morality in Paul.* Rome: Biblical Institute, 1981.

"Dental Drug 'Awakens' Man in Vegetative State." *Lexington Herald-Leader,* 29 March 1990, A3.

Dessaur, C. I., and C. J. C. Rutenfrans. "Mag de dokter doden?" Amsterdam: Querido, 1986.

Destro, Robert A. "Quality-of-Life Ethics and Constitutional Jurisprudence: The Demise of Natural Rights and Equal Protection for the Disabled and Incompetent." *Journal of Contemporary Health Law and Policy* 2 (Spring 1986): 71-130.

DeVries, William C., et al. "Clinical Use of the Total Artificial Heart." *New England Journal of Medicine,* 2 February 1984, 273-78.

De Wachter, M. A. M. "Active Euthanasia in the Netherlands." *Journal of the American Medical Association,* 15 December 1989, 3316-19.

Doukas, David J., and Laurence B. McCullough. "The Values History: The Evaluation of the Patient's Values and Advance Directives." *Journal of Family Practice* 32 (1991): 145-53.

Doukas, David J., et al. "The Living Will: A National Survey." *Family Medicine* 23 (July 1991): 354-56.

Doyle, B. Rod. "A Concern of the Evangelist: Pharisees in Matthew 12." *Australian Biblical Review* 34 (October 1986): 17-34.

Drane, James F. *Becoming a Good Doctor.* Kansas City: Sheed & Ward, 1988.

Duclow, Donald F. "Into the Whirlwind of Suffering: Resistance and Transformation." *Second Opinion* 9 (November 1988): 10-27.

Dunstan, G. R. *The Artifice of Ethics.* London: SCM Press, 1974.

Dyck, Arthur J. *On Human Care.* Nashville: Abingdon Press, 1977.

————. "The Image of God: An Ethical Foundation for Medicine." *Linacre Quarterly* 57 (February 1990): 35-45.

Dyer, Allen R. "Patients, Not Costs, Come First." *Hastings Center Report* 16 (February 1986): 5-7.

"Dying for Want of a Transplant: One Man's Plight; Society's Burden." *Medical World News,* 14 November 1983, 49-50.

"Dying Friend Extends Life through Heart Transplant." *Lexington Herald-Leader,* 17 November 1988, A10.

Edmunds, Lavinia. "The Long Wait for a New Life." *Johns Hopkins Magazine* 41 (February 1989): IX-XVI.

Eglit, Howard C. *Age Discrimination.* Colorado Springs: Shepard's/McGraw-Hill, 1987.

Ellul, Jacques. *The Ethics of Freedom.* Grand Rapids: William B. Eerdmans, 1976.

Emanuel, Linda L., and Ezekiel J. Emanuel. "The Medical Directive: A New Comprehensive Advance Care Document." *Journal of the American Medical Association,* 9 June 1989, 3288-93.

Engelhardt, H. Tristram, Jr. "The Counsels of Finitude." In *Death Inside Out,* edited by Peter Steinfels and Robert Veatch, 115-25. New York: Harper & Row, 1974.

Epstein, Aaron. "Lawyer Pleads for 'Liberty' of Coma Victim." *Lexington Herald-Leader,* 7 December 1989, 1, 6.

Erdahl, Lowell O. *Pro-Life/Pro-Peace.* Minneapolis: Augsburg Press, 1986.

"European Hospitals Less Technology-Intensive, Less Expensive than U.S." *Medical World News,* 12 March 1984, 23-24.

Evans, J. Grimley. "Age and Equality." *Annals of the New York Academy of Sciences* 530 (1988): 118-24.

Evans, Roger W. "Health Care Technology and the Inevitability of Resource Allocation and Rationing Decisions." *Journal of the American Medical Association,* 15 April 1983, 2047-53, and 22/29 April 1983, 2208-19.

————. "Money Matters: Should Ability to Pay Ever Be a Consideration in Gaining Access to Transplantation?" *Transplantation Proceedings* 21 (June 1989): 3419-23.

Evans, Roger W., and Diane L. Manninen. "Public Opinion concerning Organ Donation, Procurement, and Distribution." Results of a survey conducted for the United Network for Organ Sharing by Battelle Human Affairs Research Centers, Seattle, 1987.

Partially published in *Transplantation Proceedings* 20 (October 1988): 781-85.

Evans, Roger W., and Junichi Yagi. "Social and Medical Considerations Affecting Selection of Transplant Recipients: The Case of Heart Transplantation." In *Human Organ Transplantation,* edited by Dale H. Cowan et al., 27-41. Ann Arbor: Health Administration Press, 1987.

Evans, Roger W., et al. "National Policies for the Treatment of End-Stage Renal Disease." Seattle: Battelle Human Affairs Research Centers, 1984.

———. "The Quality of Life of Patients with End-Stage Renal Disease." *New England Journal of Medicine,* 28 February 1985, 553-59.

Farley, Margaret A. "Feminist Consciousness and the Interpretation of Scripture." In *Feminist Interpretation of the Bible,* edited by Letty Russell, 41-51. Philadelphia: Westminster Press, 1985.

Feldman, David M. *Health and Medicine in the Jewish Tradition.* New York: Crossroad, 1986.

Fenigsen, Richard. "A Case against Dutch Euthanasia." *Hastings Center Report* 19 (January/February 1989): 522-30.

———. "Mercy, Murder, and Morality." *Hastings Center Report* 19 (November/December 1989): 50-51.

———. "The Report of the Dutch Governmental Committee on Euthanasia." *Issues in Law and Medicine* 7 (Winter 1991): 339-44.

Ferrans, Carol E. "Quality of Life as a Criterion for Allocation of Life-Sustaining Treatment: The Case of Hemodialysis." In *Health Care Ethics,* edited by Gary Anderson and Valerie Glesnes-Anderson, 109-24. Rockville, Md.: Aspen, 1987.

Field, Mervin D. "California Poll: Strong Public Support for the Right to Die." *San Francisco Chronicle,* 21 July 1983, 12.

"Final Report of the Netherlands State Commission on Euthanasia: An English Summary." *Bioethics* 1 (1987): 163-74.

Fiorenza, Elizabeth Schüssler. *In Memory of Her.* New York: Crossroad, 1983.

Fish, Nina M. "Hospice: Terminal Illness, Teamwork and the Quality of Life." In *Social Work in Health Settings,* edited by Toba Kerson, 449-69. New York: Haworth Press, 1989.

Fletcher, John. "Ethical Issues." In *Current Therapy in Critical Care Medicine,* edited by Joseph Parrillo, 341-44. Philadelphia: B. C. Decker, 1987.

Fletcher, Joseph. *Situation Ethics.* Philadelphia: Westminster Press, 1966.

Foley, Kathleen M. "The Relationship of Pain and Symptom Man-

agement to Patient Requests for Physician-Assisted Suicide."
Journal of Pain and Symptom Management 6 (July 1991): 289-97.

Foner, Nancy. *Ages in Conflict: A Cross-Cultural Perspective on Inequality between Old and Young*. New York: Columbia University Press, 1984.

Fox, Renee C., and Judith P. Swazey. *The Courage to Fail*. 2d ed. Chicago: University of Chicago Press, 1978.

Frame, John M. *Medical Ethics: Principles, Persons, and Problems*. Grand Rapids: Baker Book House, 1988.

Francis, John G., and Leslie P. Francis. "Rationing of Health Care in Britain: An Ethical Critique of Public Policy-Making." In *Should Medical Care Be Rationed by Age?* edited by Timothy M. Smeeding, 119-34. Totowa, N.J.: Rowman & Littlefield, 1987.

Francis, Leslie P. "Poverty, Age Discrimination, and Health Care." In *Poverty, Justice, and the Law*, edited by George R. Lucas, 117-29. Lanham, Md.: University Press of America, 1986.

Friedland, Gerald H. "Clinical Care in the AIDS Epidemic." *Daedalus* 118 (Spring 1989): 59-83.

Friedman, Emily. "Rationing and the Identified Life." *Hospitals* 58 (May 1984): 65-66+.

Friedrich, Otto. "One Miracle, Many Doubts." *Time*, 10 December 1984, 70-77.

Fries, James F. "Aging, Natural Death, and the Compression of Morbidity." *New England Journal of Medicine*, 17 July 1980, 130-35.

Fromer, Margot J. *Ethical Issues in Health Care*. St. Louis: C. V. Mosby, 1981.

Fuchs, Victor. "The 'Rationing' of Medical Care." *New England Journal of Medicine*, 13 December 1984, 1572-73.

Fumento, Michael. "The Dying Dutchman: Coming Soon to a Nursing Home Near You." *American Spectator*, October 1991, 18-22.

Furnish, Victor P. *The Love Command in the New Testament*. Nashville: Abingdon Press, 1972.

———. *The Moral Teaching of Paul: Selected Issues*, 2nd ed. Nashville: Abingdon Press, 1985.

———. *Theology and Ethics in Paul*. Nashville: Abingdon Press, 1968.

Gaylin, Willard, et al. " 'Doctors Must Not Kill.' " *Journal of the American Medical Association*, 8 April 1988, pp. 2139-40.

Geelhoed, Glenn W. "Access to Care in a Changing Practice Environment." *Bulletin of the American College of Surgeons* 70 (June 1985): 11-15.

Geisler, Norman. *Options in Contemporary Christian Ethics*. Grand Rapids: Baker Book House, 1981.

Georgi, Dieter. *Die Geschichte der Kollekte des Paulus für Jerusalem.* Hamburg-Bergstedt: Reich, 1965.

Gerhardsson, Birger. *The Ethos of the Bible.* Philadelphia: Fortress Press, 1981.

Gervais, Karen G. *Redefining Death.* New Haven: Yale University Press, 1986.

Gillon, Raanan. "Justice and Allocation of Medical Resources." *British Medical Journal,* 27 July 1985, 266-68.

Gillund, Gary. "Memory Processes in the Aged." In *Should Medical Care Be Rationed by Age?* edited by Timothy M. Smeeding, 48-60. Totowa, N.J.: Rowman & Littlefield, 1987.

Glover, Jonathan. *Causing Death and Saving Lives.* New York: Penguin, 1977.

Godshall, Stan. "Allocating Limited Medical Resources." In *Medical Ethics, Human Choices: A Christian Perspective,* edited by John Rogers, 121-31. Scottdale, Pa.: Herald Press, 1988.

Goldhaber, Samuel Z., et al. "Cardiac Surgery for Adults with Mental Retardation: Dilemmas in Management." *American Journal of Medicine,* October 1985, 403-6.

Gomez, Carlos F. *Regulating Death: The Case of the Netherlands.* New York: Free Press, 1991.

Gooch, Paul W. "Authority and Justification in Theological Ethics: A Study in I Corinthians 7." *Journal of Religious Ethics* 11 (Spring 1983): 62-74.

Gore, Albert, Jr. "National Transplantation Network: UNOS or NBC." Loma Linda University Ethics Center *Update* 3 (January 1987): 3-5.

Gostin, Larry, and Robert F. Weir. "Life and Death Choices after *Cruzan:* Case Law and Standards of Professional Conduct." *Milbank Quarterly* 69 (1991): 143-73.

Graber, Glenn C., et al. *Ethical Analysis of Clinical Medicine.* Baltimore: Urban & Schwarzenberg, 1985.

Green, Charles. "Government Might Step into Fray, Push 'Living Wills.'" *Lexington Herald-Leader,* 12 January 1990, A2.

Greenfield, Sheldon, et al. "Patterns of Care Related to Age of Breast Cancer Patients." *Journal of the American Medical Association,* 22/29 May 1987, 2766-70.

Grisez, Germain, and Joseph M. Boyle, Jr. "The Morality of Killing: A Traditional View." In *Bioethics: Reading and Cases,* edited by Baruch Brody and H. Tristram Engelhardt, Jr., 156-60. Englewood Cliffs, N.J.: Prentice-Hall, 1987.

Grundmann, Walter. "ἀγαθός. . . ." In *Theological Dictionary of the New Testament,* vol. 1, edited by Gerhard Kittel, translated by Geoffrey Bromiley, 10-18. Grand Rapids: William B. Eerdmans, 1964.

Gruson, Lindsey. "Some Doctors Move to Bar Transplants to Foreign Patients." *New York Times,* 10 August 1985, 1, 5.

Gula, Richard M. *What Are They Saying about Euthanasia?* New York: Paulist Press, 1986.

Gunby, Phil. "Media-Abetted Liver Transplants Raise Questions of 'Equity and Decency.' " *Journal of the American Medical Association,* 15 April 1983, 1973-74+.

Gustafson, James M. "The Transcendence of God and the Value of Human Life." In *On Moral Medicine: Theological Perspectives in Medical Ethics,* edited by Stephen Lammers and Allen Verhey, 121-26. Grand Rapids: William B. Eerdmans, 1987.

Haber, Paul A. "Rationing Is a Reality." *Journal of the American Geriatrics Society* 34 (October 1986): 761-63.

Hall, David R. "Romans 3:1-8 Reconsidered." *New Testament Studies* 29 (1983): 183-97.

Halper, Thomas. "Life and Death in a Welfare State: End-Stage Renal Disease in the United Kingdom." *Milbank Memorial Fund Quarterly* 63 (Winter 1985): 52-93.

Haney, Daniel Q. "Panel Backs Doctors' Aiding in Suicides of Terminally Ill." *Lexington Herald-Leader,* 30 March 1989, 1, 5.

Hardwig, John. "Robin Hoods and Good Samaritans: The Role of Patients in Health Care Distribution." *Theoretical Medicine* 8 (February 1987): 47-59.

Harris, J. Gordon. *God and the Elderly.* Philadelphia: Fortress Press, 1987.

Harris, John. "QALYfying the Value of Life." *Journal of Medical Ethics* 13 (September 1987): 117-23.

Hastings Center. *Guidelines on the Termination of Life-Sustaining Treatment and the Care of the Dying.* Briarcliff Manor, N.Y.: Hastings Center, 1987.

Hastings Center Research Group. "Values and Life-Extending Technologies." In *Life Span,* edited by Robert M. Veatch, 29-79. San Francisco: Harper & Row, 1979.

Hauerwas, Stanley. *A Community of Character.* Notre Dame, Ind.: University of Notre Dame Press, 1981.

————. *Naming the Silences.* Grand Rapids: William B. Eerdmans, 1990.

————. "Rational Suicide and Reasons for Living." In *On Moral Medicine: Theological Perspectives in Medical Ethics,* edited by Stephen Lammers and Allen Verhey, 460-66. Grand Rapids: William B. Eerdmans, 1987.

————. "Religious Concepts of Brain Death and Associated Problems." In *Brain Death,* Julius Korein, 329-38. New York: New York Academy of Sciences, 1978.

————. *Suffering Presence.* Notre Dame, Ind.: University of Notre Dame Press, 1986.

Held, Philip J., et al. "Access to Kidney Transplantation: Has the U.S. Eliminated Income and Racial Differences?" *Archives of Internal Medicine* 148 (December 1988): 2594-2600.

Hendee, William R. "Rationing Health Care." In *Life and Death Issues,* edited by James Hamner III and Barbara Jacobs, 1-10. Memphis: University of Tennessee Press, 1986.

Henderson, Gail E., et al. "High Technology Medicine in China." *New England Journal of Medicine,* 14 April 1988, 1000-1004.

Hiatt, Howard H. *America's Health in the Balance: Choice or Chance?* New York: Harper & Row, 1987.

Hicks, John M. "The Sabbath Controversy in Matthew: An Exegesis of Matthew 12:1-14." *Restoration Quarterly* 27 (1984): 79-91.

Hilhorst, H. W. A. *Euthanasia in het ziekenhuis.* Lochem-Poperinge: De Tijdstroom, 1983.

Hinds, Stuart W. "Triage in Medicine." In *Triage in Medicine and Society,* edited by George R. Lucas. Houston: Texas Medical Center Institute of Religion and Human Development, 1975.

Holifield, E. Brooks. *Health and Medicine in the Methodist Tradition.* New York: Crossroad, 1986.

Hollinger, Dennis. "Can Bioethics Be Evangelical?" *Journal of Religious Ethics* 17 (Fall 1989): 161-79.

Holmberg, Bengt. *Paul and Power.* Lund, Sweden: C. W. K. Gleerup, 1978.

Holmes, Arthur F. *Ethics: Approaching Moral Decisions.* Downers Grove, Ill.: InterVarsity Press, 1984.

————. *Shaping Character.* Grand Rapids: William B. Eerdmans, 1991.

Horn, John L. "Comments on Gillund's 'Memory Processes in the Aged.'" In *Should Medical Care Be Rationed by Age?* edited by Timothy M. Smeeding, 61-68. Totowa, N.J.: Rowman & Littlefield, 1987.

Horsley, Richard. "Ethics and Exegesis: 'Love Your Enemies' and the Doctrine of Non-Violence." *Journal of the American Academy of Religion* 54 (Spring 1986): 3-31.

Houlden, J. L. *Ethics and the New Testament.* Baltimore: Penguin, 1973.

House, Deborah M. "Advance Medical Directives and the Role of the Church." *Christian Century,* 4 December 1991, 1137-39.

Hughes, Colin. "Call for Inquiry on Kidney Patient." *London Times,* 8 January 1985, 3.

Humphry, Derek. *Final Exit*. Eugene, Oreg.: The Hemlock Society, 1991.

Hunter, Kathryn M. "Making a Case." *Literature and Medicine* 7 (1988): 66-79.

Hutchinson, Tom A., et al. "Predicting Survival in Adults with End-Stage Renal Disease: An Age Equivalence Index." *Annals of Internal Medicine* 96 (April 1982): 417-23.

Hyman, Allen I. "Commentary on Belliotti's 'Allocation of Resources.'" *Values and Ethics in Health Care* 5 (1980): 263-65.

———. "Ethical Considerations in Intensive Care." In *Human and Ethical Issues in the Surgical Care of Patients with Life-Threatening Disease,* edited by Frederic Herter et al., 39-43. Springfield, Ill.: Charles C. Thomas, 1986.

Iglehart, John K. "Transplantation: The Problem of Limited Resources." *New England Journal of Medicine,* 14 July 1983, 123-28.

Indian Health Service. *Bridging the Gap: Report of the Task Force on Parity of Indian Health Services*. Washington: U.S. Department of Health and Human Services, 1986.

Ingman, Stanley R., et al. "ESRD and the Elderly: Cross-National Perspective on Distributive Justice." In *Ethical Dimensions of Geriatric Care,* edited by Stuart Spicker et al., 223-62. Boston: D. Reidel, 1987.

"It's Over, Debbie." *Journal of the American Medical Association,* 8 January 1988, 272.

Jackson, David L., and George J. Annas. "The Introduction of Major Organ Transplantation on the State Level: Ethical and Practical Considerations in the Development of Public Policy." In *Human Values in Critical Care Medicine,* edited by Stuart Youngner, 109-22. New York: Praeger, 1986.

Jackson, Douglas MacG., and David S. Short. "The Distinctive Christian Ethic in Medical Practice." In *Medical Ethics: A Christian View,* 2d ed., edited by Vincent Edmunds and C. Gorden Scorer, 11-27. London: Tyndale Press, 1966.

Jamieson, Dale. "The Artificial Heart: Reevaluating the Investment." In *Organ Substitution Technology,* edited by Deborah Mathieu, 277-93. Boulder: Westview Press, 1988.

Jecker, Nancy S., and Robert A. Pearlman. "Ethical Constraints on Rationing Medical Care by Age." *Journal of the American Geriatric Society* 37 (November 1989): 1067-75.

Jewett, Robert. *Christian Tolerance: Paul's Message to the Modern Church*. Philadelphia: Westminster Press, 1982.

Johnson, Timothy, et al. "Medical Miracles: Can We Afford the Bill?" ABC News Nightline, 29 August 1985.

Jonasson, Olga. "In Organ Transplants, Americans First?" *Hastings Center Report* 16 (October 1986): 24-25.

Jones, D. Gareth. *Brave New People*. Rev. ed. Grand Rapids: William B. Eerdmans, 1985.

Jonsen, Albert R., et al. *Clinical Ethics*. New York: Macmillan, 1982.

Kalb, Paul E., and David H. Miller. "Utilization Strategies for Intensive Care Units." *Journal of the American Medical Association*, 28 April 1989, 2389-95.

Kant, Immanuel. *Foundations of the Metaphysics of Morals*. Indianapolis: Bobbs-Merrill, 1969.

Kantzer, Kenneth S. "Biomedical Decision Making: We Dare Not Retreat." *Christianity Today*, 21 March 1986, 15I-16I.

Käsemann, Ernst. *Jesus Means Freedom*. Translated by F. Clarke. Philadelphia: Fortress Press, 1969.

Kass, Leon R. "Averting One's Eyes, or Facing the Music? — On Dignity and Death." In *Death Inside Out*, edited by Peter Steinfels and Robert Veatch, 101-14. New York: Harper & Row, 1974.

————. "Neither for Love Nor Money: Why Doctors Should Not Kill." Paper presented at the annual meeting of the American Association of Medical Colleges, Chicago, 13 November 1988.

Katz, Alfred H. "Patients in Chronic Hemodialysis in the United States: A Preliminary Survey." *Social Science and Medicine* 3 (1970): 669-77.

Katz, A. H., and D. M. Procter. "Social-Psychological Characteristics of Patients Receiving Hemodialysis Treatment for Chronic Renal Failure." U.S. Department of Health, Education, and Welfare, Kidney Disease Control Program. Washington: U.S. Government Printing Office, 1969.

Kayser-Jones, Jeanie S. "Distributive Justice and the Treatment of Acute Illness in Nursing Homes." *Social Science and Medicine* 23 (1986): 1279-86.

Keck, Leander E. *Paul and His Letters*. Philadelphia: Fortress Press, 1979.

Keegan, Terence J. "Paul's Dying/Rising Ethics in I Corinthians." In *Christian Biblical Ethics*, edited by Robert J. Daly. New York: Paulist Press, 1984.

Kellermann, Arthur L., and Bela B. Hackman. "Emergency Department Patient 'Dumping': An Analysis of Interhospital Transfers to the Regional Medical Center at Memphis, Tennessee." *American Journal of Public Health* 78 (October 1988): 1287-92.

Kennedy, Arthur C. "The Problem of ESRD in Developing Countries." In *Proceedings of the 8th International Congress of Nephrology*, 584-89. Athens: N.p., 1981.

Kevorkian, Jack. *Prescription: Medicide.* Buffalo: Prometheus, 1991.

Kilner, John F. "Ethical Issues in the Initiation and Termination of Treatment." *American Journal of Kidney Diseases* 15 (March 1990): 218-27.

————. "Hurdles for Natural Law Ethics: Lessons from Grotius." *American Journal of Jurisprudence* 28 (1983): 149-67.

————. "Selecting Patients When Resources Are Limited: A Study of U.S. Medical Directors of Kidney Dialysis and Transplantation Facilities." *American Journal of Public Health* 78 (February 1988): 144-47.

————. *Who Lives? Who Dies? — Ethical Criteria in Patient Selection.* New Haven: Yale University Press, 1990.

————. "Who Shall Be Saved? An African Answer." *Hastings Center Report* 14 (June 1984): 18-22.

King, Thomas C. "Ethical Dilemmas of Restricted Resources." In *Human and Ethical Issues in the Surgical Care of Patients with Life-Threatening Disease,* edited by Frederic Herter et al., 169-75. Springfield, Ill.: Charles C. Thomas, 1986.

Kirby, Michael D. "Bioethical Decisions and Opportunity Costs." *Journal of Contemporary Health Law and Policy* 2 (Spring 1986): 7-21.

Kjellstrand, Carl M. "Age, Sex, and Race Inequality in Renal Transplantation." *Archives of Internal Medicine* 148 (June 1988), 1305-9.

————. "Who Should Decide about Your Death?" *Journal of the American Medical Association,* 1 January 1992, 103-4.

Kjellstrand, Carl M., and George M. Logan. "Racial, Sexual and Age Inequalities in Chronic Dialysis." *Nephron* 45 (1987): 257-63.

Kleinig, John I. "In Organ Transplants, Americans First?" *Hastings Center Report* 16 (October 1986): 25.

————. *Valuing Life.* Princeton: Princeton University Press, 1991.

Kleinman, Arthur. *The Illness Narratives: Suffering, Healing and the Human Condition.* New York: Basic Books, 1988.

Kolata, Gina B. "Dialysis after Nearly a Decade." *Science,* 2 May 1980, 473-76.

————. "Liver Transplants Endorsed." *Science,* 8 July 1983, 139.

Koop, C. Everett. *Right to Live, Right to Die.* Wheaton: Tyndale Press, 1976.

Kopelman, Loretta M. "Justice and the Hippocratic Tradition of Acting for the Good of the Sick." In *Ethics and Critical Care Medicine,* edited by John C. Moskop and Loretta Kopelman, 79-103. Boston: D. Reidel, 1985.

Kotulak, Ronald. "Never-Say-Die Policy Prompts Rationing Call." *Chicago Tribune,* 15 July 1986, 1+.

Krabill, Willard S. "Death and Dying: Prevailing Medical Perspectives." In *Medical Ethics, Human Choices: A Christian Perspective*, edited by John Rogers, 53-61. Scottdale, Pa.: Herald Press, 1988.

Krauthammer, Charles. "Lifeboat Ethics: The Case of Baby Jesse." *Washington Post*, 13 June 1986, A19.

Kübler-Ross, Elisabeth. *Death: The Final Stage of Growth*. Englewood Cliffs, N.J.: Prentice-Hall, 1975.

Kuitert, Harry. "Have Christians the Right to Kill Themselves? From Self-Murder to Self-Killing." In *Suicide and the Right to Die*, edited by Jacques Pohier and Dietmar Mieth, 100-106. Edinburgh: T. & T. Clark, 1985.

Lambert, P., et al. "The Values History: An Innovation in Surrogate Medical Decision-Making." *Law, Medicine and Health Care* 18 (Fall 1990): 202-12.

La Puma, John, et al. "Advance Directives on Admission." *Journal of the American Medical Association*, 17 July 1991, 402-5.

Larson, Ed, and Beth Spring. "Life-Defying Acts: Do Modern Medical Technologies Sustain Life or Merely Prolong Dying?" *Christianity Today*, 6 March 1987.

Lawton, M. Powell, et al. "The Quality of the Last Year of Life of Older Persons." *Milbank Quarterly* 68 (1990): 1-28.

Lebacqz, Karen. "Bio-ethics: Some Challenges from a Liberation Perspective." In *On Moral Medicine: Theological Perspectives in Medical Ethics*, edited by Stephen Lammers and Allen Verhey, 64-69. Grand Rapids: William B. Eerdmans, 1987.

———. *Foundations of Justice*. Minneapolis: Augsburg Press, 1987.

Leenen, H. J. J. "The Definition of Euthanasia." *Medicine and Law* 3 (1984): 333-38.

———. "The Selection of Patients in the Event of a Scarcity of Medical Facilities — An Unavoidable Dilemma." *International Journal of Medicine and Law* 12 (Fall 1979): 161-80.

Lemcio, Eugene. "Pirke 'Abot 1:2(3) and the Synoptic Redactions of the Commands to Love God and Neighbor." *Asbury Theological Journal* 43 (Spring 1988): 43-53.

Levenson, S. A., et al. "Ethical Considerations in Critical and Terminal Illness in the Elderly." *Journal of the American Geriatrics Society* 29 (1981): 563-67.

Levine, Carol. "Stopping Dialysis for 'Low Quality' of Life: A Case from Britain." *Hastings Center Report* 15 (February 1985): 2-3.

Levine, Etan. "The Sabbath Controversy according to Matthew." *New Testament Studies* 22 (1976): 480-83.

Levine, Myra E. "Ration or Rescue: The Elderly Patient in Critical Care." *Critical Care Nursing Quarterly* 12 (June 1989): 82-89.

Levinsky, Norman G. "The Doctor's Master." *New England Journal of Medicine,* 13 December 1984, 1573-75.

————. "Health Care for Veterans: The Limits of Obligation." *Hastings Center Report* 16 (August 1986): 10-15.

Levison, John R. "Responsible Initiative in Matthew 5:21-48." *The Expository Times* 98 (May 1987): 231-34.

Linss, Wilhelm C. "The First World Hunger Appeal." *Currents in Theology and Mission* 12 (August 1985): 211-19.

Linzer, Mark. "Doing What 'Needs' to Be Done." *New England Journal of Medicine,* 16 February 1984, 469-70.

Lo, Bernard. "Quality of Life Judgments in the Care of the Elderly." In *Medical Ethics,* edited by John Monagle and David Thomasma, 140-47. Rockville, Md.: Aspen, 1988.

Loewen, Howard J. "The Clinic, the Church, and the Kingdom." In *Medical Ethics, Human Choices: A Christian Perspective,* edited by John Rogers, 41-51. Scottdale, Pa.: Herald Press, 1988.

Lombardi, Joseph L. "Suicide and the Service of God." *Ethics* 95 (October 1984): 56-67.

Luhrmann, Dieter. "Neutestamentliche Haustafeln und antike Okonomie." *New Testament Studies* 27 (October 1980): 83-97.

Lynn, Joanne, and James F. Childress. "Must Patients Always Be Given Food and Water?" *Hastings Center Report* 13 (October 1983): 17-21.

Lyon, Jeff. "Organ Transplants: Conundra without End." *Second Opinion* 2 (March 1986): 40-64.

McCartney, James J. "The Development of the Doctrine of Ordinary and Extraordinary Means of Preserving Life in Catholic Moral Theology before the Karen Quinlan Case." *Linacre Quarterly* 47 (August 1980): 215-24.

————. "The Right to Die: Perspectives from the Catholic and Jewish Traditions." In *To Die or Not to Die?* edited by Arthur Berger and Joyce Berger, 13-24. New York: Praeger, 1990.

McClish, Donna K., et al. "The Impact of Age on Utilization of Intensive Care Resources." *Journal of the American Geriatrics Society* 35 (November 1987): 983-88.

McCloskey, Elizabeth L. "The Patient Self-Determination Act." *Kennedy Institute of Ethics Journal* 1 (June 1991): 163-69.

McCormick, Richard A. " 'A Clean Heart Create for Me, O God': Impact Questions on the Artificial Heart." In *Medical Ethics,* edited by John Monagle and David Thomasma, 122-26. Rockville, Md.: Aspen, 1988.

————. "George and Marion: A Theological Brief." In *Christian Theology: A Case Method Approach,* edited by Robert Evans and Thomas Parker, 88-93. New York: Harper & Row, 1976.

————. "Physician-Assisted Suicide: Flight from Compassion." *Christian Century*, 4 December 1991, 1132-34.

————. "Theology and Bioethics: Christian Foundations." In *Theology and Bioethics*, edited by Earl Shelp, 95-113. Boston: D. Reidel, 1985.

McGee, Daniel B. "Issues of Life and Death." In *Understanding Christian Ethics*, 227-48. Nashville: Broadman Press, 1988.

McGinn, Paul R. "Infant Mortality Battle: Heroic Saves, Tragic Losses." *American Medical News*, 7 January 1991, 23-24.

McKevitt, Patricia M., et al. "The Elderly on Dialysis: Physical and Psychosocial Functioning." *Dialysis and Transplantation* 15 (March 1986): 130-37.

Macklin, Ruth. *Mortal Choices.* New York: Pantheon Books, 1987.

Maitland, David J. *Aging: A Time for New Learning.* Atlanta: John Knox Press, 1987.

Mandel, Stanley R. "Setting the Record Straight on Organ Sales." *Hastings Center Report* 16 (August 1986): 48-49.

Martin, Brice L. "Matthew on Christ and the Law." *Theological Studies* 34 (April 1983): 53-70.

Marty, Martin E. "The Tradition of the Church in Health and Healing." *Second Opinion* 13 (March 1990): 48-72.

Massachusetts Task Force on Organ Transplantation. *Report.* Boston: Boston University Schools of Public Health and Medicine, 1984.

May, William F. *The Patient's Ordeal.* Bloomington, Ind.: Indiana University Press, 1991.

————. *The Physician's Covenant.* Philadelphia: Westminster Press, 1983.

Mays, William C. "Christian Ethics and Biomedical Issues: A Chaplain's Perspective." In *A Matter of Life and Death.* compiled by Harry Hollis, 62-67. Nashville: Broadman Press, 1977.

Mbiti, John S. *Concepts of God in Africa.* London: SPCK, 1970.

Meeks, Wayne A. *The Moral World of the First Christians.* Philadelphia: Westminster Press, 1986.

Mehlman, Maxwell J. "Rationing Expensive Lifesaving Medical Treatments." *Wisconsin Law Review*, no. 2 (1985): 239-303.

Meilaender, Gilbert. "The Distinction between Killing and Allowing to Die." *Theological Studies* 37 (September 1976): 467-70.

————. "Euthanasia and Christian Vision." In *On Moral Medicine: Theological Perspectives in Medical Ethics*, edited by Stephen Lammers and Allen Verhey, 454-60. Grand Rapids: William B. Eerdmans, 1987.

————. "On Removing Food and Water: Against the Stream." *Hastings Center Report* 14 (December 1984): 11-13.

Meissner, Joseph. "Legal Services and Medical Treatment for Poor People: A Need for Advocacy." *Issues in Law and Medicine* 2 (July 1986): 3-13.

Menzel, Paul T. *Medical Costs, Moral Choices.* New Haven: Yale University Press, 1983.

————. *Strong Medicine.* New York: Oxford University Press, 1990.

Merriken, Karen, and Thomas D. Overcast. "Patient Selection for Heart Transplantation: When Is a Discriminating Choice Discrimination?" *Journal of Health Politics, Policy and Law* 10 (Spring 1985): 7-32.

Meyer, Eugene L. "Tax Money for Transplant Operations: Who Pays?" *Washington Post,* 12 September 1984, C1+.

Miles, John. "Protecting Patient Self-Determination." *Health Progress* 72 (April 1991): 26-30.

Miles, Steven H., et. al. "The Total Artificial Heart: An Ethics Perspective on Current Clinical Research and Deployment." *Chest* 94 (August 1988): 409-13.

Mill, John S. "Utility of Religion." In *The Philosophy of John Stuart Mill.* Edited by Marshall Cohen. New York: Random House, 1961.

Miller, Frances H. "Reflections on Organ Transplantation in the United Kingdom." *Law, Medicine and Health Care* 13 (February 1985): 31-32.

Miller-McLemore, Bonnie J. *Death, Sin and the Moral Life.* Altanta: Scholars Press, 1988.

Minnesota Coalition on Health Care Costs. *The Price of Life: Ethics and Economics.* Minneapolis: Minnesota Coalition on Health Care Costs, 1984.

Minogue, Brendan P. "The Exclusion of Theology from Public Policy: The Case of Euthanasia." *Second Opinion* 14 (July 1990): 85-93.

Misbin, Robert I. "Physicians' Aid in Dying." *New England Journal of Medicine,* 31 October 1991, 1307-11.

Molin, Lennart. "Christian Ethics and Human Life." *Covenant Quarterly* 45 (August 1987): 113-24.

Moltmann, Jürgen. *Theology and Joy.* Translated by D. E. Jenkins. London: SCM Press, 1973.

Moody, Dale. *The Word of Truth.* Grand Rapids: William B. Eerdmans, 1981.

Morgan, W. T. W. "Kikuyu and Kamba: The Tribal Background." In *Nairobi: City and Region,* edited by W. T. W. Morgan. Nairobi: Oxford University Press, 1967.

Morison, Robert S. "The Dignity of the Inevitable and Necessary." In *Death Inside Out,* edited by Peter Steinfels and Robert Veatch, 97-100. New York: Harper & Row, 1974.

Moskop, John C. "The Moral Limits to Federal Funding for Kidney Disease." *Hastings Center Report* 17 (April 1987): 11-15.

Mott, Stephen C. *Biblical Ethics and Social Change.* New York: Oxford University Press, 1982.

———. "The Use of the New Testament for Social Ethics." *Journal of Religious Ethics* 15 (Fall 1987): 225-60.

Mouw, Richard J. "Biblical Revelation and Medical Decisions." In *On Moral Medicine: Theological Perspectives in Medical Ethics,* edited by Stephen Lammers and Allen Verhey, 55-64. Grand Rapids: William B. Eerdmans, 1987.

Munley, Anne. *The Hospice Alternative.* New York: Basic Books, 1983.

Murray, John. *Principles of Conduct.* Philadelphia: Westminster Press, 1957.

Muthiani, Joseph. *Akamba from Within: Egalitarianism in Social Relations.* New York: Exposition Press, 1973.

Najman, J. M., et al. "Patient Characteristics Negatively Stereotyped by Doctors." *Social Science and Medicine* 16 (1982): 1781-89.

National Council of Senior Citizens. "For-Profit Hospital Care: Who Profits? Who Cares?" Washington: National Council of Senior Citizens, 1986.

National Heart Transplantation Study. Seattle: Battelle Human Affairs Research Centers, 1984.

National Kidney Dialysis and Kidney Transplantation Study. Seattle: Battelle Human Affairs Research Centers, 1986.

Ndeti, Kivuto. *Elements of Akamban Life.* Nairobi: East Africa Publishing House, 1972.

———. "The Role of Akamba Kithitu in Questions of Human Justice." In *Proceedings of the Fifth Annual Conference.* Nairobi: University of East Africa Social Science Council, 1969.

Nelson, J. Robert. "Live and Let Live . . . and Die When You Must." *Perkins Journal* 39 (January 1986): 1-9.

———. "The Question of Euthanasia." *Engage/Social Action* 4 (April 1976): 17-48.

Nelson, James B., and Jo Anne S. Rohricht. *Human Medicine.* Rev. ed. Minneapolis: Augsburg Press, 1984.

Neu, Steven, and Carl M. Kjellstrand. "Stopping Long-Term Dialysis." *New England Journal of Medicine,* 2 January 1986, 14-20.

Neuhaus, Richard J. "The Way They Were, the Way We Are: Bioethics and the Holocaust." *First Things,* March 1990, 31-37.

"New Poll Shows Americans Prefer Care Withdrawal in Irreversible Coma Cases." *Medical Ethics Advisor,* May 1987.

Nickel, James W. "Should Undocumented Aliens Be Entitled to Health Care?" *Hastings Center Report* 16 (December 1986): 19-23.

Niebuhr, Reinhold. *The Nature and Destiny of Man.* Vol. 1. New York: Charles Scribner's Sons, 1941.

O'Connell, Laurence J. "The Preferential Option for the Poor and Health Care in the United States." In *Medical Ethics,* edited by John Monagle and David Thomasma, 306-13. Rockville, Md.: Aspen, 1987.

O'Connell, Marvin R. "The Roman Catholic Tradition since 1545." In *Caring and Curing,* edited by Ronald Numbers and Darrel Amundsen, 108-45. New York: Macmillan, 1986.

Oden, Thomas C. "George and Marion: A Theological Brief." In *Christian Theology: A Case Method Approach,* edited by Robert Evans and Thomas Parker, 98-103. New York: Harper & Row, 1976.

————. *Should Treatment Be Terminated?* New York: Harper & Row, 1976.

O'Donnell, Michael. "One Man's Burden." *British Medical Journal,* 5 July 1986, 59.

Office of the Inspector General. *The Access of Foreign Nationals to U.S. Cadaver Organs.* Boston: U.S. Department of Health and Human Services, 1986.

Ogden, David A. "Organ Procurement and Transplantation." In *Health Care Clinics,* edited by Gary Anderson and Valerie Glesnes-Anderson, 91-108. Rockville, Md.: Aspen, 1987.

Ogletree, Thomas W. *The Use of the Bible in Christian Ethics.* Philadelphia: Fortress Press, 1983.

Okeke, G. E. "The After-Life in St. Matthew as an Aspect of Matthean Ethic." *Communio Viatorum* 31 (Summer 1988): 159-68.

Orentlicher, David. "Denying Treatment to the Noncompliant Patient." *Journal of the American Medical Association,* 27 March 1991, 1579-82.

O'Rourke, Kevin D., and Dennis Brodeur. *Medical Ethics: Common Ground for Understanding.* Vol. 2. St. Louis: Catholic Health Association of the U.S., 1989.

Orr, Robert D., et al. *Life and Death Decisions.* Colorado Springs: NavPress, 1990.

Pacific Presbyterian Medical Center. "Who Lives, Who Dies, Who Decides? — National Poll Results." San Francisco: Pacific Presbyterian Medical Center, 1987.

Parachini, Allan. "The California Humane and Dignified Death Initiative." *Hastings Center Report* 19 (January/February 1989): S10-12.

Park Ridge Center for the Study of Health, Faith, and Ethics. *Active Euthanasia, Religion, and the Public Debate.* Chicago: Park Ridge Center, 1991.

Parsons, Arthur. "Allocating Health Care Resources: A Moral Dilemma." *Canadian Medical Association Journal,* 15 February 1985, 466-69.

Parsons, Victor, and P. M. Lock. "Triage and the Patient with Renal Failure." *Journal of Medical Ethics* 6 (December 1980): 173-76.

————. "The Selection and De-Selection of Patients for Dialysis and Transplantation." In *Renal Failure — Who Cares?* edited by F. M. Parsons and C. S. Ogg, 41-47. Lancaster, England: MTP, 1983.

Paulus, Sharon M. "Suit Filed in Oklahoma Alleging Twenty-Four Infants Died after Being Denied Beneficial Medical Treatment." *Issues in Law and Medicine* 1 (January 1986): 321-30.

Payne, Franklin E., Jr. *Biblical/Medical Ethics.* Milford, Mich.: Mott Media, 1985.

Pearlman, Robert A., and Albert R. Jonsen. "The Use of Quality-of-Life Considerations in Medical Decision Making." *Journal of the American Geriatrics Society* 33 (May 1985): 344-52.

Pellegrino, Edmund. "Character, Virtue, and Self-Interest in the Ethics of the Professions." *Journal of Contemporary Health Policy and Law* 5 (Spring 1989): 53-73.

Pence, Gregory E. "Do Not Go Slowly into That Dark Night: Mercy Killing in Holland." *American Journal of Medicine* 84 (January 1988): 139-41.

Perkins, Pheme. *Love Commands in the New Testament.* New York: Paulist Press, 1982.

————. "Paul and Ethics." *Interpretation* 38 (July 1984): 268-80.

Piper, John. *Love Your Enemies.* Cambridge: Cambridge University Press, 1979.

Pirsch, John D., et al. "Orthotoptic Liver Transplantation in Patients 60 Years of Age or Older." *Transplantation* 51 (1991): 431-33.

Pledger, H. G. "Triage of Casualties after Nuclear Attack." *Lancet,* 2 September 1986, 678-79.

Plough, Alonzo L., and Susanne Salem. "Social and Contextual Factors in the Analysis of Mortality in End-Stage Renal Disease Patients: Implications for Health Policy." *American Journal of Public Health* 72 (November 1982): 1293-95.

Post, Stephen G. "Family Caretaking: Moral Commitments and the Burden of Care." *Second Opinion* 8 (July 1988): 115-27.

————. "Justice for Elderly People in Jewish and Christian Thought." In *Too Old for Health Care?* edited by Robert Benstock and Stephen Post, 120-37. Baltimore: The Johns Hopkins University Press, 1991.

President's Commission for the Study of Ethical Problems in Medicine and Biomedical and Behavioral Research. *Deciding to*

Forego Life-Sustaining Treatment. Washington: U.S. Government Printing Office, 1983.

————. *Securing Access to Health Care.* Washington: U.S. Government Printing Office, 1983.

Prottas, Jeffrey M. "In Organ Transplants, Americans First?" *Hastings Center Report* 16 (October 1986): 23-24.

Prottas, Jeffrey M., et al. "Cross-National Differences in Dialysis Rates." *Health Care Financing Review* 4 (March 1983): 91-103.

Purtilo, Ruth B. "Justice in the Distribution of Health Care Resources: The Position of Physical Therapists in the United States and Sweden." *Physical Therapy* 62 (January 1982): 46-50.

Quill, Timothy E. "Death and Dignity — A Case of Individualized Decision-Making." *New England Journal of Medicine,* 7 March 1991, 691-94.

Rabinowitz, Stanley, and Hermanus I. J. van der Spuy. "Selection Criteria for Dialysis and Renal Transplant." *American Journal of Psychiatry* 135 (July 1978): 861-63.

Rabkin, Mitchell, et al. "Orders Not to Resuscitate." *New England Journal of Medicine,* 21 August 1976, 364-66.

Ramsey, Paul. *The Patient as Person.* New Haven: Yale University Press, 1970.

————. *Ethics at the Edges of Life.* New Haven: Yale University Press, 1978.

————. "The Indignity of 'Death with Dignity.'" In *Death Inside Out,* edited by Peter Steinfels and Robert Veatch, 81-96. New York: Harper & Row, 1974.

Rapaport, Felix T. "Living Donor Kidney Transplantation." *Transplantation Proceedings* 19 (February 1987): 169-73.

"Rationing of Health Care." *Perspective* 20 (Summer 1985): 1-9.

Reed, William G., et al. "The Effect of a Public Hospital's Transfer Policy on Patient Care." *New England Journal of Medicine,* 27 November 1986, 1428-32.

Reidy, Maurice. "Distribution and Choice." In *Foundations for a Medical Ethic,* 71-81. New York: Paulist Press, 1979.

Reinhold, Robert. "Crisis in Emergency Rooms: More Symptoms Than Cures." *New York Times,* 28 July 1988, A1, A20.

Reiser, Stanley J. "The Dilemma of Euthanasia in Modern Medical History." In *The Dilemma of Euthanasia,* edited by A. Behnke and S. Bok. New York: Anchor Books, 1975.

Rennie, Drummond, et al. "Limited Resources and the Treatment of End-stage Renal Failure in Britain and the United States." *Quarterly Journal of Medicine* 56, n.s. (July 1985): 321-36.

Rescher, Nicholas. "The Allocation of Exotic Medical Lifesaving Therapy." *Ethics* 79 (1969): 173-86.

Richards, Glenn. "Technology Costs and Rationing Issues." *Hospitals*, 1 June 1984, 80-86.

Richards, Larry, and Paul Johnson. *Death and the Caring Community*. Portland: Multnomah Press, 1980.

Richardson, Peter. *Paul's Ethic of Freedom*. Philadelphia: Westminster Press, 1979.

Ridderbos, Herman. *Paul: An Outline of His Theology*. Translated by John R. de Witt. Grand Rapids: William B. Eerdmans, 1975.

" 'Right-to-Die' Case Reflects Thorny Privacy Issue." *Lexington Herald-Leader*, 25 July 1989, 2.

Rigter, Henk. "Euthanasia in the Netherlands: Distinguishing Facts from Fiction." *Hastings Center Report* 19 (January/February 1989): 31-32.

———. "Mercy, Murder, and Morality." *Hastings Center Report* 19 (November/December 1989): 52.

Robb, J. Wesley. "The Allocation of Limited Medical Resources: An Ethical Perspective." *Pharos* 44 (Spring 1981): 29-35.

Robbins, Christopher. "The Ethical Challenge of Health Care Rationing." In *The End of an Illusion: The Future of Health Policy in Western Industrialized Nations*, edited by Jean de Kervasdoue et al., 110-33. Berkeley and Los Angeles: University of California Press, 1984.

Robertson, John A. "Supply and Distribution of Hearts for Transplantation: Legal, Ethical, and Policy Issues." *Circulation* 75 (January 1987): 77-87.

Rodgers, Joann. "Life on the Cutting Edge." *Psychology Today* 18 (October 1984): 58-67.

Roper Organization of New York City. "The 1988 Roper Poll on Attitudes toward Active Voluntary Euthanasia." Los Angeles: National Hemlock Society, 1988.

Rosner, Fred. "Allocation of Scarce Medical Resources." *New York State Journal of Medicine* 83 (March 1983): 353-58.

Ross, W. David. *The Right and the Good*. Oxford: Oxford University Press, 1973.

Rothman, David J. "Ethical and Social Issues in the Development of New Drugs and Vaccines." *Bulletin of the New York Academy of Medicine* 63 (July-August 1987): 557-68.

Royal Dutch Society of Medicine. "Reactie op vragen Staatscommissee Euthanasie." *Medisch Contact* 31 (1984): 999-1002.

Sage, William M., et al. "Intensive Care for the Elderly: Outcome of Elective and Nonelective Admissions." *Journal of the American Geriatrics Society* 35 (April 1987): 312-18.

———. "Is Intensive Care Worth It? — An Assessment of Input and

Outcome for the Critically Ill." *Critical Care Medicine* 14 (September 1986): 777-82.

Samet, Jonathan, et al. "Choice of Cancer Therapy Varies with Age of Patient." *Journal of the American Medical Association,* 27 June 1986, 3385-90.

Sanders, David, and Jesse Dukeminier, Jr. "Medical Advance and Legal Lag: Hemodialysis and Kidney Transplantation." *UCLA Law Review* 15 (February 1968): 366-80.

Sanders, Jack T. *Ethics in the New Testament.* Philadelphia: Fortress Press, 1975.

Sanders, John B. "ICU Admission and Discharge Screening Criteria." *Nursing Administration Quarterly* 10 (Spring 1986): 25-31.

Sapp, Stephen. *Full of Years: Aging and the Elderly in the Bible and Today.* Nashville: Abingdon Press, 1987.

Saul, D. Glenn. "The Ethics of Decision Making." In *Understanding Christian Ethics,* edited by William Tillman, Jr., 79-99. Nashville: Broadman Press, 1988.

Sawyer, Tom. Written text of interview by authors of "Scarce Medical Resources" conducted 29 August 1968, on file at Columbia Law Library.

"Scarce Medical Resources." *Columbia Law Review* 9 (April 1969): 620-92.

Schaeffer, Francis A., and C. Everett Koop. *Whatever Happened to the Human Race?* Old Tappan, N.J.: Fleming H. Revell, 1979.

Schemmer, Kenneth E. *Between Life and Death.* Wheaton, Ill.: Victor Books, 1988.

Schiff, Robert L., et al. "Transfer to a Public Hospital: A Prospective Study of 467 Patients." *New England Journal of Medicine,* 27 February 1986, 552-57.

Schlier, Heinrich. "ἐλεύθερος." In *Theological Dictionary of the New Testament,* vol. 2, edited by Gerhard Kittel, translated by Geoffrey Bromiley, 487-502. Grand Rapids: William B. Eerdmans, 1964.

Schnackenburg, Rudolf. "Neutestamentliche Ethik im Kontext heutiger Wirklichkeit." In *Anspruch der Wirklichkeit und christlicher Glaube: Festschrift für A. Auer,* edited by H. Weber and D. Mieth, 193-207. Düsseldorf: Patmos, 1980.

Schneider, Andrew, and Mary P. Flaherty. "The Challenge of a Miracle: Selling the Gift." *Pittsburg Press,* 3-10 November 1985.

Schneider, Johannes. "ὅμοιος. . . ." In *Theological Dictionary of the New Testament,* vol. 5, edited by Gerhard Kittel and Gerhard Friedrich, translated by Geoffrey Bromiley, 186-99. Grand Rapids: William B. Eerdmans, 1967.

Schottroff, Luise, and Wolfgang Stegemann. "The Sabbath Was Made for Man." In *God of the Lowly*, edited by Willy Schottroff and Wolfgang Stegemann, 118-28. Maryknoll, N.Y.: Orbis Books, 1984.

Schrage, Wolfgang. *Ethik des Neuen Testaments*. Grundrisse zum Neuen Testament, NTD 4. Göttingen: Vandenhoeck & Ruprecht, 1982.

Schroeder, David. "Life and Death: Biblical-Theological Perspectives." In *Medical Ethics, Human Choices: A Christian Perspective*, edited by John Rogers, 63-72. Scottdale, Pa.: Herald Press, 1988.

Schwartz, Robert, and Andrew Grubb. "Why Britain Can't Afford Informed Consent." *Hastings Center Report* 15 (August 1985): 19-25.

Schwartz, William B., and Daniel N. Mendelson. "Hospital Cost Containment in the 1980's — Hard Lessons Learned and Prospects for the 1990's." *New England Journal of Medicine*, 11 April 1991, 1037-42.

Schwartz, William B., and Henry J. Aaron. "Rationing Hospital Care: Lessons from Britain." *New England Journal of Medicine*, 5 January 1984, 52-56.

Schweizer, Eduard. *The Good News according To Matthew*. Atlanta: John Knox Press, 1975.

Scitovsky, Anne A. "Medical Care Expenditures in the Last Twelve Months of Life." Final Report to the John A. Hartford Foundation, March 1986.

Scitovsky, Anne A., and Alexander M. Capron. "Medical Care at the End of Life: The Interaction of Economics and Ethics." *Annual Review of Public Health* 7 (1986): 59-75.

Scroggs, Robin. *Paul for a New Day*. Philadelphia: Fortress Press, 1977.

Sehgal, Ashwini, et al. "How Strictly Do Dialysis Patients Want Their Advance Directives Followed?" *Journal of the American Medical Association*, 1 January 1992, 59-63.

Shannon, Thomas A. "What Guidance from the Guidelines?" *Hastings Center Report* 7 (June 1977): 28-30.

Shelp, Earl E. "Justice: A Moral Test for Health Care and Health Policy." In *Justice and Health Care*, edited by Earl Shelp, 213-29. Boston: D. Reidel, 1981.

Sherer, Paul. *The Plight of Freedom*. New York: Harper, 1948.

Short, David S. "The Persistent Vegetative State." *Ethics and Medicine* 7 (Autumn 1991): 39.

Showalter, J. Stuart, and Brian L. Andrew. *To Treat or Not to Treat: A Working Document for Making Critical Life Decisions*. St. Louis: Catholic Health Association of the United States, 1984.

Siegler, Mark. "Should Age Be a Criterion in Health Care?" *Hastings Center Report* 14 (October 1984): 24-27.

Simmons, DebbieLynne. "Created for Life." *The Plough,* March-April 1985, 13.

Simmons, Paul D. *Birth and Death: Bioethical Decision-Making.* Philadelphia: Westminster Press, 1983.

Simmons, Roberta G., and Richard L. Simmons. "Sociological and Psychological Aspects of Transplantation." In *Transplantation,* edited by J. S. Najarian and R. L. Simmons, 361-87. Philadelphia: Lea & Febiger, 1972.

Smedes, Lewis B. "Respect for Human Life: 'Thou Shalt Not Kill.' " In *On Moral Medicine: Theological Perspectives in Medical Ethics,* edited by Stephen Lammers and Allen Verhey, 143-49. Grand Rapids: William B. Eerdmans, 1987.

Smeeding, Timothy M. "Artificial Organs, Transplants and Long-Term Care for the Elderly: What's Covered? Who Pays?" In *Should Medical Care Be Rationed by Age?* edited by Timothy M. Smeeding, 140-55. Totowa, N.J.: Rowman & Littlefield, 1987.

Smith, Alwyn. "Qualms and QALYs." *Lancet,* 16 May 1987, 1134-36.

Smith, George P., II. "Death Be Not Proud: Medical, Ethical and Legal Dilemmas in Resource Allocation." *Journal of Contemporary Health Law and Policy* 3 (Spring 1987): 47-63.

Smith, Harmon L. "Dying with Style." *Anglican Theological Review* 70 (October 1988): 327-45.

Smith, William B. "Judeo-Christian Teaching on Euthanasia: Definitions, Distinctions and Decisions." *Linacre Quarterly* 54 (1987): 27-42.

Snyder, Graydon F. *Tough Choices.* Elgin, Ill.: Brethren Press, 1988.

Somerville, Margaret A. "Justice across the Generations." *Social Science and Medicine* 29 (1989): 385-94.

———. "Should the Grandparents Die? Allocation of Medical Resources with an Aging Population." *Law, Medicine and Health Care* 14 (September 1986): 158-63.

Sommers, Christina H. "Once a Soldier, Always a Dependent." *Hastings Center Report* 16 (August 1986): 15-17.

Stambaugh, John E., and David L. Balch. *The New Testament in Its Social Environment.* Philadelphia: Westminster Press, 1986.

Starr, T. Jolene, et al. "Quality of Life and Rescuscitation Decisions in Elderly Patients." *Journal of General Internal Medicine* 1 (November/December 1986): 373-79.

Starzl, Thomas E., et al. "Equitable Allocation of Extrarenal Organs: With Special Reference to the Liver." *Transplantation Proceedings* 20 (February 1988): 131-38.

————. "Liver Transplantation in Older Patients." *New England Journal of Medicine*, 19 February 1987, 484-85.

Steinbock, Bonnie. "Recovery from Persistent Vegetative State? The Case of Carrie Coons." *Hastings Center Report* 19 (July/August 1989): 14-15.

Steinfels, Peter. "Beliefs: In Cold Print, the Euthanasia Issue Can Take on Many Shades of Color." *New York Times*, 9 November 1991, A8.

Stiller, C. R. "Ethics of Transplantation." *Transplantation Proceedings* 17, no. 6, Suppl. 3 (December 1985): 131-38.

Stith, Richard. "Toward Freedom from Value." In *On Moral Medicine: Theological Perspectives in Medical Ethics*, edited by Stephen Lammers and Allen Verhey, 127-43. Grand Rapids: William B. Eerdmans, 1987.

Strauss, Michael J., et al. "Rationing of Intensive Care Unit Services: An Everyday Occurrence." *Journal of the American Medical Association*, 7 March 1986, 1143-46.

Stob, Henry. *The Christian Concept of Freedom*. Grand Rapids: Grand Rapids International Publications, 1957.

"Suicide Device for Terminally Ill Raises Legal, Ethical Concerns." *Lexington Herald-Leader*, 29 October 1989, E6.

Sutherland, D. E. R., et al. "The High-Risk Recipient in Transplantation." *Transplantation Proceedings* 14 (March 1982): 19-27.

Task Force on Organ Transplantation. *Organ Transplantation: Issues and Recommendations*. Rockville, Md.: U.S. Department of Health and Human Services, 1986.

Taube, David H., et al. "Successful Treatment of Middle Aged and Elderly Patients with End Stage Renal Disease." *British Medical Journal*, 25 June 1983, 2018-20.

Ten Have, Henk A. M. J. "Euthanasia in the Netherlands: The Legal Context and the Cases." *HEC Forum* 1 (1989): 41-45.

Thielicke, Helmut. "The Doctor as Judge of Who Shall Live and Who Shall Die." In *Who Shall Live?* edited by Kenneth Vaux, 146-94. Philadelphia: Fortress Press, 1970.

————. *The Freedom of the Christian Man*. New York: Harper & Row, 1963.

Thomasma, David C. The Basis of Medicine and Religion: Respect for Persons." In *On Moral Medicine: Theological Perspectives in Medical Ethics*, edited by Stephen Lammers and Allen Verhey, 288-92. Grand Rapids: William B. Eerdmans, 1987.

————. *Human Life in the Balance*. Louisville: Westminster/John Knox Press, 1990.

————. "Quality of Life Judgments, Treatment Decisions and Medical Ethics." *Clinics in Geriatric Medicine* 2 (February 1986): 17-27.

Thomasma, David C., and Glenn C. Graber. *Euthanasia: Toward an Ethical Social Policy.* New York: Continuum, 1990.

Thompson, Mark E. "Selection of Candidates for Cardiac Transplantation." *Heart Transplantation* 3 (November 1983): 65-69.

Thurston, Bonnie B. "Matthew 5:43-48." *Interpretation* 41 (April 1987): 170-73.

"A Time to Die: The Cases of Nancy Cruzan and Janet Adkins." *Bulletin of the Park Ridge Center* 5 (September 1990): 16-31.

Toombs, S. Kay. "The Meaning of Illness: A Phenomenological Approach to the Physician-Patient Relationship." *Journal of Medicine and Philosophy* 12 (August 1987): 219-40.

Tournier, Paul. *A Doctor's Casebook in the Light of the Bible,* translated by Edwin Hudson. New York: Harper & Row, 1960.

Transplantation Society (Council). "Commercialisation in Transplantation: The Problems and Some Guidelines for Practice." *Lancet,* 28 September 1985, 715-16.

Twycross, Robert. "Decisions about Death and Dying." In *Decision Making in Medicine: The Practice of its Ethics,* edited by Gordon Scorer and Antony Wing, 101-15. London: Edward Arnold, 1979.

Uddo, Basile J. "The Withdrawal or Refusal of Food and Hydration as Age Discrimination: Some Possibilities." *Issues in Law and Medicine* 2 (July 1986): 39-59.

UNICEF. *The State of the World's Children 1988.* New York: Oxford University Press, 1988.

United Nations Secretary General. "Human Rights and Scientific and Technological Developments." 30th Session, Item 70 of the Provisional Agenda, 28 July 1975.

United Network for Organ Sharing (UNOS). "Memorandum on UNOS Policy regarding Utilization of the Point System for Cadaveric Kidney Allocation," 11 November 1988.

————. "The Nursing Shortage." *Transplant Perspectives,* February 1989, 1-3.

U.S. Congress Office of Technology Assessment, "Intensive Care Units: Clinical Outcomes, Costs, and Decisionmaking." Health Technology Case Study 28, November 1984.

————. *Life-Sustaining Technologies and the Elderly.* OTA-BA-306. Washington: U.S. Government Printing Office, 1987.

U.S. Department of Commerce. *1992 U.S. Industrial Outlook.* Washington: U.S. Government Printing Office, 1992.

U.S. Department of Health and Human Services, Task Force on Organ Transplantation. "Report to the Secretary and the Congress on Immunosuppressive Therapies." Rockville, Md.: U.S. Government Printing Office, 1985.

U.S. House of Representatives, Committee on Science and Technology, Sub-Committee on Investigations and Oversight. "Procurement and Allocation of Human Organs for Transplantation." Hearings of 2 and 9 November 1983. Washington: U.S. Government Printing Office, 1983.

Van den Beld, A. "Killing and the Principle of Double Effect." *Scottish Journal of Theology* 41 (1988): 93-116.

Van der Maas, Paul J., et al. "Euthanasia and Other Medical Decisions concerning the End of Life." *Lancet,* 14 September 1991, 669-74.

Van Wijmen, F. C. B. *Artsen en zelfgekozen levenseinde.* Maastricht: Vakgroep Gezondheidsrecht Rijksuniversiteit Limburg, 1989.

Vaux, Kenneth L. "Debbie's Dying: Euthanasia Reconsidered." *Christian Century,* 16 March 1988, 269-71.

———. "The Theologic Ethics of Euthanasia." *Hastings Center Report* 19 (January/February 1989): 19-22.

———. "Theological Foundations of Medical Ethics." In *Health/Medicine and the Faith Traditions,* edited by Martin Marty and Kenneth Vaux, 215-28. Philadelphia: Fortress Press, 1982.

Veatch, Robert M. "Death and Dying: The Legislative Options." *Hastings Center Report* 7 (October 1977): 5-8.

———. *Death, Dying, and the Biological Revolution.* Rev. ed. New Haven: Yale University Press, 1988.

———. "Distributive Justice and the Allocation of Technological Resources to the Elderly." Contract report prepared for the U.S. Congress Office of Technology Assessment, Washington, December 1985.

———. "Ethical Foundations for Valuing Lives: Implications for Life-Extending Technologies." In *A Technology Assessment of Life-Extending Technologies,* Supplementary Report, vol. 6, 196-242. Glastonbury, Conn.: Futures Group, 1977.

———. *The Foundations of Justice.* New York: Oxford University Press, 1986.

———. "From Fae to Schroeder: The Ethics of Allocating High Technology." *Spectrum* 16 (April 1985): 15-18.

———. "Justice and Valuing Lives." In *Life Span,* edited by Robert M. Veatch, 197-224. San Francisco: Harper & Row, 1979.

Velez, Ramon, et al. "Treatment of End-Stage Renal Disease." *New England Journal of Medicine,* 5 February 1981, 356.

Verhey, Allen. *The Great Reversal: Ethics and the New Testament.* Grand Rapids: William B. Eerdmans, 1984.

———. "The Doctor's Oath — and a Christian Swearing It." In *On Moral Medicine: Theological Perspectives in Medical Ethics,* edited by Stephen Lammers and Allen Verhey, 72-82. Grand Rapids: William B. Eerdmans, 1987.

"View of Suicide as a Right Disturbs Philosophers." *Bulletin of the Park Ridge Center* 5 (September 1990): 6-7.

Voelker, Rebecca. "Weighing Costs, Benefits in Neonatal Care." *American Medical News,* 7 January 1991, 22.

Waldholz, Michael. "Cost of Using Kidney Device Sparks Debate." *Wall Street Journal,* 5 February 1981, 23, 32.

Wanzer, Sidney H., et al. "The Physician's Responsibility toward Hopelessly Ill Patients: A Second Look." *New England Journal of Medicine,* 30 March 1989, 844-49.

Ward, Elizabeth. "Death or Dialysis — A Personal View." *British Medical Journal,* 22/29 December 1984, 1712-13.

Warmbrodt, Jane. "Who Gets the Organs?" *Midwest Medical Ethics* 1 (Summer 1985): 3-4.

Washington Health Choices. *Executive Report.* Seattle: Puget Sound Health Systems Agency, 1986.

Wauters, J., et al. "Selection Criteria and Physician Bias in the Treatment of End-Stage Renal Failure: Results of a National Survey." Report presented at the Fourth Congress of the International Society for Artificial Organs, Kyoto, Japan, 1983.

Weckman, George, and Richard W. Willy. "Descriptive Medical Ethics and Allocation." *Listening* 22 (Winter 1987): 12-21.

Wehr, Elizabeth. "National Health Policy Sought for Organ Transplant Surgery." *Congressional Quarterly,* 25 February 1984, 453-58.

Weller, John M., et al. "Analysis of Survival of End-Stage Renal Disease Patients." *Kidney International* 21 (January 1982): 78-83.

Wenham, David. "Paul's Use of the Jesus Tradition: Three Samples." In *The Jesus Tradition outside the Gospels,* edited by David Wenham. Sheffield, England: JSOT Press, 1985.

Wennberg, Robert N. *Terminal Choices.* Grand Rapids: William B. Eerdmans, 1989.

Wesley, John. "An Israelite Indeed." In *The Works of the Reverend John Wesley,* vol. 2, edited by John Emery. New York: J. Emery and B. Waugh, 1831.

————. "On Working Out Our Own Salvation." In *The Works of the Reverend John Wesley,* vol. 2, edited by John Emery. New York: J. Emery and B. Waugh, 1831.

Westerholm, Stephen. "Letter and Spirit: The Foundation of Pauline Ethics." *New Testament Studies* 30 (April 1984): 229-48.

Westlie, L., et al. "Mortality, Morbidity and Life Satisfaction in the Very Old Dialysis Patient." *Transactions of the American Society for Artificial Internal Organs* 30 (1984): 21-30.

Wetle, Terrie. "Age as a Risk Factor for Inadequate Treatment." *Journal of the American Medical Association,* 2 July 1987, 516.

Wetle, Terrie, and Sue E. Levkoff. "Attitudes and Behaviors of Service Providers toward Elder Patients in the VA System." In *Older Veterans: Linking VA and Community Resources,* edited by Terrie Wetle and John Rowe, 205-30. Cambridge: Harvard University Press, 1984.

White, Margot L., and John C. Fletcher. "The Patient Self-Determination Act." *Journal of the American Medical Association,* 17 July 1991, 410-12.

White, R. E. O. *Biblical Ethics.* Atlanta: John Knox Press, 1979.

Wikler, Daniel. "Comments on Battin's 'Age Rationing.'" In *Should Medical Care Be Rationed by Age?* edited by Timothy M. Smeeding, 95-98. Totowa, N.J.: Rowman & Littlefield, 1987.

————. "Not Dead, Not Dying? Ethical Categories and Persistent Vegetative State." *Hastings Center Report* 18 (February/March 1988): 41-47.

Wildes, Kevin W. "Health Care Rationing and Insured Access: Does the Catholic Tradition Have Anything to Say?" *Linacre Quarterly* 58 (August 1991): 50-58.

Wilkerson, Isabel. "Rage and Support for Doctor's Role in Suicide." *New York Times,* 25 October 1991, A1.

Wilson, William C., et al. "Ordering and Administration of Sedatives and Analgesics during the Withholding and Withdrawal of Life Support from Critically Ill Patients." *Journal of the American Medical Association,* 19 February 1992, 949-53.

Winslade, William J., and Judith W. Ross. *Choosing Life or Death.* New York: Free Press, 1986.

Winslow, Gerald R. *Triage and Justice.* Berkeley and Los Angeles: University of California Press, 1982.

Wogaman, J. Philip. "Economics and Medicine: Theological Reflections." *Second Opinion* 8 (July 1988): 66-85.

Working Group on Mechanical Circulatory Support, National Heart, Lung and Blood Institute. *Artificial Heart and Assist Devices: Directions, Needs, Costs, Societal and Ethical Issues.* Bethesda, Md.: National Institutes of Health, 1985.

World Bank. *Poverty in Latin America.* Washington: World Bank, 1986.

Young, Robert. "Some Criteria for Making Decisions concerning the Distribution of Scarce Medical Resources." *Theory and Decision* 6 (November 1975): 439-55.

Zaner, Richard M. *Ethics and the Clinical Encounter.* Englewood Cliffs, N.J.: Prentice-Hall, 1988.

Zaner, Richard M. (ed.). *Death: Beyond Whole-Brain Criteria.* Hingham, Mass.: Kluwer, 1989.

Zawacki, Bruce E. "ICU Physician's Ethical Role in Distributing Scarce Resources." *Critical Care Medicine* 13 (January 1985): 57-60.

Ziegler, Jesse H. "Prolonging Life, Prolonging Death." In *Medical Ethics, Human Choices,* edited by John Rogers, 83-91. Scottdale, Pa.: Herald Press, 1988.

Index

Ability-to-pay criterion, 147,
155, 157, 204, 205-6, 211, 213,
214-20, 228, 233, 235, 239
Access to health care, 26, 63,
178, 237, 238, 302n.5
Advance directives, 88-93, 155
Age criterion: equal-opportunity
justification, 177-78, 180-82; in-
appropriateness of, 160, 161-64;
length-of-medical-benefit justification, 165-66; life-span justification, 178, 182-83; likelihood-
of-medical-benefit justification,
169-71; medical-benefit justification, 172-75, 210, 224, 233;
productivity-oriented justifications, 176-77, 179-80, 183, 188-
91, 193; prudential justification,
178, 184-87, 191, 192-93; quality-
of-medical-benefit justification,
166-69, 183; support for, 155-58,
187-88, 190, 235, 236
AIDS, 300n.6
Alcoholism, 212, 300n.6
Allocating resources, 1, 55, 146,
153-55, 163-64, 217, 220, 236-
39, 243, 244n.1

American Medical Association,
90-91
American Protestant Health As-
sociation, 89
Anesthesia, 142
Animals, 37, 251n.10
Antibiotics, 154, 230, 231
Autonomy, 24, 58-59, 81, 111,
248n.21. See also Freedom

Baptism, 21
Benefit/Burden of treatment, 83,
86, 94, 123, 125, 133, 135, 141,
142-49, 240
Best interests of patients, 81, 84,
91, 199-200
Bible: Jesus' teaching, 30-40,
251n.8; Paul's teaching, 15-29,
42-43, 247n.15; as source of
ethical insight, 2, 3, 7-8, 14-15,
37, 39, 45, 48, 50, 51, 94, 100,
185, 222, 242, 246n.10
Biblical persons/places:
Abimelech, 272n.5; Abraham,
42; Adam, 98, 100-101, 246n.5;
Ahithophel, 271n.5;
Corinth(ians), 18-19, 23, 63,

147, 248n.22; David, 59, 67,
99, 268n.18; Elijah, 99; Elisha,
59, 60, 61; Enoch, 99; Eve, 21,
106, 121; Galatia(ns), 23;
Gethsemane, 107, 120;
Israelites, 61, 63; Jacob, 59, 60;
Jerusalem, 147, 259n.23; Jesus'
disciples, 67, 98, 121, 139;
Joab, 99; Job, 103, 105; Joshua,
59, 60, 61; Judas, 271n.5; Mace-
donia(ns), 24, 147; Matthew,
30; Paul, 15, 105, 268n.17;
Peter, 121; Pharisees, 36, 37,
38, 62, 70, 259n.23; Philemon,
25; Puah and Shiphrah, 59,
60, 61; Rahab, 59, 60; Samson,
271n.5; Samuel, 59, 60, 61;
Saul, 60, 61, 268n.18, 271n.5;
Stephen, 121; Timothy, 29;
Titus, 29; Zimri, 271n.5. See
also Jesus Christ
Body, human, 23, 35, 100, 124
Body of Christ, 22, 23, 25,
265n.41

Cancer, 13, 140
Care, comfort, 5, 69, 115, 128-29,
134, 139-42, 178, 184, 187, 239-
40, 243, 277n.11
Caregiver-patient relationship,
49, 61, 80-83, 112, 122-23, 164,
171, 199-200, 229; contract
model of, 80-81, 81-82; covenant model of, 81, 82; family
model of, 80, 81, 82; war model
of, 80, 81, 87, 134, 138, 143
Catholic Health Association, 89
Character. See Virtue
Charisma, 195
Chemotherapy, 13, 143
Children, 93, 154, 203, 212, 213,
220, 238-39, 265n.43
Choice, 25, 97, 104, 155, 163,
215, 223. See also Freedom;
and Wishes

Churches, 93, 147, 237, 240
Circumcision, 29
Clergy, 4-5
Coercion, 85, 88, 114, 133, 134,
135, 143, 146-47, 187, 202, 217-
18, 219, 223, 224, 236, 300n.6
Committees, 197
Common good, 48, 200. See also
Community
Communication, 123, 133, 135,
284n.16. See also Informed con-
sent
Community, 28, 53, 59, 63, 66,
70-71, 111-13, 116, 119, 129,
146, 147, 148-49, 161, 189, 192-
93, 222, 243, 253n.23
Compassion, 140, 170. See also
Love
Competence, mental. See Mental
capacity
Compliance, 199, 209, 235
Conscience, 22, 246n.10
Consequences: bad, 101, 229;
good, 28, 121; significance of,
39, 45-46, 101-2, 160, 162, 188,
195, 200. See also Ethics of con-
sequences
Convenience, 168, 173, 176-77,
179, 203-4, 209
Cost-benefit analysis, 41, 170,
176, 179, 203, 217, 237, 238, 241
Cost of health care, 1, 2, 6, 78,
114, 128, 153, 154, 155, 179.
See also Money
Counsel, 93, 94, 159, 189, 210,
240, 246n.10
Courage, 47
Courts of law, 93, 117, 130
Covenant, 49, 81, 87
Creation: in the image of God,
47, 53, 54, 98, 124, 160; of life,
35, 54, 55, 56, 122, 126, 128,
146; of moral-spiritual reality,
20, 57, 71, 94, 115, 128, 129,
222; of people, 23, 25, 49, 59,

67, 96, 100, 101, 111, 115, 147, 191, 199, 258n.18; of the world, 22, 32, 37, 38, 42, 43, 65, 70, 120, 127, 222, 242
Criminals, 199

Death: desire to control, 109-10, 241; with dignity, 111, 119; as disaster, 102-3, 143, 177; as enemy, 80, 99, 102, 103, 109, 119, 122, 133; intending, 79, 80, 96-97, 110, 113, 118, 120-21, 125, 130, 131, 133, 137, 141, 144, 146, 189, 243; nature of, 75, 97-103, 109, 110, 115, 124-25, 127, 128, 162-63, 202; as opportunity, 103, 121-22, 128, 177, 180; origin of, 97-98, 99; overcome by God, 98, 99, 102, 103, 109, 128; right to, 110-11; as tool of the devil, 99. *See also* Jesus Christ, death of
Deontological ethics. *See* Principles, ethics of
Dependence, 104
Dialysis, 154, 155, 156-57, 158, 165, 166, 174, 177, 181, 187-88, 196-97, 201, 210, 211, 215, 218, 228, 230, 260n.5, 295n.15
Dignity, 111, 199. *See also* Life, significance of
Disabled persons, 78, 114, 115, 198, 199, 210
Discernment, 22, 23-24, 28, 44, 51, 52, 53, 61, 129, 134, 145, 146, 147-48, 214, 242, 243, 246n.10
Diversity: economic, 8; ethnic, 8; gender, 7
Double effect, principle of, 275n.8
Durable power of attorney, 89-91, 93
Duty, 25, 43, 44, 45, 110-11, 165-66, 191, 248n.22, 303n.9

Efficiency, 170, 173, 199. *See also* Consequences; Ethics of consequences
Elderly people: assertiveness of, 158, 177; disproportionate need for health care, 78, 158, 177, 179-80, 236; diversity of, 192, 280n.6; and end-of-life treatment decisions, 78, 114, 115, 155, 236; goals of, 183, 190; limited access to health care, 2, 33, 155-58, 216, 235; protection of, 160; respect for, 159-60, 168, 173, 189, 192; righteousness of, 159, 161; services provided by, 190; the very old, 158; virtues of, 173, 175, 190; weakness of, 159, 161, 174, 179, 216; wisdom of, 159, 160, 189, 190
Emergency care, 204, 215
Empowerment, 17-18, 19, 44, 47, 53, 104, 107, 148, 198, 228
Ending someone's life: ethical unacceptability of, 97, 243; justifications of, 79-80, 106-16, 140; pressures toward, 1-2, 235, 236; requests for, 4-5, 13, 75, 95; support for, 76, 77-78; social significance of, 49, 56-57, 111, 112, 115, 244n.1, 270n.31. *See also* Forgoing treatment; Suicide
Equality, 25-26, 32, 39, 62, 63-64, 65, 71, 160, 161, 165, 168-69, 170, 172, 177-78, 179, 192, 198, 206, 227, 229-30, 239, 259n.21
Equal opportunity, 177-78, 180-82, 185, 208, 227
Eschatology, 21, 22, 23, 33, 34, 35, 42, 43, 246n.14
Eternal life, 20, 55, 63, 75, 100, 102, 107, 120, 128, 162-64, 168, 197, 223, 266n.5
Ethical guides, 51-52, 53-54, 66,

67, 68, 70, 71, 81, 94, 147, 195, 222, 223
Ethical norms, conflict between, 39-40, 45-46, 61, 65-69, 145, 195
Ethics of consequences, 16-17, 19, 21, 41-43, 47, 48, 49, 106, 108, 109, 110, 114, 115, 122, 139-40, 158, 164, 178, 179, 183, 186, 189-91, 194-200, 208, 222, 230. *See also* God-centered ethics
Euthanasia, 78-80, 117, 241-42, 271n.2. *See also* Ending someone's life
Evil, 21, 106, 121, 245n.3
Experience, 44-45, 52, 65, 108, 124, 128, 129, 137, 138, 142, 143-44, 148, 158, 159, 167, 181-82, 185, 197, 211, 218, 222, 240. *See also* Discernment
Experimentation, 201-3

Faith: as recognizing all of reality, 35, 40, 108, 161; as reliance on other people, 111, 112, 122-23, 171, 199-200; as trust in God, 18, 20, 26-27, 34, 40, 47, 60, 103, 104, 108, 119, 135, 228, 241
Faithfulness, 18, 49, 67, 69, 86, 104, 105, 107, 108, 115, 116, 122, 140, 144, 146
Fallenness. *See* Sin
Family: biological, 4-5, 23, 66, 68, 75, 87, 92, 93, 123, 134, 142, 144, 145, 146, 159, 169, 212, 214, 216, 217, 219, 223-24, 239, 240, 241; spiritual, 22, 23, 31, 32, 66, 93, 147, 189; as surrogate decision-makers, 75, 92, 93, 123, 124
Favored-group criterion, 157, 199, 203-7, 233
Fear, 75, 90, 102, 112, 123, 140, 240

Feeding: artificial, 117, 143, 276n.11; non-artificial, 37, 145, 164, 211, 300n.6
First-come first-served, 228-29
Forgiveness, 20, 47, 53, 119
Forgoing treatment: as a common option, 75, 76; as different from intentionally ending life, 78, 121, 125-29, 131-32, 275n.5; as a form of suicide, 121; justifications of, 49, 53, 56, 67, 92, 121, 123-24, 125-49, 183, 223, 236, 237; support for, 4, 13, 75-76, 130, 239, 243; as a test of caregiver support, 123, 133
Freedom: to follow Christ, 19, 23-25, 28; as a guide, 57-59, 67-68, 81, 83-84, 85, 86, 87, 92, 168, 169, 186, 195, 201-2, 203, 205, 215, 218, 223-24, 232, 237, 274n.3; as a principle, 43, 111, 120; from restrictions, 57-59, 215, 223; to be wrong, 59, 83-84, 87-88, 92, 133, 149. *See also* Slavery
Fruit of the Spirit, 27, 47, 86
Futile treatment, 117, 214, 237, 241. *See also* Forgoing treatment, justifications of
Future. *See* Eschatology

Genetic disabilities, 185. *See also* Disabled persons
Gentleness, 86
Giving, 24, 33, 38, 161, 196
God: as basis of moral authority, 51, 52, 57; character of, 27, 46, 200, 254n.28; determining the will of, 18, 27-28, 37, 52, 106, 242, 246n.10; as example, 56, 69, 160, 171; faithfulness of, 26, 31, 34, 105, 115; glory of, 42, 53, 105, 115; goodness of, 104; grace of, 18, 20, 40, 43,

47, 104, 105; as healer, 134-35;
incarnation of, 51, 55, 255n.32;
intentions of for people, 48,
69, 99, 100, 111, 185, 191, 200,
232, 254n.28; intentions of for
the world, 27, 39, 42, 57, 61,
66, 68, 194, 198, 222; involvement in the world, 16-17, 27,
45, 52, 200; as judge, 17, 195;
justice of, 16, 44, 62, 63, 64,
254n.4; love of, 26, 27, 38, 69,
103, 160, 161, 179, 240; mercy
of, 17, 38; as moral leader, 18;
omniscience of, 195, 197, 201,
208, 212; power of, 105, 119;
presence of in the believer, 18;
purposes of, 67, 96, 98, 103,
107, 109, 122, 126, 197, 243; reality of, 22, 242; righteousness
of, 16, 36; as ruler, 34, 35, 36,
37, 44, 66, 98, 200, 251n.9;
timing of, 101; transcendence
of, 51, 109, 198, 222; truthfulness of, 59; as victor, 21; will
of, 20, 24, 51, 54, 60, 93, 97,
108, 115, 119, 121; wisdom of,
47, 94. *See also* Creation; Image of God
God-centered ethics: compared
with other approaches, 41-42,
44, 46, 47, 114, 194-95, 245n.3;
and elderly people, 158, 185;
and ending life, 120, 127, 145;
explanation of, 15, 16-20, 51-
53; and faith, 33-34, 102; and
love, 31-32, 38, 69, 116; other
aspects of ethics defined by,
27, 29, 66; and suffering, 102,
106, 108, 116
Good, 21, 26, 64, 80, 109, 121,
245n.3, 248n.23
Gospel, 29
Guilt, 68-69, 197, 268n.20

Happiness. *See* Well-being

Harm, 71, 85, 86, 103, 125, 136,
137-38, 147, 236, 238
Hate, 32, 34, 71
Health care costs, 1, 2, 6, 78, 114,
128, 153, 154, 155, 179
Health maintenance. *See* Life-
style
Hermeneutical ethics, 45
Hippocratic Oath, 111
Holiness, 20, 22, 47, 53, 96
Holy Spirit, 18, 20, 21, 27, 46, 47,
53, 59, 66, 71, 86, 148, 159
Honoring God, 18, 42
Hope, 71, 112, 119, 268n.16
Hospice, 140
Humility, 47, 148
Humor, 196

Idolatry, 17, 115, 127, 128, 134
Image of God, 47, 52-53, 54-55,
98, 124, 128, 160, 254n.28,
256n.5
Imagination, moral, 66
Imminent-death criterion: for allocating resources, 225-26,
229, 233; for forgoing treatment, 132-36, 137, 141, 144,
173, 277n.11
Impartial-selection criterion,
157, 202, 227-30, 233, 243
Informed consent, 81-82, 84-85,
133, 134, 138, 202, 215, 223
Insulin, 295n.15
Intensive care, 153, 154, 155,
166, 174, 177, 211, 215, 218, 233
Intentions, 49, 71, 96-97, 110,
118, 126, 185, 255n.31, 276n.8
Intuition, 43, 179, 222
Isolation, 75, 99

Jesus Christ: as the center of
ethics, 15, 18-19, 22, 27, 31-32,
43; death of, 21, 25, 43, 53, 55,
67, 68, 69, 70, 120, 145, 146,
160, 191, 224; example of, 53,

67, 69, 71, 107, 120, 140, 145-46, 224; as Lord, 36, 37, 107; mind of, 23; resurrection of, 21, 43, 55, 128; return of, 21, 99, 200, 246n.14; as the "Son of Man," 36; truthfulness of, 59; as unifier, 161. *See also* Bible: Jesus' teaching

Justice: compensatory, 198, 228-29; as a guide, 61-65, 81, 124, 125, 158, 168-69, 171, 172, 173, 177, 179, 184, 192, 195, 203, 204, 208, 209, 212, 213, 215, 216, 217, 218, 220, 224, 227, 228, 229, 232, 237; importance of, 20, 46, 62, 70, 108, 170, 184, 186, 258n.18; as a principle, 43, 164; retributive, 190, 204, 227; as a virtue, 47

Justification, 20, 23

Killing, 52, 54-55, 109, 111-12, 113, 121, 137, 268n.20. *See also* Ending someone's life

Kingdom of God. *See* God, as ruler

Law, written religious/moral, 18, 19, 20, 27, 29, 36, 37, 38, 39, 66, 246n.9, 249n.25, 249n.26, 253n.23

Length-of-benefit criterion, 156, 165-66, 207, 224-25

Life: equal regard for everyone's, 65, 165-66, 170, 181, 229, 232; full span of, 164, 174, 178, 182-83, 185; as a gift, 67-68, 110; as a guide, 54-57, 67-68, 81, 96, 97, 103, 115, 124, 125, 131-32, 133, 158, 168, 169, 177, 179, 195, 208, 217, 219, 223, 229, 232, 237, 276n.8, 302n.14; as an idol, 57, 102, 126-27, 128, 134; as life-years, 178, 180-81, 188; as a loan, 67-68, 110, 127, 146; nature of, 34-35, 54, 67, 97-102, 109, 127, 128, 161-64; as an orientation, 97-98, 113; as a principle, 43; respect for, 37, 47, 49, 52, 70, 92, 111, 145, 160, 162, 191, 192, 199, 206, 216, 229, 232, 239; as special by God's design, 22, 25, 46, 54-55, 122, 138, 188, 199, 224, 229; special significance of, 44, 48, 54-57, 61, 67, 102, 127, 170, 216, 217, 243; as spiritual, 161-62, 168; sustained by God, 97, 99, 100, 109, 111, 119, 122, 161, 229; uniqueness of each, 165, 170; value of, 37, 56, 63-64, 109, 114, 115, 122, 190-91, 199, 227, 230, 270n.30; the worthlessness of, 119, 122, 125, 144, 179. *See also* Eternal Life

Lifestyle, 200, 213, 237, 300n.6

Likelihood-of-benefit criterion, 156, 166, 169-71, 207-8, 224-25, 229-30, 232

Living wills, 88-89, 90-91, 92, 143

Lottery, 228-29, 233, 302n.14

Love: as action, 70, 124, 130; as comprehensive, 38; as edification, 26; toward enemies, 31-33, 36, 56, 71; as essence of moral life, 26, 66; toward God, 26-27, 38-40, 42, 59, 66, 70, 115, 135, 146; toward neighbors, 26-27, 28, 31, 36, 38-40, 47, 53, 59, 66, 69, 70, 115, 135, 146, 147-49, 195, 233, 249n.26, 254n.25; nourished by God, 148; as right motivations, 38, 44, 59, 223; as right thinking, 38, 46; toward self, 118; and suffering, 46, 115, 140, 240, 254n.27; universal, 28, 33, 35, 63-64; as a virtue, 47, 148, 254n.27

Love-impelled ethics: compared with other approaches, 41, 45-46, 47, 48, 114, 168, 222; egalitarian nature of, 33, 192; and elderly people, 158-59; and ending life, 120, 128-29, 133-34, 144, 145; explanation of, 15-16, 26-29, 69-72; and faith, 26, 36; God-oriented vs. people-oriented, 27, 39-40, 66, 168, 195, 222, 232-33; and mercy, 38; situational nature of, 28, 41, 50, 94, 133-34, 145, 222, 242; and suffering, 106, 108, 116

Marriage, 23
Meat offered to idols, 18, 28-29
Media appeals, 13, 216-17, 219, 220
Medical-benefit criterion, 133, 137, 138, 156, 171, 172-75, 180, 205, 207, 210, 211, 214, 224-25, 226, 233, 243
Medicine, the profession of, 112, 169. See also Caregiver-patient relationship
Mental capacity, 77, 84, 85, 88, 90, 93, 113, 133, 135-36, 142
Mercy killing. See Ending someone's life
Mercy, 37
Money, 33-36, 145-47, 148
Motivations, 38, 46, 47, 67, 71-72, 96-97, 108, 109, 110, 114, 119, 126, 276n.8

Narrative ethics, 45, 52
Natural laws, 22, 40, 102
Nazi Germany, 78-79, 114
Need: differing perceptions of, 85, 134, 140, 171, 173, 192, 202, 277; dimensions of, 135, 164, 173; God's concern over, 37, 63, 64, 69, 224, 258n.18; importance of people responding to, 38, 69, 70-71, 134, 146, 172-74, 179, 211, 213, 216, 224; life-or-death nature of, 63, 64-65, 67, 145, 146, 154, 172, 214, 217, 225, 241; as a standard of justice, 62, 64-65, 172, 179, 192, 213, 216, 217, 227, 258n.18. See also Weakness
Netherlands, The, 77

Obedience, 18, 19, 25, 27, 44, 59, 68, 69, 71, 98-103, 104, 107, 109, 110, 126, 127, 197, 249n.26
Obligation. See Responsibility
Ordinary/Extraordinary treatment, 142-44. See also Benefit/Burden of treatment
Organs: donation of, 90, 205, 216, 217, 218-19; transplantation of, 4, 13, 124, 145, 153, 154, 155, 156-57, 174, 201, 203, 204, 205, 206-7, 215, 216, 218-19, 220, 228, 230, 233, 243, 301n.9, 302n.15

Pain. See Care, comfort; Suffering
Patience, 86
Patient Self-Determination Act, 92-93
Peace, 135
Perfection, 31, 32, 33, 255n.32
Perseverance, 104
Persistent vegetative state, 123-24, 273n.9. See also Unconscious patients
Personhood, 52, 53, 55, 56, 191
Phenomenological ethics, 45
Playing God, 127, 197-98, 200, 201, 208, 241
Pleasing God, 18, 119
Pneumonia, 4
Politically undesirable people, 78, 199, 204, 217
Poor people: attitudes toward,

189, 198, 216, 280n.6; limited access to health care of, 2, 33, 65, 168, 198, 204, 216, 218, 235; warrant special care, 24, 64-65, 198, 204, 215

Power, 160, 199, 227, 228. *See also* Empowerment; Weakness

Praise, 105

Prayer, 32, 52, 66, 146, 147-48, 222

Preventive care, 178, 220, 237, 238-39

Pride, 20, 44, 70, 110, 209

Principles, ethics of, 43-46, 47, 48, 49, 52, 126, 253n.23, 255n.1, 256n.2

Progress-of-science criterion, 156, 200-203

Prudence, 178, 184-87

Psychological-ability criterion, 156, 208-11, 213, 224, 233

Public policy, 48-49

Punishment, 21, 63

Quality-of-benefit criterion, 155, 156, 166-69, 183, 207, 212-13, 224-25

Quality of life, 54, 56-57, 83, 121-25, 132, 144, 146, 181-82, 183, 188, 192, 209

Racism, 161, 177, 180, 185, 199, 213, 217, 238, 239

Radiation treatment, 13

Random selection, 202, 227-29, 243

Reality-bounded ethics: discernment required by, 23, 28, 66, 71, 145, 242; explanation of, 15, 20-26, 50-51, 53-69; God's intentions for the world reflected by, 27, 37-38, 43-44, 49, 53-54, 61, 68, 94, 120, 127, 170, 173; limits of love defined by, 27, 29, 32-33, 38-39, 42, 46, 48,

66, 70, 115, 128, 129, 144, 168, 179, 195, 217, 232-33; nonmaterial aspects of, 24-25, 34-35, 40, 60, 108, 168, 242; not always definitive, 28, 29, 45, 49, 133; people's identity reflected by, 22-23, 25, 32-33, 37, 38-39, 42-43, 49, 53-57, 63-64, 114, 128, 147, 158, 179, 185; and suffering, 106, 107, 108, 115, 116

Reason: distorted, 17, 19, 23, 43-44, 197-98; limited, 52, 158; self-deceived, 17, 255n.31; as a source of knowledge, 14, 222, 242; transformed by God, 17, 18, 19, 23, 28

Reconciliation, 99

Redemption, 38, 53, 102, 106

Repentance, 20

Resources-required criterion, 156, 230-31, 232, 233

Respirators, 4, 13, 130, 137-38

Responsibility, 18, 24, 27, 45, 68, 71, 85, 113, 117, 118, 119, 127, 141, 147, 149, 171, 189, 191, 193, 206, 219, 253n.23, 291n.36

Resurrection, 100, 128. *See also* Jesus Christ, resurrection of

Reverence toward God, 159-60

Reward, 21, 33, 63

Righteousness, 19-20, 27, 62, 159, 161, 251n.7

Rights, 25-26, 67, 110-11, 165-66, 177-78, 191-93, 248n.22

Sabbath, 36-38, 63, 67, 71

Sacrifice, 145-47, 161, 224

Salvation, 19

Satan, 17, 19, 105

Self-centeredness, 17, 24, 32, 33, 38-39, 42, 46, 58, 68, 104, 109, 113, 126, 147, 185, 194, 197, 199. *See also* Sin

Sex criterion, 157

Sexism, 177, 180, 185, 199, 206

Sexuality, 23

Sin, 16, 17, 19, 20, 21, 22, 24, 29, 39, 43, 48, 58, 61, 65, 66, 68, 97-103, 106, 119, 183, 184-85, 188, 246n.5, 246n.10. *See also* Self-centeredness

Situational ethics, 41, 214, 222, 232, 233-34, 242, 246n.10. *See also* Discernment

Slavery: to another person, 57, 63, 161, 257n.8; to death, 58; to false teaching, 58; to religious law and custom, 20, 29, 58, 249n.26; to righteousness, 24; to Satan, 20, 58; to self-deception, 58; due to sin, 17, 24, 58; to worry, 36. *See also* Freedom

Smoking, 300n.6

Social Security, 186

Social-value criterion, 19, 40, 154, 157, 168, 170, 176, 195-200, 201, 203, 210, 212-13, 227, 232, 235, 238, 243

Spiritual perspective, 35, 134-35, 142, 161-62, 189

Standard medical practice, 226

Stewardship, 67, 124, 191, 229, 241

Subjectivity, 18, 167

Suffering: of the caregiver, 105, 113, 123, 126; importance of removing, 19, 40, 104, 106-8, 109, 115, 119, 139; instances of, 4-5, 13, 105, 107, 109, 159, 239; mystery of, 103, 107, 109; nature of, 46, 87, 101-2, 103-8, 111; sometimes increased by treatment, 49, 75, 81, 115, 125-26, 127, 128, 132, 137, 144, 240, 241; as unqualifiedly evil, 103-6, 109; value of, 101-2, 103-4, 105-6, 108, 115, 139, 267n.12; victory over, 104, 122

Suicide: caregiver-assisted, 76, 95, 111-13, 178, 187, 191; problems associated with, 118-21, 191; social impact of, 112, 119, 187, 240; support for, 95, 120, 178

Support, 93, 113, 115, 134, 142

Supportive-environment criterion, 13, 155, 156, 211-14, 224, 233

Surrogate decision makers, 75, 77-78, 87-88, 89-94, 143

Symbols, 277n.11, 284n.18

Taxes, 217

Technology, 49, 126, 137-38, 142-43, 175, 206, 237, 241

Terminal/nonterminal distinction, 80, 131-36, 141

Thankfulness, 18

Trial, therapeutic, 138, 172, 175, 211

Trust. *See* Faith

Truth: as a guide, 59-61, 65, 81, 86, 87, 237; the importance of, 112, 171, 183, 200; as a principle, 43; as reality, 19, 21, 22, 255n.31; as a virtue, 47; the whole, 59-61

Uncertainty, 93, 102, 103, 105, 112, 125, 136, 146, 165, 166, 170-71, 172, 195-97, 201, 207-9, 211, 212, 213, 214, 225, 226, 230-31

Unconscious patients, 76, 117, 123-25, 130, 272n.7. *See also* Mental capacity

Understanding, 86-87, 129, 133, 138, 140, 159, 211, 300n.6

Uniqueness of described approach, 40-49

Unproductive people, 2, 33, 168, 198

Unrighteousness. *See* Sin

Utilitarian ethics. *See* Ethics of consequences

Vaccines, 145, 154, 228
Values: cultural, 158, 160, 162, 165, 175, 187-91, 193, 195-97, 209, 213, 223, 228; worldly, 19, 20, 21, 35
Values history, 92
Veterans, 203, 206
Virtue: ethics of, 21, 46-47, 48-49; importance of, 20, 32, 38, 41, 42, 44, 71, 86-87, 96, 104, 114, 126, 148, 161, 173, 183, 196, 242
Vision, 48, 71
Vital-responsibilities criterion, 156, 231-32, 233
Voluntariness. *See* Coercion

Weakness: 85, 104, 111, 112, 113, 118, 120, 123, 135, 141, 159, 160, 161, 174, 179, 204, 216, 232
Well-being: concern for people's, 47, 66, 70, 87, 128, 144, 222, 232, 254n.25; enhanced by observing ethical guides, 58, 59, 62, 71, 232; apart from God, 35, 44, 122; health care and, 83, 125, 186, 240; material vs. nonmaterial, 35, 104, 107-8, 109, 182; maximizing, 42, 45-46, 106, 194-95; pursuit of limited by ethical guides, 42, 46, 66, 70, 81, 222, 232, 254n.25
Will, human. *See* Wishes
Willingness criterion, 133, 138, 156, 161, 183, 208, 211, 223-24, 233. *See also* Wishes
Wisdom, 19, 42, 43-44, 51, 99, 104, 159, 189, 197, 198, 243
Wishes: of the family, 117; of the patient, 5, 49, 59, 77, 78, 79, 81, 82, 83-94, 114, 123, 133, 135, 143, 186, 223-24, 243, 277n.11; of people, 19, 24, 64, 215, 223
Withdrawing/Withholding treatment, 136-38. *See also* Forgoing treatment

Youth, 158, 160, 162, 163-64, 179-80, 187-90, 193